The Heart of Long-Term Care

The Heart of Long-Term Care

Rosalie A. Kane
Robert L. Kane
Richard C. Ladd

New York   Oxford
OXFORD UNIVERSITY PRESS
1998

Oxford University Press

Oxford   New York
Athens   Auckland   Bangkok   Bogotá   Buenos Aires   Calcutta
Cape Town   Chennai   Dar es Salaam   Delhi   Florence   Hong Kong   Istanbul
Karachi   Kuala Lumpur   Madrid   Melbourne   Mexico City   Mumbai
Nairobi   Paris   São Paulo   Singapore   Taipei   Tokyo   Toronto   Warsaw

and associated companies in
Berlin   Ibadan

Library of Congress Cataloging-in-Publication Data
Kane, Rosalie A.
The heart of long-term care / Rosalie A. Kane, Robert L. Kane, Richard C. Ladd.
p.   cm.   Includes index.   ISBN 0-19-512238-0
1. Long-term care of the sick—United States.
2. Aged—Long-term care—United States.
I. Kane, Robert L., 1940– .
II. Ladd, Richard C.
III. Title.   RA997.K36   1988   362.1'6'0973—dc21   98-5831

2 3 4 5 6 7 8 9

Printed in the United States of America
on acid-free paper.

Preface

This book is motivated by a strong urge on the part of all three authors to say something true and compelling about long-term care and long-term care service systems. All three of us have made statements about long-term care before. Why, then, did we—a physician, a social worker, and a public administrator—come together to write this book at this time? What was our intention, and how does this work differ from other books that Rosalie and Robert Kane have already written about long-term care?

For more than two decades, two of us—Rosalie and Robert Kane—have conducted research—sometimes together and sometimes separately—to illuminate various facets of long-term care: who needs it, how to assure its quality, how to finance it, and what effects various long-term care arrangements have on various groups of consumers. Over the years, Robert Kane has given particular consideration to the need to align payment incentives with desired outcomes, and to forge a genuine integration between acute care and long-term care, using management information systems as a tool. Rosalie Kane has explored roles and responsibilities of family members, and the question of how public policy should strike a balance between protecting vulnerable older people and fostering sometimes risky opportunities for people with disabilities—mostly seniors—to live meaningful, dignified, and autonomous lives! Both Rosalie and Robert Kane have been preoccupied with developing and testing quality assurance systems for nursing home care and for home- and community-based care.

The third author—Richard Ladd—has spent the last two decades actually developing and administering long-term care programs at the state level, particularly in Oregon and, later, in Texas. His work has tested and expanded the definition of the possible in long-term care, both programmatically and fiscally. He envisaged and has put into practice long-term care programs for people in their homes and in new group residential settings that maximize independence, choice, dignity, and normal lifestyles, and he has pioneered nonmedical approaches to long-term care. Most of all, he has insisted on using the language of human values in arenas dominated by professional rhetoric and cold cost accounting, all the while managing to escape charges of naivete or romanticism because the programs he stimulated proved affordable and desirable. Over the years, Rosalie and Robert Kane have had the opportunity to evaluate some of the programs launched by Richard Ladd and have found that, although naturally not perfect, they seem to produce better benefits for their clientele at lower costs than the programs they replaced.

In the fall of 1995, we three began to work together on a project funded by the United States Administration on Aging to stimulate home- and community-based long-term care programs in states and local areas. The overriding goal of that work was to shift the balance of long-term care provision and funding from nursing home care to care in people's own homes or in group residential settings sufficiently homelike that they do not make a mockery of the term "home." We still subscribe passionately to that goal and over the last 2 years undertook fact-finding about long-term care at the state level, where much long-term care policy is forged. In the course of this collaboration, we came to believe that yet another book about long-term care is needed.

This book, then, is a product of the interchange among the three of us on the subject that has been central to much of our careers. It draws heavily on both the statistical work and the case studies that we undertook as part of our recent Administration on Aging project, but also attempts to provide a comprehensive vision of long-term care based on our accumulated experiences. Because we think the subject needs demystification, we attempt to write about long-term care in a way that a layperson can understand. We approach the topic with a minimum of jargon and lapsing into acronyms. To preserve the narrative flow, references are minimized and, when needed, assigned to reference notes at the end of each chapter. A glossary is provided to help the reader keep the welter of terms in mind.

Besides trying to write in a way accessible to a wide range of readers, we further aspired to write a practical book, one that could provide an antidote to the despair and pessimism that often seem to prevail among those who develop long-term care policies and those who deliver services. We believe that problems in provision of long-term care can be solved and that ideas of how to do so can be found all over the United States. The technology is available, and, if the issues are formulated in a convincing way, perhaps the political will can also be mustered.

In 1987, Rosalie and Robert Kane published a book, *Long-Term Care: Principles, Programs and Policies,* which united conceptual discussions about long-term care with a detailed review and critique of existing research on the need for long-term care and on the effectiveness of a wide variety of home-based and institutional long-term care programs. This new book updates and adds to the ideas of the earlier volume, taking into account a decade of new research. However, this book does not replace the 1987 volume, nor does it aspire to present a similar comprehensive compendium of relevant research. Research and demonstration projects in long-term care have abounded in the past 10 years, and each of us has been associated with these general activities. In this book, however, we step back from separate studies to look at long-term care more generally. We believe there is a compelling need to go beyond technocratic efforts, such as measuring the needs of older people and the so-called case-mix characters of those who get long-term care or evaluating the cost-effectiveness of specific policy or program changes. This book reconsiders the very nature of the long-term care enterprise in an effort to envision what it should be like and what it can achieve.

We hope we have provided sufficient historical and factual material so that this book can serve as a text on long-term care. At the same time, we have not avoided expressing our own opinions and interpretation. We believe that long-term care in the United States can and must be improved. We are not proud of the prevailing patterns of long-term care, though we have no interest in allocating blame. Indeed, long-term care programs and policies in the United States arose by happenstance— some as by-products of trying to achieve something else, such as more efficient hospital care. The status quo has also been sustained by professional orthodoxies that require challenging. We believe that it is possible to develop much improved long-term care programs at an affordable cost. We also believe that positive examples that now exist in various parts of the country can help point the way to sensible and progressive strategies to provide long-term care for the American citizenry.

Exemplary long-term care programs such as we highlight in this book will hardly cure all the difficulties of the human predicament. Better approaches to long-term care cannot dispel the pain, sadness, or loneliness that accompanies disease and loss. They cannot eradicate the guilt or distress experienced by family members when the needs of their relatives exceed their own capacity to help. Good long-term care policies do not mask the insult and tragedy of Alzheimer's disease and other conditions that rob people of memory, ability to express themselves, even personality. But exemplary long-term care programs do help to cushion these tragedies. They sometimes result in improvements in the functioning and perceived well-being of the people needing care. Equally important, they avoid making things worse. To our great regret, we believe that many long-term care programs and policies, however well-intentioned, result in unnecessary misery for the people receiving the help and for their families.

One of the knottiest problems that we take up again and again in this book relates to the goals of long-term care and how its success or lack of success should be defined. We shy away from unrealistic, grandiose goals for long-term care. These end up making providers feel a sense of failure and futility or, worse, a resentment toward those whom they cannot help according to the terms laid out. On the one hand, some goals, such as improved social well-being, are too often claimed to be satisfied in counter-intuitive ways—for example, putting people in double rooms in nursing homes so they have companionship, or sending people off to homogenized day centers for "socialization" without regard to what they consider pleasant or interesting. On the other hand, we do believe that long-term care providers should be held responsible for some outcomes related to the people they serve. Although good long-term care cannot, in the words of soap operas, bring happiness and fulfillment, it should do something that is observable to others and that separates it from mediocre or inadequate long-term care. The three of us have been preoccupied with finding that elusive gold standard for a set of services that, by their very nature, are inextricably intertwined with everyday life.

Structure of the Book

Part I, constituting the first four chapters, lays out issues and describes the backdrop of current policies and programs. Chapter 1 defines long-term care and discusses its goals, always a difficult subject because of the heterogeneity of services and clientele in programs that fly under the long-term care banner. Chapter 2 presents an overview of the current system for long-term care in the United States, highlighting the dominant patterns for funding and for service delivery. Chapter 3 goes to the heart of the long-term care policy predicament: that is, the seeming inability to develop a system of long-term care in the United States that is consistent with the kinds of services and provisions that people of all ages with disabilities value and seek. The chapter recognizes the domination of the nursing home in United States long-term care and discusses logistical, political, and strategic barriers to achieving more balanced, user-friendly long-term care programs. Chapter 4 follows with a discussion of how state long-term care expenditures actually vary from state to state. In this variation, we see substantial promise. If some states and communities have been able to alter the emphasis of their long-term care programs, others should be able to follow suit.

Part II reviews programs that will be important planks of revised long-term care systems, concentrating on desirable and often new policy and program directions. Chapter 5 looks at home-based services, exploring options for greater consumer direction and greater service capacity for the persons receiving long-term care in their own homes. This leads to discussion of home health care, personal assistant services, voucher and cash options, and case management. Chapter 6 examines models of residential care that almost make a 180° reversal in the premises of nursing home care as we know it. It also looks at best practices in existing nursing homes. In Chapter 7, we discuss models of accountability and quality assurance for long-term care, including case management, which was previously discussed in Chapter 5 as a service in home care. In Chapter 8 we discuss the kind of acute health care programs needed to undergird long-term care, emphasizing ways to provide some continuity of health care between acute care and long-term care. This leads naturally to Chapter 9, devoted to the relationship of long-term care to managed care, given that increasing numbers of seniors receive health care in general from managed care organizations. Moreover capitation and managed care for long-term care is the subject of much discussion on some experimentation in the United States as we approach the twenty-first century. In Chapter 10, we briefly consider models from other developed countries that could be pertinent to the United States.

Part III summarizes our thoughts about how to approach long-term care in the United States. In framing the recommendations in Chapter 11, we touch on unresolved policy issues, including the role of private long-term care insurance, the proper blend of public and private financing, the relationship between family care and paid care, and the relationships among federal, state, and local governments. Although we favor some solutions over others, we maintain that whatever level of government is in charge and whatever the blend between private and public dollars, we can, should, and must provide more efficient, effective, and, above all, humane, long-term care for the sake of the millions of Americans with long-term disabilities whose quality of life depends on it.

Acknowledgments

We are grateful to the Administration on Aging, which funded us to work together on a National Long-term Care Mentoring Project. This set in motion the collaboration, the fact-finding and profiling work, and the discussions that led us to write this book. Alfred Duncker and James Steen of the Administration on Aging were associated with the project management at the initial stages. We are also grateful to the Office of the Assistant Secretary for Planning and Evaluation (ASPE) of the United States Department of Health and Human Services, which funded continued profiling and to the Robert Wood Johnson Foundation for funding our continuing efforts in a project called *Balancing LTC Systems*. Thank-you to Pamela Doty from ASPE and James Knickman from the Robert Wood Johnson Foundation for the support of our work.

Among our immediate colleagues, we owe special thanks to Wendy Nielsen Veazie, not only for her substantial research assistance related to Chapter 4 but for the many times she pulled information out of the hat to assist us. We were also dependent on Jennifer Koehn, who bore the lion's share of the clerical work associated with the many iterations of this book over a two-year period. At the end game, we also were grateful for the help of Lynette Sylvain and Aleta Johanssen.

R.A.K.

Minneapolis, Minn.   R.L.K.

Austin, Tex.   R.C.L.
March 1998

Contents

I
PRINCIPLES OF LONG-TERM CARE

1.

Nature and Purpose of Long-Term Care

Starting at the beginning demands a definition of long-term care, the subject of this book. Long-term care is an odd term, which emerged to mark a distinction from acute health care. To define long-term care clearly, therefore, we must first define acute care. Acute care presumes an active illness or health problem that needs attention. The term *acute care* refers to health care typically offered in hospitals and doctors' offices to diagnose and treat health conditions. Primary health care (a component of acute care) refers to the overall, first-order responsibility for managing an individual's health, usually in an outpatient setting; primary care providers have responsibility for performing periodic health maintenance activities as well as treating or arranging for the treatment of active or acute illnesses. Typically, those who receive acute care, whether from hospital personnel or primary care practitioners, view themselves and are viewed as *patients*. To make the distinction between long-term care and acute care more complicated, most acute care for older people is directed at managing chronic, long-term health problems.

So, what is long-term care? First, and foremost, it is a response to disability and functional impairment. As a result of illnesses, accidents, or conditions developed at birth or during developmental stages, some people experience long-term or even permanent inability to perform tasks associated with everyday living. Some of these impairments affect basic self-care activities that are taught to infants and that most people take for granted—for example, eating, moving in and out of bed, using the toilet, dressing, and bathing. In the jargon of long-term care, these fundamental tasks have been labeled activities of daily living, or ADLs.

Other regular tasks that are less elemental also call for combinations of physical dexterity, strength, energy, speech, hearing, vision, and memory, which those needing long-term care may lack. These tasks could include cooking, cleaning, shopping, doing laundry, driving an automobile, using a telephone, reading mail, or following instructions. Again in the jargon of long-term care, such activities (and the list could be extended) are sometimes known as instrumental activities of daily living (IADLs).

The temporal implications of the terms acute care and long-term care are confusing. They refer to the length of an episode of contact, but even then are imprecise. A chronically ill person may receive acute care over a period of more years than he or she receives long-term care. Thus, a time dimension is only one part of the definition of long-term care; the nature of the services is also intrinsic to the definition.

Long-term care, then, may be defined as assistance given over a sustained period of time to people who are experiencing long-term inabilities or difficulties in functioning because of a disability. Long-term care services are those services needed to compensate for the individual's functional impairments, such as were just described, or those services designed to restore or improve functional abilities. Long-term care services could entail cooking, cleaning, driving, shopping, bathing, dressing, assistance in using the toilet, mobility assistance, and even spoon-feeding or other help with eating and drinking. They could also entail assessment, rehabilitation, and treatments to reduce disability and functional impairment as much as possible. Finally, long-term care services include environmental assessment and modification, and provision of equipment and devices; these strategies improve functional abilities by rendering the environment easier for the consumer to manage.

Long-term care is not an extension of acute care—it is distinctive in its very nature. Because long-term care continues for prolonged periods, it becomes enmeshed in the very fabric of people's lives. Unlike the situation with acute care, where lifestyles may be temporarily disrupted in pursuit of tangible gains in health (for example, by an admission to the hospital), the predominant strategy in long-term care emphasizes integration of treatment and living. The point is not to ignore or undervalue health care for those getting long-term care, but to incorporate health care into the context of daily life. Ironically, this principle is most dramatically violated in the most visible embodiment of long-term care, the nursing home. Because nursing homes were created as miniature hospitals, they were designed in that image and adopted many hospital traits. As nursing homes are increasingly used for active convalescence of patients who were formerly cared for in hospitals, this hospital-like treatment philosophy has become even more pervasive in the nursing home.

Of course, people who need long-term care also need primary health care and other acute care services when they are ill. In particular, older people needing long-term care are highly likely to have chronic illnesses that require ongoing medical management. Older people with disabilities use about twice as much Medicare money per person as does the general population of Medicare beneficiaries. Thus, thinking about long-term care and acute care as alternatives to each other is inaccurate and counterproductive. People who need long-term care will also need acute care from time to time. The focus of this book is long-term care, but inevitably we are led into discussions of acute care for long-term care users.

Deciding what to call people who use long-term care is somewhat perplexing. They are usually *patients* of one or more physicians or nurses, but as long-term care users, they are often referred to as *consumers, customers* (especially if they pay their own bill), *clients* (in the language of the professionals, the agencies, or public programs that have sprung up to provide service), *recipients* (with reference to clientele of public benefit programs for low-income people), and *beneficiaries* (with reference to Medicare). Doubtless, few people receiving long-term care even know how to refer to their relationship with those who give them long-term care.

For those who live in nursing homes or board and care homes, the nomenclature problem is often finessed by the term *resident*. This is hardly a solution, however; people who reside in nursing homes and other residential settings are *patients* with reference to their health care providers and, as we suggest in later chapters, they might better be considered residents or (our preferred term) *tenants* merely in relation to those who supply their housing. We acknowledge that people needing long-term care often must move into new living quarters to get the care and services they need. This is particularly true of very old people who may have no relatives able to provide the mainstay of in-home care. But, phrases such as "nursing home care," "residential care," "day care," and "home care" conflate the place where care is given with the care itself, leading to a simplistic notion that a certain set of care processes and capabilities are inevitably linked to the site where care is offered. In fact, in this book we argue that distinguishing the place of care from the care received in a particular place is conceptually useful and can lead to practical policy directions regarding payment and accountability.

The lack of a well-accepted noun for the person who receives long-term care is in part a reflection of the ambiguity of programs that provide a social service at their core but, in the United States, are funded out of health dollars through means-tested, health-related welfare programs (described further in the next chapter). In Britain and some European countries, much of long-term care falls under the general umbrella of personal social services, many of which tend to be available free or at minimal cost (heavily subsidized) to all citizens.[1] In the United States, the term *social services* has a pejorative connotation; those who need social services have somehow failed in life's tasks and are most properly allowed to land in a safety net of services. Since long-term care needs fall unpredictably upon individuals because of health problems, accidents in life, or accidents of birth, long-term care has escaped the full stigma that adheres, say, to welfare services for younger people. Nonetheless, societal ambivalence is everywhere strong regarding the extent to which governments are responsible for ensuring that long-term care needs are met. This ambivalence is more pronounced in the United States, where the issues of private versus public responsibility for health care are still unsettled.

For lack of a better word, we will generally use the term *consumer* to refer to those using long-term care, unless the context cries out for a different term. We will reserve the term *patient* for direct relationships with those responsible for preventing or treating illnesses, and we will use the term *resident* or *tenant* to refer to direct relationships with housing providers. We avoid the word *customer* to help combat the currently popular inference that health care and long-term care should be construed as products like all others traded in the marketplace.

Who Needs Long-Term Care?

Age
People well over 65 are the most likely group to need long-term care. Indeed, people who are in good health when they reach the landmark of statistical aging, which in the United States is usually construed as age 65, are unlikely to be at risk for needing long-term care until they are age 80 or over. On the other hand, many people under the age of 65 do need long-term care. Societal costs for long-term care in the aggregate are mostly attributable to the care of people over age sixty-five, but the average lifetime costs for long-term care of a given person with a disability are much higher for people who begin receiving that care under age 65. This is because many younger people need long-term care for decades, whereas older people who come into old age without a disability tend to need long-term care for shorter periods in the months or years before their deaths.

Another factor may also contribute to the higher *public* per-person costs of long-term care for younger consumers: Different goals and expectations are held out for younger people than for old people. Many younger people with disabilities are supported by sophisticated technologies and extensive services which allow them to function in the community. Under the pressure of strong lobbying from people with physical disabilities themselves and family members of adults with both physical and developmental disabilities, many younger disabled persons are actively engaged in the mainstream of life—for example, at school, college, or work. In turn, this has required that social supports be promoted to all them to participate in regular activities. In contrast, older people with disabilities are more likely to remain isolated. Even arranging transportation to allow them to participate in community activities can be a major undertaking. Given that differences exist between provisions for younger and older long-term care consumers, it is reasonable to ask if this differential cost *should* be present, and, if not, which standard is the correct one? Or perhaps, distinctions in the amount, type, and cost of long-term care are valid but should be based on criteria other than age. We will return to this discussion later in the chapter and throughout the book.

Functional Impairment
Estimates of the population with functional impairments vary from study to study, depending on the precise definitions used.[2] Using somewhat conservative definitions (neither the most stringent nor the least stringent in the literature), analysts

of the 1991 Survey of Income and Program Participants estimated that in 1991 about 4.5 million civilians over age 65 living in the community had difficulties performing one or more ADL functions.[3] Figure 1.1 shows the prevalence of functional impairment by age, rising from 9.2% of the population aged 65–69 to 49.5% of the population aged 85+. In contrast, only 2.4% of the population between ages 15 and 64 met the criteria for functional impairment. In 1991, there were also about 1.6 million older people in nursing homes, or 5% of the population over age 65.

The relationship between aging and the prevalence of disability fuels the repeated forecasts of economic crisis in long-term care when the baby boom generation becomes elderly around the year 2030. But, simple linear extrapolations that multiply current disability rates for age-specific and gender-specific groups times the expected numbers of persons in each group are precarious at best. Figure 1.2 shows such a progression for the population over 85, which was less than 1 million in each decennial census until 1970, was 3 million in 1990, and is extrapolated to almost 18 million in 2050. However, birth rates are hard to predict and changes in disability rates over the next few decades also seem likely. Even official population projections are imprecise at best. For example, Figure 1.3 displays projections of

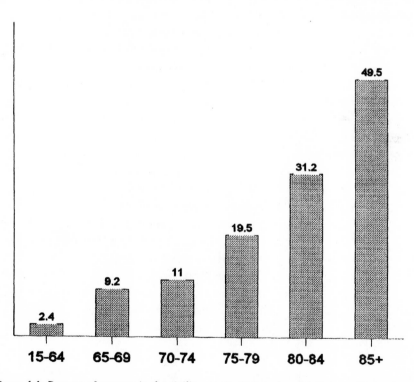

Figure 1.1. Percent of persons in the civilian noninstitutional population needing assistance with everyday activities by age in 1991 [Source: U.S. Bureau of the Census, 1990 and 1991 panels of the Survey of Income and Program Participants (SIPP) files.].

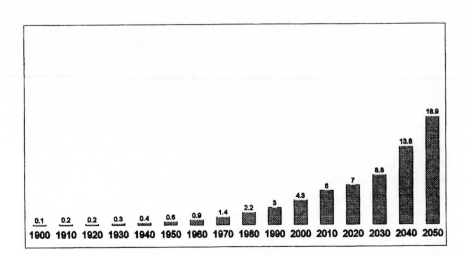

Figure 1.2. Population age 85+ years from 1900 to 2050 (in millions) [Source: U.S. Bureau of the Census, Decennial Censuses for specified years and Population Projections of the United States by Age, Sex, Race, and Hispanic Origin: 1993 to 2050, *Current Population Reports, P25-1104, U.S. Government Printing Office, Washington, DC, 1993. Data for 1990 from* 1990 Census of Population and Housing, CPH-L-74, Modified and Actual Age, Sex, Race, and Hispanic Origin Data.].*

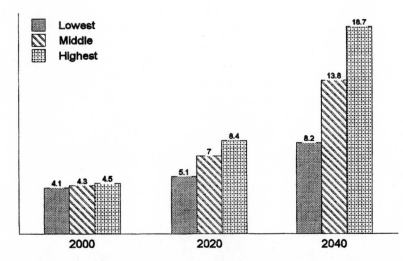

Figure 1.3. Population age 85+ under alternative assumptions from 2000 to 2040 (in millions) [Source: U.S. Bureau of the Census, Population Projections of the United States, by Age, Sex, Race, and Hispanic Origin: 1993 to 2050, *Current Population Reports, P25-1104, U.S. Government Printing Office, Washington, DC, 1993. Adapted from Hobbs, FB and Damon, BL. (1996).* 65+ in the United States *Washington, DC: Government Printing Office (U.S. Bureau of the Census).].*

8

the population over 85 by the Bureau of the Census under three different assumptions about survival of the population and disability rates; note that the estimate for 2040 ranges from 8.2 million people over 85 to 18.7 million.

Using a survey with a somewhat less restrictive definition, Hing & Bloom estimated that 6.7 million noninstitutionalized elderly people had difficulty with performing one or more of seven ADL and IADL activities in 1985. All of the then–1.3 million nursing home residents also fell into the impaired category, resulting in an estimate of 8 million elderly persons with functional impairments in the United States in 1985. When inability to do heavy housework was omitted from the IADL list the number of community dwelling older people with functional impairments dropped to 5.5 million.[4]

Regardless of the actual measures used (which change the prevalence of functional impairment), studies tend to agree on the correlates of functional impairment. Women are more likely to be functionally impaired than men, and blacks are more likely to be functionally impaired than whites. Most notably, the prevalence of functional disability rises sharply with advancing age. Table 1.1 shows a fuller breakdown of impairment data for older community- dwelling elderly in 1991; for each task, the impairment levels rise dramatically with age, as do the proportions getting help with the function.

Health

Older long-term care users often suffer from the diseases that are the major killers of older people—for instance, heart disease, cancer, stroke, diabetes, and pulmonary disease. Such diseases are chronic in nature and their complications may result in fatigue, weakness, and general impairments that necessitate long-term care services. But, just as likely, older people needing long-term care have highly prevalent conditions such as arthritis, which affects mobility and stability. Or, they may have urinary or gynecological problems that cause incontinence and require long-term care as a response. They may have eye diseases and related visual impairments that are the primary cause of the need for long-term care services, or that complicate other conditions. And older people are at much higher risk for Alzheimer's disease, which over time has a devastating effect on overall functioning.

Using 1993 data, federal analysts stated that the most frequently occurring chronic conditions of older people were as follows: arthritis (49%), heart disease and hearing impairments (31% for each), orthopedic impairments (18%), cataracts and sinusitis (15% for each), and diabetes, tinnitus, and visual impairments (10% for each).[5] This is consistent with 1990 national survey data stating that the most common conditions creating a need for long-term care among the elderly were arthritis, coronary heart disease, visual impairments, stroke, and respiratory conditions. In contrast, leading conditions causing a need for long-term care among children included mental retardation and other developmental disabilities, mental illnesses, and respiratory conditions.[6] Some people who need long-term care may, of course, have had the bad fortune to contract one of the chronic diseases affecting

Table 1.1. Functional Limitations of Persons 65 Years and Over by Age and Gender in the 1991 Civilian Noninstitutional Population

Functional limitations	Persons 65 years +	Persons 65 to 74 years		Persons 75 to 84 years		85 years +
		Male	Female	Male	Female	
	30,748	8,264	10,133	3,906	6,014	2,430
% WITH DIFFICULTY[a]						
Walking	14.3	7.4	10.5	16.2	20.4	34.9
Getting outside	15.9	5.9	10.9	15.9	26.4	44.8
Bathing/showering	9.4	4.0	7.0	8.6	13.0	30.6
Transferring from bed or chair	9.0	4.8	6.9	9.3	13.1	21.9
Dressing	5.8	3.4	4.1	5.3	8.1	16.1
Using toilet	4.2	1.5	2.5	4.2	6.8	14.2
Eating	2.1	0.8	1.7	3.1	3.1	4.1
Preparing meals	8.6	4.0	4.9	8.7	13.6	27.6
Managing money	7.1	2.6	3.0	8.1	11.7	26.2
Using the telephone	7.1	5.2	2.7	12.3	8.0	21.4
Light housework	11.4	5.3	7.7	12.4	17.5	30.8
% OF TOTAL RECEIVING HELP[a]						
Walking	5.9	2.9	3.5	8.4	8.0	16.8
Getting outside	13.2	3.7	8.5	13.4	22.3	42.3
Bathing/showering	5.9	2.6	3.8	6.2	7.5	20.9
Transferring from bed or chair	3.9	2.2	2.7	3.9	5.4	11.0
Dressing	3.9	2.3	2.3	4.2	5.5	11.1
Using toilet	2.6	1.0	1.5	3.4	4.1	7.8
Eating	1.1	0.4	0.6	2.2	1.7	2.5
Preparing meals	7.5	3.7	3.5	8.5	11.7	25.4
Managing money	6.4	2.2	2.7	7.5	10.1	24.6
Light housework	8.9	3.9	5.6	9.3	14.0	27.3

[a] Numbers are in thousands

Source note: U. S. Bureau of the Census (1996). *65+ in the United States*, Washington, DC: U.S. Government Printing Office. Data derived from 1992 Survey of Income and Program Participation.

older people at an early age. Coronary heart disease and respiratory conditions are also among the top reasons that people age 18–64 need long-term care. But, the top causes of long-term care needs in 1990 for these younger adults were, in order, bad back, mental retardation, and mental illness.

Service structures have arisen to meet the particular constellation of needs that arise as a combination of life-stage and disease. Among identifiable long-term care populations are people with developmental disabilities, such as cerebral palsy, that can affect physical functioning, mental abilities, or both; people with spinal cord injuries resulting in paraplegia or quadriplegia, who often sustain this injury in their teens or young adulthood; people with progressive neurological diseases such as multiple sclerosis, muscular dystrophy, amyotrophic lateral sclerosis (ALS) also known as Lou Gehrig's disease; people who sustain brain injuries that affect their physical or cognitive abilities; and, increasingly in the 1980s and 1990's, people who have acquired immunodeficiency syndrome (AIDS) or human immunodeficiency virus (HIV). By dint of age of onset and nature of the disability, people under 65 with some conditions, for example, multiple sclerosis, are likely to have spouses in a position to provide or coordinate long-term care.

Researchers have examined the relationship among three major health events: death, disease, and disability. They recognize that changes in the rates of one will affect the others and that the period of disability (and thus the period for needing long-term care) can be influenced by a number of factors. Figure 1.4 shows the hypothetical relationship between survival curves for each of these three elements. The curves are drawn to show the rate that a population loses life or health. At birth, almost everyone is alive and few are disabled or ill. Over time, people acquire disability and disease. In general the onset of disease comes before the development of disability. Although some diseases lead directly to death, most entail a period of disability. Thus, if the age of death is postponed and other factors are unaffected, more people will be in a disabled state longer. Likewise, if the onset of disease can be postponed with no change in the death rate, the period of illness (known as morbidity) and disability can be compressed. The view that morbidity is indeed becoming compressed into later years has been actively championed by James Fries,[7] who argues that preventive actions can create this state, wherein most ill nesses and disabilities of older people are concentrated in a short period before their death. On the other hand, reducing the incidence of diseases that cause disability will also reduce death rates from these conditions, leaving people in the population who can develop other diseases that in turn lead to disability requiring long-term care. Thus, as Chad Boult and colleagues argue,[8] it is possible that the overall number of people with disabilities might increase even if the overall health of the older population improves.

Cognition
One cannot write about who needs long-term care without alluding to the large population with Alzheimer's disease and similar cognitive impairments accompa-

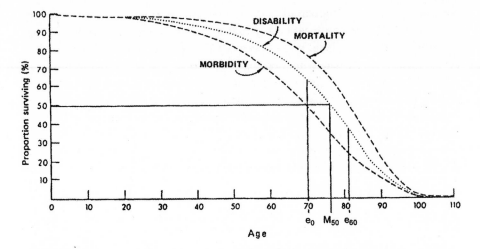

Figure 1.4. The observed mortality and hypothetical morbidity and disability survival curves for females in the United States of America in 1980. NOTE: e_0 *and* e_{60} *are the number of years of autonomous life expected at birth and at age 60, respectively;* M_{50} *is the age to which 50% of females could expect to survive without loss of autonomy. [Source: World Health Organization.* The Uses of Epidemiology in the Study of the Elderly: Report of a WHO Scientific Group on the Epidemiology of Aging. *Technical Report Series No. 706. Geneva, 1984.].*

nied by pervasive memory loss. Alzheimer's disease is a specific condition that cannot be definitively diagnosed except at autopsy, so statistics cannot easily be developed for Alzheimer's disease alone. The term *senile dementia* is used to group a wide-range of disorders that are characterized by irreversible and increasing memory loss, sometimes accompanied by personality change and disturbing behavior and, at the end stage, resulting in almost complete loss of function. Dementia accounts disproportionately for people in nursing homes and people receiving formal long-term care, but it is important to recognize that dementing illnesses typically have a long time horizon and a gradual progression. At early stages, long-term care may not be needed.

How prevalent is dementia? A 1996 consensus panel convened by the Agency for Health Care Policy and Research examined all the estimates of dementia from population studies worldwide and concluded that the rate of moderate-to-severe dementia (the stage at which long-term care is definitely needed) is about 2% in people aged 65–69, 4% in people aged 70–74, 8% in people aged 75–79, and 16% in people over 85. In contrast, a study of older people in East Boston that used less restrictive criteria (and, thus, counted people with mild dementia and no functional disability) concluded that 10% of the population over 65 and 47% over 85 had some degree of dementia. The panel estimated that at least 2 million Americans, and possibly as many as 4 million, suffer from cognitive decline related to dementia.[9] Many in this group have measurable ADL and IADL impairment. The extent to which common measures of functional impairment adequately pick up the need for care of people with dementia is vigorously debated. However, the current trend is to include within estimates of people with functional impairment those people who can perform the function physically but need to be reminded about it and supervised because of cognitive disability.

Alzheimer's disease is not the only cause of cognitive impairment. Large numbers of people with intellectual impairment due to developmental disability also need long-term care, as do some people who have sustained brain injuries leading to difficulties in problem solving, exercising judgment, and memory.

Mental Illnesses and Chemical Dependency

Chronic mental illnesses rarely in themselves create a need for long-term care. Typically, people with schizophrenia, manic depressive illness, or personality disorders need good primary care and periodic acute care in hospitals. They may have difficulty finding affordable housing, partly because of income limitations and partly because of eccentricity. In the 1960s, when large numbers of people were discharged from mental hospitals to the community, efforts were made to create less restrictive, more affordable housing options for them. As a consequence, many people with chronic mental illness received outpatient psychiatric care and were passed from program to program. Public policy associated with their care was coupled with long-term care concepts, yet many people were lost to follow-up.

As this population develops physical problems requiring long-term care, their psychiatric problems may be exacerbated, and they will return to restrictive care settings. Similarly, although alcohol and drug problems rarely necessitate long-term care, people with chemical dependency pose special difficulties when long-term care becomes necessary.

Poverty

Poverty is not in itself a reason to need long-term care. However, older people with low income and few assets are most likely to rely on public financing for the care they need. The press has recently promulgated the idea that elderly people are wealthy in contrast to children. Indeed, the Social Security Program, combined with individual pensions and savings, have reduced official poverty statistics among old people. Based on 1992 data, the median income for white males over age 65 was $15,276, and white females $8,579; the figures for blacks were $8,031 and $6,220, respectively. Looking at the income another way, by examining the proportions of elderly people living alone with incomes of less than $10,000, 33.7% of elderly men and 44% of elderly women fell into that category. After age 75, 39.8% of elderly men and 56.8% of elderly women had incomes under $10,000. Of married-couple households, 7.2% of whites and 21.9% of blacks had a house-

hold income under $10,000.[10] Thus, although social security produced overall im-
provements in income for older people, we approach the twenty-first century with
substantial poverty among elderly people. Poverty is more likely among elderly
women, very old elderly, black elderly, and elderly people living alone. It is unlikely that any of these individuals could finance their own long-term care without
substantial public subsidy.

Older people, at least in the birth cohorts presently old, tend to own their own
homes; of 20.3 million persons living outside institutions in 1993, 77% owned their
homes, and 82% of these owned their homes free and clear, without mortgage.
Older people (72% of elderly householders) tended to live in single-family homes;
6%, a full 1.2 million elderly householders, lived in mobile homes. Often the major
asset of the older person is his or her home, however; the 1991 median value of
these homes was $70,418. Policy-makers have spent considerable energy trying to
determine ways that older people needing long-term care could parlay the value of
their homes—for example, by taking out loans on the home, by reverse-mortgage
arrangements, or even by home-sharing or live-in help arrangements.

Diversity

This section has discussed target groups needing long-term care in a way that
suggests that all people needing long-term care share common characteristics. In
fact, people who need long-term care are first and foremost individuals. In factors
unrelated to the need for long term care, each consumer has his or her own unique
social milieu, personal history, accomplishments, interests, preferences, and wishes,
so one cannot generalize a long-term care plan.

There is simply no substitute for getting to know each long-term care consumer
and to gain appreciation for them. The consumer may be in mourning for a deceased loved one. He or she may have had satisfying recent self-affirming experiences, or may feel neglected and disrespected. The people most important to this
consumer may be minutes away and in close contact or half way across the world.
Since long-term care concerns the betterment of everyday life for people with
functional disabilities, and since what constitutes meaning and pleasure is such an
individual matter, those who provide and plan long-term care cannot neglect the
enormous diversity among those who receive it. By the time we consider all the
potential variations that can be combined in a long-term care consumer, we can
conclude that, almost like snowflakes, each person needing long-term care differs
from each other person in a way that should help shape a long-term care plan.

Who Gives Long-Term Care?

Ordinary people living out their lives and doing what needs to be done to assist
family members with disabilities are hardly likely to see themselves as long-term
care providers. In fact, however, most long-term care is given by family members

and friends, and most such care is given without financial compensation. When the person needing long-term care lives with a husband or wife or some other relative, distinguishing the added long-term care activities may be difficult. A woman who has always done the family laundry and cooking may simply have a bit more to do. A retired person who typically spent her evenings with her sister in their shared household may now *need* to be on hand to supervise that sister's safety given the latter's stroke, Alzheimer's disease, or unsteady gait. On the other hand, some family members find themselves undertaking completely new long-term tasks. A man who never cooked or managed a household is suddenly doing so for himself and his spouse with a disability. A spouse, daughter, or other relative is suddenly called upon to assist a family member with bathing, dressing, getting in and out of bed, and taking medicines. If these family long-term care providers live in different households from the people they are helping, the time commitments are somewhat easier to calculate than in the case of shared households. In both scenarios, the time commitments and responsibilities can become formidable, although difficulties remain in separating the discretionary time spent with relatives from time spent doing long-term care tasks.

According to data from the 1990 Survey of Program Participants, which samples noninstitutionalized people with chronic disabilities, nearly 83% of such people under age 65 and 73% of such 65 and older relied *exclusively* on help from family and friends, whereas only 9% relied exclusively on care from professionals and other paid helpers.[11] A national 1985 survey held that about 4.2 million Americans were giving long-term care to a spouse or parent with a physical disability or illness that impaired functional abilities and that 2.6 million of these were deemed "primary caregivers," meaning that they had the major responsibility for providing the assistance.[12] Most of these family caregivers were providing care to a person over age 65, and many of them were, themselves, in their retirement years. People under 65 also received substantial help from family members, including from their parents, as well as spouses, brothers and sisters, and children. Despite the popular appeal of the image of a "sandwich generation," which must balance child care and work with care of older relatives, the reality is that most family caregivers are themselves old.

Long-term care is also provided by people who are paid to do the job—professionals and other workers who are employed by organizations, employed by clients directly, or self-employed. (The distinction between being self-employed and employed by the client is a technical one; in fact, given recent rulings of the Internal Revenue Service, it may be inappropriate to construe many home-care workers as self-employed because of the repetitive, supervised nature of their work.[13]) Such long-term care is sometimes called *formal care*, to distinguish it from *informal care* provided by unpaid family members. Some family members are also paid directly by their relatives who receive the care, or by public authorities subsidizing that care. This steady trend toward payment of family members is muddying the distinction between family care and paid care.

A plethora of job titles are used for those who provide hands-on long-term care services as an occupation: nursing aide, nursing assistant, home health aide, home-maker, practical nurse, personal care assistant, attendant, chore worker, driver. By and large, the people who literally provide ongoing long-term care services are not and need not be professionals such as nurses, social workers, occupational thera-pists, physical therapists, or speech therapists. Many of the services are, after all, the same services that people provide for themselves when they can and that family members often provide without any special credentials.

Although many tasks of long-term care are ordinary and well within the abilities of people without formal credentials, nevertheless, professionals do have crucial roles. Professionals may be needed to plan long-term care services, to teach family members or paid providers, or to perform particular specialized tasks (for example, a nurse to do some skin care or catheter insertion, or to teach family members and paid personnel to do so).[14] But, by and large, the labor-intensive tasks that consti-tute long-term care can be done by nonprofessionals. If regulations require that various long-term care be performed by professionals or be supervised by profes-sionals at frequent, prescribed intervals, the cost of the care is likely to soar and perhaps become impractical to be provided in private homes for all but the very wealthy. Paradoxically, informal care of even great complexity can legally be per-formed by just about anyone, whereas once payment for the service is involved, professional and other regulations often require specific credentials.

One of the recurrent themes in this book addresses the thorny issue of the extent to which long-term care can and should be provided by generalist, nonprofessional personnel and how to achieve a standard of safety that is acceptable to the person receiving care and to the public. We believe that it is possible, desirable, and necessary to take explicit steps to render long- term care less professional. We also believe such steps can be taken without compromising the quality of long-term care and the competence of those who provide it, or belittling the contributions of professionals.

Places for Long-Term Care

Too often long-term care has been circumscribed by service settings. Thus, neo-phytes are likely to define long-term care as care given to people in nursing homes, home health care clients, day care clients, and so on. It is imperative that long-term care services be distinguished from the places where long-term care is pro-vided. Even hospitals, those bastions of acute care, sometimes provide long-term care services to their long-stay patients—and perhaps they *should* do so more often. And increasingly staff of nursing homes and home health agencies provide acute care to chronically ill people who have active illnesses. Although it is often difficult to distinguish a long-term care service from an acute care service, the attempt is worth making.

As mentioned earlier, most people who receive long-term care in the community rely exclusively or extensively on family members for these services. Those outside nursing homes who receive paid help—in the jargon, *formal care*—usually live in private homes or apartments in the community. Some live in boarding homes, small group homes, foster homes (which have now sprung up for adults as well as children), and various kinds of retirement homes, congregate housing, or assisted living settings. The minority of seniors receiving long-term care—estimated variously as 1 in 3, 1 in 2, or 1 in 1.5—live in nursing homes. Here the presumption has been that the care is all formal, but some data are available to show that many family members continue to provide hands-on care and also monitor the facility care for older relatives who live in nursing homes.[15] Such relatives do not merely visit; they help.

Details on where long-term care users under age 65 live are harder to come by because fewer governmental programs exist for their care. Again, the vast majority seem to live in the community, though some adults with developmental disabilities do live in small group homes and residential care facilities. Some people with developmental disabilities and mental retardation also live in specialized intermediate care facilities (that is, nursing homes) or even in nursing homes largely serving older people.

Policy analysts at the Department of Health and Human Services used 1990 Census data to estimate where people who need long-term care reside. They calculated that 64% of the 262,000 children under 18 who needed long-term care, 86% of the 5 million people aged age 18–64 who needed long-term care, and 78% of the 7.3 million people over 65 who needed long-term care lived in the community. Among the elderly, more than 1.6 million people lived in nursing homes; about 50,000 were scattered in other kinds of institutional accommodations. Those between 18 and 64 who lived in institutions were more likely to live in special intermediate care facilities for mental retardation (118,000), other facilities for mental retardation (109,000), or facilities for the mentally ill (144,000), though 181,000 lived in nursing homes. Also, the census also found a scattering of other institutions housing people needing long-term care, including prisons and jails (119,000 under 65 and 3,000 over 65) and homeless shelters (29,000 under 65 and 3,000 over 65).[16] Ordinarily, all those who live in institutions are counted as receiving formal as opposed to informal care. However, as we already indicated, some family members do provide ADL and IADL help to older people living in nursing homes.

Goals of Long-Term Care

Goals for long-term care can be seen at two levels—the level of the individual consumer and the community or societal level. In either case, the goals are difficult to articulate, let alone measure.

Goals for Individual Consumers

What should long-term care achieve for the long-term care consumer? This question is as perplexing as it is crucial. Many goals have been attributed to long-term care programs, in general. Although extremely long lists could be generated, most goals can be subsumed under the following major categories:

- Improve or maintain health
- Improve or slow deterioration of functional abilities
- Meet needs for care and assistance (sometimes called "unmet needs")
- Enhance psychological well-being
- Enhance social well-being
- Maximize client independence and autonomy
- Permit clients to live in the least restrictive settings feasible
- Promote a meaningful life

Most of these categories, with some variation from author to author, have been combined to describe the phenomenon labeled "quality of life." This term addresses the range of attributes that affect a client's perception of his or her situation and its impact on his or her daily existence. Let us consider each separately.

Improve or maintain health. This goal, which is consistent with general goals for health services, emphasizes prevention of diseases (for example, through flu vaccines); timely and accurate diagnosis of diseases; provision of treatments that cure disease and ease pain or alleviate symptoms; and rehabilitation of physical conditions to restore as much functional ability as possible. This also entails minimizing iatrogenic problems—that is, health problems caused by the treatments themselves. Although some complications of treatment are inevitable, it has become a classic problem of geriatric medicine that older people have been unnecessarily harmed by medical care, particularly medication errors (inappropriate medicine, too much medicine, not enough medicine, or incompatible medicines).[17] The achievement of health goals can be measured in conventional terms by morbidity and mortality rates, complication rates for existing conditions, and low rates of untreated treatable conditions found in the target population. Other approaches include measures of bed-days and use of hospitals, or scores on measures of pain and discomfort.

Since these are also the goals of acute care (to which, we argue, each long-term care client needs access), postulating health goals for long-term care may seem redundant. But, long-term care clients often receive perfunctory, haphazard, or poor-quality acute care, and it is, thus, important to institute some system to monitor health outcomes for those getting long-term care. Chapter 8 deals in detail with the challenge of providing excellent medical care to those who receive long-term care. Certainly goals could and should be established for that enterprise. The goals of long-term care would ordinarily (but perhaps not always) be consistent with the goals of acute health care.

Health goals could be at the heart of long-term care even though long-term care is not about health per se. Although the paramount goal of long-term care is likely not directed at improving health, good long-term care can have a positive effect on health. For example, close monitoring of clients' status can detect problems early and bring them into effective treatment. Giving good long-term care is often associated with avoiding untoward events, such as pressure sores, infections, and falls. By that standard, protecting the client from injury and falls, maintaining sterile conditions to minimize infections, making sure that diets are followed, and making sure medicines are taken as ordered would seem to be important long-term care efforts. Although good long-term care can enhance health, the pursuit of health should not become the primary obsession of long-term care. Just as other people do, long-term care consumers make choices every day about pursuing practices that are pleasurable but unhealthy or risky. We argue that long-term care consumers should be allowed to take the same risks as others. Indeed, some might argue that since many older long-term care clients are already at substantial risk for premature death, they might want to maximize their enjoyment of what pleasures life can afford them, even if such actions compromise their longevity.

All Americans are routinely exhorted to maintain healthy lifestyles, and long-term care consumers who are highly dependent on assistance with everyday living too often are forced to live according to some official (though ever-changing) view of how to be healthy and safe. Yet most long-term care clients are nearing the ends of their lives and have no expectations of preventing death in the relatively near future. They may have strong negative reactions to living their lives by prescription, in subservience to a rigid plan for health and safety.

Functional abilities. The relationship between health and functioning is intertwined. A schema developed by the World Health Organization[18] to address this connection describes a continuum, as shown below:

Disease → Impairment → Disability → Handicap

A disease can produce a physiological impairment that makes a person less healthy. This impairment, in turn, can lead to a disability, that is, a limitation in functioning. This limitation may or may not create a handicap in that person's performance of various social roles. The existence and extent of handicap depends on the demands made and the environmental supports (including human assistance) available. Thus, many people with quadriplegia can hold down jobs and travel if they have sufficient personal assistance.

As already stated, functional limitations are the trigger and the reason for long-term care. Considerable consensus exists that long-term care programs should aspire to help people regain the capacity to perform self-care tasks and other functional tasks and to help them retain their existing abilities. This requires a rehabilitative stance, especially pertinent for those who have just left a hospital or are recovering from a period of illness and bed rest. It entails attention to vision care, foot care, medication regimens, prosthetic devices, and environmental changes, all of which can affect functional abilities and some of which requires involvement of health care personnel. Improving or maintaining functional abilities also requires an attitude that encourages clients to do things for themselves and by themselves to the extent that they wish. Sometimes long-term care providers find it difficult (and time-consuming) to watch, stand by, and assist a little bit rather than simply to make the bed, prepare the meal by themselves, and generally perform tasks for the consumers.

Although aiming for improvements or maintenance in functional status seems sensible, working toward the goal is by no means simple. Functional behavior is determined by a combination of forces, including physical abilities, intellectual abilities, emotional state, and social circumstances. Functional behavior—which is another way of saying "what people do"—is also determined by people's own preferences and choices. A person who prepares meals must be physically capable of doing so, must remember it is mealtime, must have some rudimentary cooking abilities, must have food on hand and money to replenish it, must have cooking equipment that is accessible and in working order, and must be motivated to use it. The same kind of list could be developed for any of the functional problems for which long-term care is given. We have sometimes expressed the multiple forces affecting functioning in a conceptual equation:

$$\text{Function} = \frac{\text{physical ability} + \text{intellectual ability} + \text{psychological state}}{\text{social resources} + \text{social support} + \text{social expectations}}$$

In this formulation, psychological states include both mood states such as depression and anxiety, and the person's motivation to perform the particular function. Note, too, that efforts to improve functioning can be directed to any of the elements in the equation.

Functional abilities are sometimes measured by the answers to "can you" questions. Can you move from your bed to a chair without assistance? Can you bathe or shower without assistance? A further step in the "can you" approach is to observe the behavior being performed. (Show me, please, how you would put on this shirt.) In contrast, sometimes functional abilities are measured by "do you" questions. Do you bathe without assistance? Dress yourself? Prepare meals? Of course, each of these functions also needs to be specified if reliable information is to be gathered.

Beyond operational definitions for each task, the distinction between "can" and "do" is pivotal. Sometimes people fail to do what they *can* do, either because of opportunity or preference. Sometimes the reason for underachievement is found in the environment. For example, I can drive, but do not have access to a car and never do drive. I can prepare meals, but am not permitted to do so in my lodgings. In my opinion, I can bathe myself, but rules require that all baths be supervised by staff in this nursing home. In my opinion, I can take my medicines, but a nurse at the assisted living program administers all medications. On the other hand, consumers who say that they cannot perform a task and then say that they actually perform it (a seemingly illogical position of exceeding one's capacity) may be setting lesser standards for performance, may be exerting themselves heroically, or may be using creative efforts to perform (e.g., attaching tools for house-cleaning or painting to a cane).[19] Some would argue that the goal is to improve capacity, whereas actual behavior is a matter of private choice and, sometimes, organizational policy. But we contend that it makes sense generally to emphasize actual performance—what consumers *do*, taking into account, of course, what they want to do. The capacity to bathe is irrelevant if the person who cherishes a private bath at the time of her choosing is never allowed to exercise the ability. On the other hand, it is important to understand the client's ability in order to interpret the effect of the environment; permissive rules will be of little avail to someone who is unable to perform the task.

Functional inability usually establishes the eligibility for long-term care programs in the first place (at least those that require public money). This means that the way functional impairment is defined and assessed is fraught with political and economic significance. Making the need for assistance the criterion for obtaining support can create perverse incentives for emphasizing dependency.

Meeting need. However hard-hearted a society, at some level it responds to human need and suffering. Needs such as eating, eliminating bodily wastes, and being clean are easily identified as necessary. If a community enjoys good long-term care programs, one can argue, no people with disabilities would be isolated and incommunicado for lack of help in getting out of bed. No people suffering from Alzheimer's disease would be left to survive in their homes and community by luck alone. Presumably some unmet need would always be present in society because some problems evolve in social isolation, but once the unmet need is identified, long-term care would be the response.

Thus, the long-term care literature is replete with references to "unmet need," which presumably a good program strives to eliminate. An "unmet need" standard is hard to apply, however; commentators might well disagree about what constitutes a need or how to distinguish needs from "wishes." If needs are defined closer to wishes, meeting needs is an impossible quest. Few of us really expect to have all our desires met. If we try to adhere to a need standard, some long-term care providers might overzealously identify needs based on professional or personal standards that exceed those of the potential client—for example, unless the house is spotless, an unmet need for housekeeping exists. Others might have an extraordinarily high threshold before they perceive an unmet need. A key factor in defining need concerns the way family activities are considered. Ordinarily, long-term care programs that use public dollars recognize unmet need only if no family member is currently providing or able to continue to provide the service. The devil here is in the details. If family members wish to give up the tasks but haven't yet done so, can unmet need be said to exist?

Measuring unmet need is also difficult. It often is approximated by asking older people about whether they get as much help as they feel they need with an enumerated list of tasks that they have previously indicated they cannot perform in-

dependently. More promising are recent efforts to measure adverse events associated with unaddressed or inadequately addressed functional impairment. For
example, being unable to bathe as often as I would like, having fallen while getting
out of bed or a chair, or waiting more than a specified time to be helped to the
toilet. On the IADL front, those who cannot cook independently could be asked
whether they go without eating when hungry, those who have transportation problems could be asked about missed doctor's appointment or being unable to go
places for fun, and those with inability to wash laundry might be asked about
wearing dirty clothes in the last month.[20]

In some ways *unmet need* is a phrase with built-in contradictions. We cannot
imagine addressing a *met need*, which would mean no need existed. Long-term
care needs at the level of eating, drinking, and basic hygiene cannot readily go
unmet without death or some crisis ensuing. Thus, one presumes that before the
moment that unmet need was identified, most clients were somehow managing
through their own and their family efforts. Once help is provided some clients will,
by definition, decrease their functional abilities in the sense of what they ordinarily
do, and such a change is often highly appropriate and desirable.

Some tension exists between the goal of improving functioning and the goal of
meeting need. Those who emphasize the latter fear belittling the goal of providing
necessary services that make people's lives bearable and allow them to pursue
whatever happiness and meaning they can. They rail against turning a simple mission into rehabilitation and resist requirements that help be justified in terms of
therapeutic efficacy. An overemphasis on therapy, for example, leads to unrealistic
goals for memory improvement for people with advanced Alzheimer's disease.
Those who prefer to emphasize functional improvement, in contrast, fear that as-
piring to meet needs and compensate for impairment will lead to therapeutic nihilism and overly modest goals. Difficult as this stance is, we think that long-term
care programs must aspire both to meet existing need and, when feasible, to
improve or maintain functioning. In Chapter 5, we reintroduce this tension between
therapeutic and compensatory goals in the context of home care.

It is important to recognize that it is virtually impossible to meet all perceived
needs associated with long-term care. The resources required would bankrupt society. Moreover, the demand for more services would likely be stimulated by the
services supplied, presuming such services are viewed as acceptable and helpful.
Thus, *need* takes on a professional aura, relying on the judgment of experts as to
what services are required in the actual circumstances. This decision is often complicated. As noted already, some people can perform a task but with great difficulty,
considerable pain, and excruciatingly slowly. What does it mean to say a person
cannot perform a task? How much suffering or effort is required to merit assistance?

Some observers worry that providing services may exacerbate dependency. In
the context of nursing home care, for example, the pressure to accomplish the
service as efficiently as possible often means that people who could feed or dress

themselves with sufficient time and encouragement are fed or dressed instead. People with Alzheimer's disease or other dementias, who require extensive reminding and cuing, are particularly vulnerable to these short-cuts. Altruistic motives could lead devoted caregivers to adopt a similar anti-rehabilitation strategy. Provision of maximal assistance may lead to increased functional dependency over time for the person who has had things done for him or her. Because many measures of functional impairment are expressed in terms of the extent to which the person gets help from someone to perform the particular ADL or IADL activity, the availability of help may have the paradoxical effect that more people are classified as functionally impaired.

Psychological well-being. Depressive mood and anxiety often accompany long-term care. Their roots may well be in the conditions that gave rise to needing long-term care in the first place (for example, illnesses and disabilities, and loss of family and friends who could help informally). Long-term care personnel may not have the responsibility or even the skill to alleviate these aspects of the human condition. However, some programs consider that their mission includes offering long-term care in such a way that depression and anxiety are reduced and that clients express positive moods (for example, pleasure and good outlooks about the future). Furthermore, long-term care programs themselves can produce or exacerbate negative emotional states (for example, a home care worker frightens the client, or the client feels a bewildering and demoralizing loss of identity in the nursing home milieu); arguably, therefore, long-term care programs could be examined and compared based on the extent of psychological well-being in their clientele, and programs should be held accountable for not making things worse.

Psychological well-being in the sense of positive and negative mood states should be distinguished from depression and other psychological conditions that fall into the purview of psychopathology. Such conditions need to be recognized and treated appropriately. The management of psychiatric conditions in long-term care presents a number of paradoxes. Examples abound of both insufficient and excessive treatment. Psychoactive drugs are often used inappropriately to quiet disruptive consumers, even those without a diagnosed psychiatric problem. (The use of drugs for such presumed convenience of caregivers has become known as "pharmacological restraint.") On the other hand, serious psychiatric problems may go unrecognized and untreated. Especially common is the failure to recognize and treat major depressive episodes, or to identify and treat alcohol abuse that begins late in life with no prior history to alert professionals.

Long-term care providers may themselves lack the skill for such differential diagnoses. Sometimes these determinations can be made by physicians, hospital discharge planners, and case managers who arrange long-term care initially. However, care providers also need to be alert to changes in psychological well-being that signal the need for expert attention. The highest suicide rates in the nation are among men over age 65.

Although depression is underdiagnosed and undertreated among older people,

one cannot exonerate long-term care programs that perpetuate conditions fostering depression with the view that older people are, in any event, often depressed.
For example, in getting feedback on care for quality assurance purposes, some
commentators would discount dissatisfaction if the informant is also depressed
on the grounds that this would distort their perceptions. We disagree with that
position. People who are depressed can also vary in their satisfaction with services, and discontent with services and life conditions can induce or exacerbate
depression.

Social well-being. Social well-being can further be subdivided into measures of
social involvement (for example, social activities), measures of role performance
(such as family roles, community roles, avocational roles, and vocational roles),
and measures of social relatedness (for example, engagement with family members and friends in interactions that give the client a sense of belonging and purpose). As with psychological well-being, long-term care programs vary as to
whether or not their goals include helping clients improve or maintain social well-
being. If a long-term care program takes the affirmative course on this issue, the
implications might be that the program would provide functional assistance so that
the clients could participate in activities of their choice and interact with companions of their choice. Although nursing homes typically have activity programs and
are attentive to "socialization needs," one doubts that social well-being is truly
synonymous with being channeled to organized social activities. The ability to
sustain and develop intimate relationships may be hampered by placing people in
unnatural group living situations. Similarly, one cannot be sanguine that social
well-being has been improved for community clientele merely by referring those
who appear socially isolated to day care programs, where they mingle with many
other people with disabilities. For some people, a referral to day care might improve social well-being, whereas for others it might well underscore their loss of
meaningful activity.

Autonomy and choice. In the last ten years or so, the long-term care field has
consciously valued client autonomy and client personal choice. Autonomy implies
control over one's situation. For example, even a person who is completely paralyzed can direct his or her life if able to direct what caregivers do.[21] Autonomy
and choice are different in kind from outcomes of care such as health and functional
outcomes, and indeed client's exercise of personal freedoms and choice may some-
time be associated with worse outcomes on other dimensions. Yet, arguments can
be made to include as goals of long-term care that clients retain their rights to
control their everyday lives and larger destinies, and to make choices about how
and where they live. This emphasis is an antidote to paternalistic modes of long-
term care that are particularly likely to prevail where older people have been concerned. Too often, frail elderly clients have been protected against their will, or
relocated summarily. Too often, the safety and physical health of the long-term
care client has been viewed as the dominant goal with no regard for the client's
own preferences.

Other chapters in this book describe initiatives at the state and program level that substantially emphasize values such as client autonomy, choice, dignity, and normal lifestyles. In several states, notably Oregon, Wisconsin, and Indiana, such values have been enacted into state law. Once a commitment has been made in principle to client autonomy and choice, long-term care programs are then constrained to achieve their other results (e.g., improved functioning, meeting unmet need) without undue compromise of those principles.

Least restrictive settings. The notion of "least restrictive settings" is also often incorporated into many state laws or policy documents. This idea is related but not identical to the issue of autonomy discussed above. The goal would be that no person be required to receive care in a setting that restricts personal freedom and control more than necessary. This principle is typically applied by creating a hierarchy of restrictiveness (e.g., a small group home or foster home is more restrictive than home care but less restrictive than a nursing home). If the more restrictive settings also tend to be more expensive (though that relationship is not necessarily causal), public payers have an economic interest in the "least restrictive setting" criteria.

The position we develop in this book, opposes assigning clients to settings deemed "appropriate" for them based on their level and type of need. In fact, the long-term care needs of a particular person can be met in quite a wide range of settings. Personal choice should be relevant when this overlap occurs. Very few people "need" a nursing home in the sense that they could not be cared for in another setting. Price, of course, is an object for most private and public purchasers, but we also argue that the relationship between the characteristics of a residential setting and the reimbursement rates they require or can obtain from the public sector can be arbitrary. Furthermore, the restrictiveness of a setting is less related to the services offered there (which do affect the price) than to other conventions of the setting (for example, locked doors to the outside, unlocked space inside for ease of staff surveillance, rules restricting privacy, use of physical restraints). We firmly endorse the goal that long-term care clients should not be unnecessarily restricted, but would apply that to the care plan that is developed in any setting rather than to attributing restrictiveness to a particular setting.

Sometimes, the goal of achieving least restrictive settings is a code word for avoiding nursing homes. As we will discuss throughout this book, we view the nursing home models of the 1970s and 1980s as anachronistic. We expect and hope that the kind of care institution known as a nursing home, the avoidance of which has been the focus of so much policy effort, will gradually largely disappear to be replaced by a variety of different kinds of living settings, characterized by privacy and residential character, where care can readily be attained. Clients who need long-term care for the foreseeable future and who cannot remain in their own homes, will, we believe, gravitate to these new kinds of apartment-type or family settings. Some long-term care clients who are in nursing homes for the short run to convalesce or be rehabilitated may also end up either at home or in a totally revamped nursing home.

Meaningful lives. It sounds unrealistic and even sophomoric to hold out a sense of meaning in life as a goal of long-term care. It is also a difficult and inescapably subjective goal to measure. But we want to flag this idea because there is all too much reason to believe that many long-term care consumers experience a sense that life is not worthwhile, that their value as people has ended. Sheldon Tobin[22] refers to maintenance of a sense of identity as the key challenge for nursing home residents, and Rosalie Kane's study of more than 800 community-dwelling long-term care consumers found that at least 25% could think of nothing to which they looked forward.[23] Jaber Gubrium found a chilling expression of this phenomenon while interviewing an elderly nursing home resident about the quality of her life.[24] She repeatedly and pleasantly asserted that the quality of life was poor but "it doesn't matter." When pressed for an explanation, she said, "my life is over." We lack the data to compare these reactions to those of older people in the community who do *not* receive long-term care; they, too, may experience a diminishment in life's meaning and quality of life. Nonetheless, one has to believe that some of these reactions represent societal failure to find meaningful roles and lifestyles for older people, particularly those receiving long-term care. Worse, such notions could be a response to the compromises in lifestyle that public long-term care policies demand. The work of Helen Kivnick and her colleagues on "elder role models in long-term care" profiles ordinary older people with severe long-term care needs whose lives, nonetheless, are replete with plans, self-perceived meaning, and even productivity.[25] Given the possibilities for fulfillment in later life, it is perhaps incumbent on a long-term care program to be aware of the extent to which consumers believe their lives are over and to try to rectify the situation. At least long-term care should not reinforce this hopeless mindset.

Societal and Community Goals

Long-term care serves the community as well as individual long-term care clients. Social decisions about long-term care provision, therefore, incorporate decisions about the expectations for family members of people with disabilities and the responsibilities of one generation to another. Some basic resolution is needed about what we expect of each other as fellow citizens and neighbors, in contrast to what we expect of each other as family members. The answers to these questions will determine what professionally provided services will be developed and the extent to which family members will be expected to finance long-term care before publicly subsidized programs come into play. Sometimes societal goals are couched in terms of reducing overall costs or reducing public costs. Sometimes they are described in terms of creating a system that is equitable in meeting need or that minimizes waiting times for getting help.

Family members will continue to be involved in providing direct long-term care services in the foreseeable future—because they want to do so, because they cannot afford to do otherwise, and also because many long-term care services are the kinds of activities that constitute doing what comes naturally in the family unit (e.g., cooking, cleaning, laundry). Some long-term care programs incorporate goals related to the well-being of family members who inevitably will be drawn into providing care, arranging care, and purchasing care for their relatives. Typically, the long-term care program may hold out as a goal that family members feel confident and competent as caregivers, that they are continue providing uncompensated help, or that they experience no undue burden as a result of caregiving activities. Some long-term care programs count as an achievement that family members continue to provide substantial, uncompensated care for their clients. Some programs aspire simultaneously to decrease family burden and to sustain the existence of family care (although these goals may at times be contradictory).

In the rest of Part 1, we turn to a discussion of long-term care programs as they are currently organized and financed. However, we will repeatedly revert to a discussion of the goals of the long-term care enterprise, an obviously critical matter when we try to evaluate how well long-term care programs are doing or to hold long-term care programs to quality standards. Our ideal is a long-term care program that aspires to identify, correct, and compensate for health problems so that the long-term care client's functional abilities can be maintained at the highest possible level. Equally important, our ideal requires that necessary assistance with daily living be rendered in such a way that the person with the disability can live as meaningfully and fully as possible. At a minimum, the way we offer long-term care should not detract from the long-term care client's social and psychological well-being; at a maximum, the long-term care programs should be designed to enhance the clients' perceived well-being, participation in family and community, and personal identity.

Notes

1. Kahn AJ & Kamerman SB (1976). *Social Services in International Perspective: The Emergence of the Sixth System*. (U.S. Department of Health, Education, and Welfare, SRS 76-05704). Washington, DC: Government Printing Office.
2. Wiener JM, Hanley RJ, Clark R, & Van Nostrand JF (1990). Measuring the activities of daily living: comparisons across outcome surveys. *Journal of Gerontology* 45: S229–S237.
3. Hobb FB & Damon BL (1996). *65 + in the United States*. (U.S. Bureau of the Census. Current Population Reports, Special Studies). Washington, DC: Government Printing Office. For the estimates reported here ADLs included were bathing, dressing, eating, getting out of bed or chairs, walking, using the toilet, and continence. IADLs included were preparing meals, shopping, managing money, using the telephone, doing light housework, and getting outside. We note, however, that a different national study done the same year, the 1991 Health Interview Survey, produced substantially lower estimates of functional impairment in older people using the same items.
4. Hing E & Bloom B (1990). Long-term care for the functionally impaired elderly. (Vital and Health Statistics, Series B; No. 104, DHHS Pub. No. PHS 90-1765). Hyattsville, MD: National Center for Health Statistics.
5. Adler M (1995). Population estimates of disability and long-term care. *ASPE Research Note*, United States. (Department of Health and Human Services, Assistant Secretary

for Planning and Evaluation, Office of Disability, Aging, and Long-Term Care, February).

6. Alder (1995). See note 5.

7. See Fries JF. (1980). Aging, natural death and the compression of morbidity. *New England Journal of Medicine* 303:130–135; Fries, JF. (1983). The compression of morbidity. *Milbank Memorial Fund Quarterly* 3: 397–419; and Fries JF & Crapo LM (1981). *Vitality and Aging: Implications of the Rectangular Curve*. San Francisco: Freeman.

8. Boult C, Altman M, Gilbertson D, Yu C, & Kane RL (1996). Decreasing disability in the 21st century: the future effects of controlling six fatal and nonfatal conditions. *American Journal Public Health* 86(10):1388–1393.

9. Costa PT, Williams TF. Albert MS, Butters, NM, Folstein, MF, Gilman S, Gurland BJ, Gwyther LP, Heyman A, Kaszniak AW, Katz IR, Levy LL, Emerson, NL, Orr-Rainey NK, Phillips LR, Storandt M. Tangelos EG, & Wykle, ML. *Recognition and Initial Assessment of Alzheimer's Disease and Related Dementias*. (Clinical Practice Guideline, Number 1, Agency for Health Care Policy and Research, U.S. Department of Health and Human Services, AHCPR Publication No. 97-0702, November 1996). Washington, DC: AHCPR.

10. The income figures cited here are found in Hobb & Damon (1996). pp. 4.8–4.17. See note 3.

11. Stone RI (1995). Foreword. In RA Kane & JD Penrod (Eds.), *Family Caregiving in an Aging Society*. Thousand Oaks, CA: Sage.

12. Stone RI & Kemper P (1989). Spouses and children of disabled elders: how large a constituency for long-term care reform? *Milbank Quarterly* 67:486–506.

13. See Flanagan S (1994). *Consumer-Directed Attendant Services: How States Address Tax, Legal, and Quality Assurance Issues*. Cambridge, MA: SysteMetrics; Sabatino CP & Litvak S (1995). *Liability Issues Affecting Consumer-Directed Personal Assistance Services: Report and Recommendations*. Oakland, CA: World Institute on Disability.

14. The rules governing exclusive areas of nurse practice that cannot be performed by lay persons are established at the state level. These vary widely and are under reconsideration in many states because some of the tasks typically reserved for nurses are routinely done by family members and are likely within the capability of unlicensed paid personnel who may already be on the scene providing help that does not require a nursing licence. A strategy whereby nurses delegate nursing functions to people who do not hold a license could dramatically reduce the cost of long-term care. See Kane RA, O'Connor C, & Baker MO (1995). *Delegation of Nursing Activities: Implications for Patterns of Long-Term Care*. Washington, DC: American Association of Retired Persons.

15. Many family members literally perform long-term care such as feeding, transferring, dressing, and bathing for their relatives in nursing homes. They also do laundry, prepare foods, and generally supervise care. Although such family care is hard to monetize because it is uncertain that nursing home costs would increase if families ceased volunteering care, family members assert that their vigilant efforts are needed to achieve the kind of care they wish, given under staffing in nursing homes.

16. Adler (1995). See note 5.

17. Kane RL, Ouslander JG, & Abrass IB (1994). *Essentials of Clinical Geriatrics* (3rd ed.). New York: McGraw Hill.

18. World Health Organization. (1980). *International Classification of Impairments, Disabilities, and Handicaps: a Manual of Classification Relating to the Consequences of Disease*. Geneva, Switzerland: World Health Organization.

19. Glass TA (1998). Conjugating the tenses of function: discordance among hypothetical, experimental, and enacted function in older adults. *The Gerontologist*, 38(1):101–112.

20. This line of work was pioneered in a community study in Springfield, MA. See Allen SM & Mor V (1997). Unmet need in the community: The Springfield study. In SL Isaacs & JR Knickman (Eds.), *To Improve Health and Health Care, 1997: The Robert Wood Johnson Foundation Anthology*. San Francisco: Jossey-Bass, and Allen SM & Mor V (1997). The prevalence and consequences of unmet need. *Medical Care*, 35 (11): 101–172.
21. For example, biblical scholar Franz Rosenzweig (1886–1929) lived for eight years in an advanced and progressive state of impairment because of ALS. Although completely dependent in all ADLs, unable to speak, unable to turn a page in his book, his physician, nevertheless, describes him as follows: "he was never simply a passive object of medical treatment and feminine nursing, but always the master of the house, whose wish, after the question had been discussed from every side, finally prevailed. F.R. was the dominant, active center of all domestic affairs—at least to the extent that a man is concerned with such things—as well as of all social contacts. In this regard, too, he planned and organized everything in advance." A nurse turned the pages of his books; his wife assisted him in a painstaking communication system where he indicated by pointing to letters of the alphabet what he wanted to say. This account from Rosenzweig's physician is found in Galtzer NN (Ed.) (1953). *Franz Rosenzweig: His Life and Thought* (pp. 138-143). New York: Schocken Books.
22. Tobin SS (1991). *Personhood in Advanced Old Age: Implications for Practice*. New York: Springer.
23. Degenholtz HD, Kane RA, & Kivnick HQ (1997.) Care-related preferences and values of elderly community-based LTC consumers: can case managers learn what's important to clients? *Gerontologist* 37(6):767–776.
24. Gubrium JF (1993). *Speaking of Life: Horizons of Meaning for Nursing Home Residents*. Hawthorne, NY: Aldine de Gruyter.
25. Kivnick HQ (1993). Everyday mental health: a guide to assessing life strengths. *Generations* 17(1):13–20.

2.

Spectrum of Care

For many Americans, long-term care is synonymous with the nursing home—so much so that some commentators use long-term care to mean nursing home. This usage causes great confusion, such as when some writers contrast long-term care with home care, whereas others (including us) perceive home care as a *form* of long-term care. Indeed, the spectrum of long-term care features a large array of services and programs, which are discussed in this chapter. The chapter also touches on financing because long-term care programs cannot be discussed intelligibly apart from the funding programs that created them, gave them shape, and, through eligibility criteria, defined their clientele.

Challenges of Long-Term Care Provision

As with many social programs, long-term care was unplanned. Most countries including the United States drifted into programmatic responses to an aging society and to the unprecedented survival of persons with disabilities. The public policy challenge facing societies at the turn of the twentieth century is to reorganize and rationalize programs that have evolved in bits and pieces.

Long-term care poses a special problem because it covers so many aspects of life. As care in response to chronic dependency, it crosses many programmatic boundaries and categories sometimes seen as mutually exclusive: for example, physical versus mental health, health care versus social care, social services versus housing. In the context of the federal system that prevails in the United States, responsibilities for defining and financing long-term care occur at both federal and state levels, and to some extent at local levels. The structure of the long-term care funding programs is, in part, the result of jurisdictional decisions. These allocations of responsibility to social or health agencies have determined the professional nuance of the care provided and its underlying value system.

In the United States, as elsewhere, the major determinant of care has been the funding source. Although long-term care was never formally designed as a residual welfare program for low-income people, it evolved that way in the United States when universal entitlements were directed toward acute care while long-term care was essentially left to be financed privately or in means-tested programs for the poor. The characteristics of organizations that provide care is also a result of historical happenstance. Nursing homes and home health agencies and, later, personal care agencies and case management agencies developed in response to the availability of public payment under Medicare (a program that is perceived as a universal entitlement), Medicaid (a program that is perceived as a welfare program for the poor), and state programs, which vary in their entitlement status (usually they are for low-income people, though some serve a broader groups, often with sliding-scale fees to consumers). Once in place, however, these organizations manifested a strong, vested interest in maintaining the funding streams that are their life's blood.

Previously we defined long-term care as assistance over a sustained period of time to people who have difficulties in functioning because of a disability. This definition leaves the boundaries of long-term care somewhat imprecise. Long-term care has a time dimension, but no one seems exactly sure when it begins, and fewer seem to recognize if and when it ends. At the same time, transitions certainly occur, at least to and from acute care. For older people, their first need for long-term care often begins while in a hospital. But where does acute care stop and long-term care begin? In the United States, the terms *transitional care* and *subacute care* have emerged to describe a set of services that seem to continue the work of the hospital after discharge. Such services are sometimes funded under Medicare, yet at least some of the services the clients receive resemble the routine maintenance and assistance associated with chronic long-term care.

In contrast to acute care, long-term care uses relatively little expensive or complex technology. Long-term care relies largely on the efforts of generic personal caregivers or homemakers who serve as nursing assistants or personal care providers and, of course, relatives of the consumer. These key long-term care personnel are largely nonprofessionals who often have the designation *aide* or *assistant* in their job titles. Yet, important roles are also needed for nurses who plan and supervise long-term care plans, monitor health regimens, and, from time to time, perform complex procedures. Social workers are also needed to help long-term care clients make and implement decisions about their care and to forge the social and familial relationships necessary to cope with disability. Physical therapists, occupational therapists, and pharmacists may have distinct roles in helping a given long-term care client to maximize his or her potential. Physicians and other primary care personnel (e.g., nurse-practitioners) are critically needed for ongoing management of the health conditions of those who receive long-term care.

Nonprofessionals are the backbone of long-term care, but professional involvement is crucial: These two axioms spell out a systemic problem. Each professional discipline involved in long-term care can readily become a lobby group, however well-meaning, for its own perpetuation and expansion, resisting policies that would permit less expensive nonprofessionals to perform any of its activities. Multidisciplinary team models are further advanced to make use of each discipline in a coordinated effort without much thought to the high costs of such teamwork. Meanwhile, the nonprofessional long-term care worker (for whom no good name yet exists) is often poorly paid and works without benefits, such as retirement benefits, health insurance, or even paid vacations and sick leave. Funding programs for long-term care have created a situation where the client has too little access to a generic long-term care worker and where such generic workers cannot forge acceptable careers. When long-term care frontline workers are construed merely as aides or adjuncts to someone else, they find themselves in jobs with enormous responsibility and no authority. Moreover, a disproportionate amount of the long-term care dollar may be spent on professionals who supervise and organize the people who do the actual work as opposed to compensating the frontline workers better and creating viable career ladders for them.

A related challenge is to find a way for the long-term care consumers themselves to achieve greater control over their care. Much of long-term care is far from mysterious. It involves tasks such as cooking, cleaning, shopping, and chauffeuring, which long-term care consumers or their agents (in the case of cognitively impaired consumers) are supremely capable of directing and evaluating. Even when personal care is at issue, the client is typically the best judge of when a care routine is administered painlessly, courteously, and in a timely fashion. When formal organizations with hierarchical structures and formal division of labor undertake assisting with everyday life, the danger is that the client's control over the care will be at the level of lip service only. The difficulty is how to structure services so that the person getting help has a direct and, for the most part, directing, relationship with the person providing the help, yet both have access to professional expertise as needed.

This book focuses on the elderly population, and only secondarily on adults with physical disabilities. Progress cannot really be claimed for long-term care programs unless the improvements affect older people, who, after all, comprise the single largest group requiring long-term care. However, many people under the arbitrary age of 65 also need and use long-term care, including people of all ages with chronic mental illnesses or developmental disabilities and children with physical disabilities. Although some commentators recommend treating all people needing long-term care as a single class, the different needs related to developmental stage, social role, and particular condition, as well as the separate funding and service streams already established to deal with diverse target groups, complicate such conceptual lumping. Perhaps, in the end, long-term care entitlements will be structured with functional impairment as the key to eligibility for benefits, regardless of age or the etiology of the disability. But ultimately, services themselves will need to be individualized, and this process of individualization is best done against a backdrop of considering what the dominant needs are likely to be for specific target populations.

History

Long-term care, as a concept and a service sector, has become important gradually. Indeed, we cannot with any confidence identify who first used the phrase. The growth of public concern about how to organize care and services for people with disabilities is associated with the dominance of chronic as opposed to acute illness; the emergence of the expensive, modern hospital; and the concentration of disability in later years. In some ways, long-term care reflects the triumphs of a health care system that permits survival of persons who, a century ago, would have died. Scottish geriatrician Bernard Isaacs coined the phrase "survival of the unfittest" to highlight this phenomenon.[1] At the same time as older people in the United States are enjoying longer life expectancy at 65 and greater vigor in old age, survival of people with substantial impairments is also occurring at all ages, from newborns to centenarians. The relative growth is greater with each decade. Thus, 80-year-olds are increasing faster than 70-year-olds, but more slowly than 90-year-olds.

The modern history of long-term care in the United States—that is, post-1965—is largely dominated by the nursing home. Since then policy discussions about long-term care have tended to focus on how to improve nursing homes or prevent their use. The American nursing home as it emerged after 1965 has a mixed heritage. Put harshly, nursing homes might be considered the mongrel offspring of the almshouse and the hospital. Like the hospitals at the turn of the century, nursing homes are disproportionately concerned with care of the poor. Nursing homes also have origins in boarding homes and convalescent arrangements that could be purchased by individuals of varying incomes since colonial times.

In large measure, the present nursing home is a creature of the 1965 federal legislation that created Medicare and Medicaid. Both these health financing programs were designed so that those people disenfranchised from health care because of its costs could purchase care available to the more affluent and better insured. These programs are sketched briefly below.

Medicare

With the landmark Medicare legislation, older people, who had been gradually priced out of the private health insurance market by the shift from community rating to risk rating, were covered by a virtually universal program appended to Social Security. Although the Medicare program has changed in various details over its 30-year history, its basic architecture remains constant. Older people and people with permanent and total disabilities that preclude employment (that is, virtually everyone who receives Social Security income from his or her own labor or that of a spouse) is eligible without regard to their income or assets. Benefits include the full range of hospital care, limited post-hospital rehabilitation and skilled nursing home care, and home health care. Hospital care and other costs of Medicare Part A are financed through the Medicare Trust Fund, which is made up of contributions from employers and employees. Physician and related care (Part B) is paid for in part by consumer charges, but also are heavily subsidized from general tax revenues. Consumer charges include premiums, substantial deductibles, and ongoing *coinsurance* charges, the latter amounting to 20% of all reasonable and customary physician fees. About 90% of seniors buy supplemental insurance to wrap around Medicare benefits, covering the deductibles and coinsurance and some services Medicare does not cover. Notable among the latter uncovered services are out-patient medications, most long-term care, and some preventive services. However, these so-called Medigap policies do not cover long-term care. Medicare is administered federally through fiscal intermediaries (i.e., insurance companies), which pay claims made by certified Medicare providers.

Initially, most policy analysts expected that the health needs of the elderly would be met by Medicare. However, the Medicare program was modeled closely on what was available in the private health insurance sector at that time. Hence, its center was the hospital and its epicenter the physician. Other modalities were considered only to the extent that they provided services to extend the period of recuperation after hospitalization or offered services that might be used in lieu of hospitals. In that spirit, Medicare covered some rehabilitation and nursing home care (the latter initially known as Extended Care Facility care) and some home health care to people with rehabilitation potential who needed skilled services. As discussed below, the home health provisions in Medicare were expanded substantially in 1990, leading to a more widespread coverage of home health than originally intended.

Major changes in Medicare occurred in the early 1980s with changing reimbursement patterns whereby Medicare paid hospitals a flat sum per episode of care based on the average cost of hospitalizations for people with that discharge diagnosis. Hospitals were previously paid their actual costs and had an incentive to provide more services and encourage longer stays. After the advent of payment by diagnosis-related groupings (DRGs), hospitals had an incentive to shorten Medicare hospital stays and provide the minimum amount of service needed. This in turn led to so-called quicker-and-sicker discharges, leaving a long-term care population with more health needs, and accentuating the importance of good communication between acute care and long-term care. (See Chapter 8.)

Another change in Medicare, occurring in 1982, made it possible for Medicare beneficiaries to transfer their Medicare coverage to a managed care organization (MCO). The MCO then would undertake to provide all Medicare-covered services for a single capitated fee. The beneficiaries making that choice would no longer have the inconvenience and possible high costs of finding their own Medicare-certified providers. Chapter 9 discusses how managed care under Medicare has affected long-term care consumers.

Medicaid

Enacted as almost an afterthought to Medicare, Medicaid is a state-administered program that covers health care costs for the poor. The program is financed by federal and state dollars on a formula basis with the federal government picking up at least half and often much more of the costs. Within broad parameters, states have the option to define eligibility and benefits, although the federal government shares heavily in Medicaid costs. Initially, eligibility was directed at those receiving benefits from categorical income-support programs, now dubbed "welfare" in the press and undergoing radical reform. At the time Medicaid was enacted, categorical welfare income-support programs consisted of Aid to the Blind, Aid to the Disabled, Aid to the Elderly, and Aid to Families with Dependent Children, all programs for which states set their own poverty thresholds.

The benefits under Medicaid were made broader than those under Medicare because the framers recognized that the low-income Medicaid recipients would have no other means of purchasing care. By rule, Medicaid pays only for services that are deemed medically necessary, which means ordered by physicians. For eligible low-income seniors who cannot afford Medicare's premiums, deductibles, and coinsurance, the Medicaid program serves the same "wrap-around" function as private supplemental insurance does for more well-to-do Medicare beneficiaries. For poor elderly persons, Medicaid benefits were shaped by Medicare's omissions (for example, medications, preventive procedures, eyeglasses). Medicaid also pays the Medicare deductibles, premiums, and copayments for seniors on Medicaid. No one at the time, however, anticipated that Medicaid might become the major payer for a dramatic Medicare omission, namely, long-term care in nursing homes.

The sleeper in the Medicaid program was a provision that permitted but did not require states to include "the medically needy" among those eligible for the program, meaning persons who became poor because of their high medical costs. When medical bills exceeded a state-determined percentage of monthly income, such bills could, at state option, be covered under a "medically indigent" provision. In a number of states this eligibility criterion became the major vehicle for coverage of older persons with heavy health care expenditures because of nursing home care. Medically indigent elderly, many in nursing homes, became significant items in state budgets. Soon, too, the Medicaid program became bifurcated into two types of expenditures: acute care services for children and families who were poor or near poor and nursing home care for older people who became poor because of their expenditures in nursing homes. By the early 1990s, the Medicaid program as a whole comprised about a third of each state's budget, with higher education and corrections being the other large items, and long-term care for seniors averaged almost a third of state Medicaid costs. (If long-term care for all populations including younger people with physical or development disabilities is counted, then long-term care expenditures account for 50% or more of state Medicaid costs.)

Because the cost of nursing home care can be reasonably well estimated in advance (in contrast to that of home care, which may vary in intensity and price from day to day), nursing home costs can be used as the basis for predicting a person's financial eligibility for Medicaid in advance of incurring the expenses. Thus, residents in a nursing home whose monthly costs of nursing home care can be calculated to exceed their incomes can be deemed eligible for Medicaid. This available income of older people must be spent fully; much of it comes from Social Security retirement pensions. In contrast, persons accruing home care costs prospectively will reach the same state only *after* they have first spent all their own funds. This situation creates a subtle but real incentive to use nursing homes for those at or near medical poverty.

If the framers of Medicare and Medicaid thought at all about long-term care at the time, they pictured chronic care facilities or intensive home care programs in which elderly patients could recuperate after hospitalization at a lower daily cost than had they remained in the hospital. Medicare's nonhospital institutional sites were called "extended care facilities" to emphasize their role of providing posthospital service. Home health care under Medicare was specifically targeted at those with rehabilitation potential needing intermittent rather than full-time care. The Medicaid program made provisions for "skilled nursing homes," which were intended, as the name implies, to provide care requiring nursing attention. Home care was included in a set of optional benefits states might provide, and most states selecting this option mirrored Medicare in their definitions of home health benefits. Little thought was given to those needing assistance on a permanent or long-term basis. Eventually, largely to address the long-term care needs of younger populations, most state Medicaid programs did introduce some benefits for personal assistant services (discussed below) as part of their state Medicaid plans. This has led to the oddity in many states that some low-income people under 65 can gain access to flexible personal assistant services with relatively low unit costs, whereas older people in the same state may be able to gain access to similar services only through a home health agency certified for Medicare.

Nursing Homes
Some form of residential care for people needing personal care, nursing services, and general help with daily life has existed back to colonial times in the form of boarding homes and other ad hoc arrangements. Old-age homes, many founded by religious denominations to respond to the needs of low-income elderly people in their communities, predated the modern nursing home. Indeed, some old-age homes are well over one hundred years old. Also county institutions along the lines of the poorhouse provided an all-purpose form of *indoor relief* for people with a wide

range of psychiatric, medical, and social problems. Typically, these institutions provided only a limited amount of medically oriented care, and payment was through private fees, philanthropy, and tax dollars.

The passage of Medicaid dramatically changed where frail older people received care. Before 1950, most dependent elderly who were unable to remain at home were housed in either state mental institutions (especially if they had dementia) or in the homes for the aged, which resembled boarding homes. The percentage of elderly people in all mental institutions fell from 23% of the mental institution census in 1950 to 10% in 1970, and this proportion, as well as the absolute numbers, has declined markedly since. The number of for-profit nursing homes expanded and the sectarian homes for the aged sector, many of which retained the designation "homes for the aged," upgraded their capacity and became Medicare and (Medicaid)-certified nursing homes.

Burton Dunlap credits the initial growth of nursing homes to a provision in the 1935 Social Security Act that prohibited Social Security payments to people in public institutions,[2] but the modern nursing home is a product of the second half of the century. The growth of the aged population, the increasing need for more sophisticated health care, and the public payment source guaranteed under Medicaid fueled the growth of the industry. In the 1950s, governments made available generous construction loans to encourage development of nursing homes and the most rapid growth of nursing home stock actually predated 1965. After 1965, Medicaid reimbursement policies that covered all the owner's capital costs encouraged expansion and, for that matter, real estate deals where nursing homes frequently changed hands. The scandals that resulted from exposing these manipulations and associated poor care led to major system changes in the mid-1980s.[3]

Figure 2.1 traces the number of nursing homes in this country from 1963 to 1995. Some care must be taken in interpreting the pattern because of differences in definitions before and after Medicaid and Medicare. Overall, there is a general pattern of growth with a drop around 1971 (probably associated with the introduction of more stringent standards), and indications of a recent reduction between 1985 and 1995 despite the aging of the population. In 1995 there were only 16,700 nursing homes compared to 19,100 a decade earlier.

Although the numbers of nursing home residents fell over the last decade, the numbers of admissions increased, suggesting more, but shorter, nursing home stays. As shown in Figure 2.2, the number of residents in nursing homes has increased but the rate of increase has slowed considerably. This perhaps indicates greater use of nursing homes for post-hospital cases. The net result of these changes has been a recent downturn in nursing home occupancy. Whereas the occupancy rate had held steadily between 91% and 92% through 1985, it fell to 87% in 1995. It is not clear if this decrease represents the effects of greater use of community-based care, but such a conclusion is consistent with the continuing growth of the population that would be most likely to use nursing homes. The actual ratio of nursing home

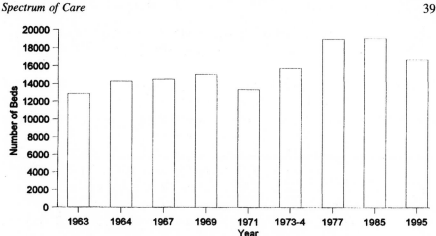

Figure 2.1. Number of nursing homes in the United States between 1963 and 1995 [Source: Dollard, KJ. (1997). Facts and Trends: The Nursing Facility Sourcebook. American Health Care Association. Washington, DC.].

residents to the population 65 years and older fell substantially from 46.2 per 1,000 in 1985 to 41.3 in 1995.[4] This drop may indicate a shift to other modalities of care, largely home-based. Some of this care corresponds to the increase in home health care use; another portion may reflect more personal care at home.

Figure 2.3 traces the growth in nursing homes from another perspective by examining the changes in the amount and sources of funding. The growth in expenditures is enormous; it comes about equally from Medicaid and out-of-pocket payments. The increase in spending from private insurance grows but remains modest. In 1995 private insurance paid only 3.3% of their nursing home bill of $77.9 billion. (This proportion is actually lower than 1990, when private insurance covered 3.7%.[5]) In contrast to hospitals, the large majority of nursing homes are operated as profit-making businesses; at least 75% of the beds and 80% of the facilities have been under for-profit ownership since the 1970s. Over time, nursing homes have also become larger and chain ownership in both the for-profit and nonprofit sector has become more prevalent.

The rate of nursing home use increases dramatically with age. Whereas less than 1% of the population aged 65 are in nursing homes, this rate increases to about 5% at age 75 and over 20% at age 85. Although there are equally frail persons living in the community, on average nursing home residents are older, more often female, less often married, and less often members of a minority group than older persons living in the community. Table 2.1 illustrates this contrast.

Nursing home residents have become more disabled over time. Figure 2.4 shows a discernible increase in the average number of ADL dependencies in activities

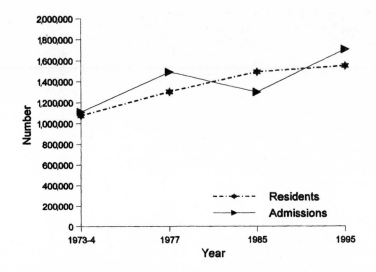

Figure 2.2. Growth in nursing home residents and admissions to nursing homes from 1973 to 1995 [Source: Strahan, GW. (1997). An Overview of Nursing Homes and Their Current Residents: Data from the 1995 National Nursing Home Survey. *(Advance Data from Vital Statistics: No. 280) Hyattsville, MD: National Center for Health Statistics.].*

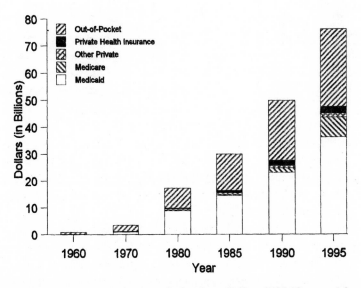

Figure 2.3. Growth in nursing home expenditures from 1960 to 1995 [Source: Adapted from Table 14 in Levit, KF, Lazenby, HC, Braden, BR, Cowan, CA, McDonell, PA, Sivarajan, L, Stiller, JM, Won, DK, Donham, CS, Long, AM, & Stewart, MW. (1996). Data View: National Health Expenditures, 1995. Health Care Financing Review, *18 (1): 175–214.].*

Table 2.1. Characteristics of Nursing Homes Residents and Noninstitutionalized People 65+ in the United States in 1995

Characteristics	Nursing home residents (N=1,385,400)	Noninstitutionalized populations (N=33,532,000)
AGE		
65–74	8%	56%
75–84	42	33
85 years and over	40	11
SEX		
Male	25	41
Female	75	59
RACE		
White	90	90
Black	9	8
Other	2	2
MARITAL STATUS		
Married	17	57
Widowed	66	33
Divorced/Separated	5	6
Never married/single	11	4
Unknown	1	—

Source note: National Nursing Home Survey, 1995; U.S. Census, 1990. See Strahan GW (1997). *An Overview of Nursing Homes and Their Current Residents* (Advance Data from Vital Statistics: No. 280) Hyattsville, MD: National Center for Health Statistics. Census data came from *Statistical Abstract of the United States,* 1996. *The National Databook,* Tables 21 and 48. Percents may not add up to 100 because of rounding.

among nursing home residents from 1977 to 1995; over this period fewer residents had no ADL dependencies and more had five. This pattern stands in contrast to that seen in the surveys of noninstitutionalized older persons. As shown in Table 2.2, the prevalence of chronic disability among the elderly population actually decreased between 1982 and 1989.[6]

Medicare and Medicaid did more than stimulate the growth of nursing home. The programs influenced the very nature of nursing homes through the rules that facilities needed to comply with to become certified to receive payments. The tremendous variation in nursing home supply from state to state is, in large part, a product of state decision making about who is eligible for Medicaid, and, later, the efforts made by states to control the supply of nursing homes. State moratoriums on new construction and state certificate-of-need rules for newly certified providers were a feature of public policy in many states in the 1980s and 1990s, partly to stimulate alternative forms of care, and also out of a belief that beds built and

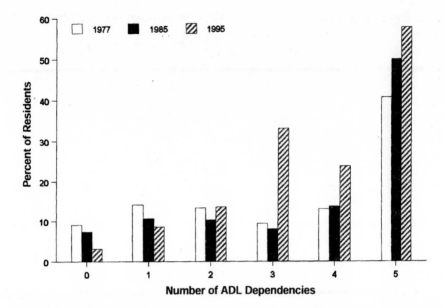

Figure 2.4. Average number of dependencies of daily living in nursing home residents from 1977 to 1995 [Source: Vital Health Statistics, Series 3: No. 30 Trends in the Health Care of Older Americans: United States, 1994, and Strahan, GW. (1997). An Overview of Nursing Homes and Their Current Residents; Data from the 1995 National Nursing Home Survey. *(Advance Data from Vital Statistics: No. 280) Hyattsville, MD: National Center for Health Statistics.].*

Table 2.2. Prevalence of Chronic Disability, 1982, 1984, and 1989 in the Noninstitutionalized Elderly Population

	1982	*1984*	*1989*
Nondisabled	76.3%	76.3%	77.4%
IADLs only	5.3%	5.7%	4.4%
1–2 ADLs	6.5%	6.5%	6.5%
3–4 ADLs	2.7%	2.8%	3.5%
5–6 ADLs	3.5%	3.1%	2.7%
Institutional	5.7%	5.5%	5.5%

Source note: Manton KG, Corder LS, & Stallard E (1993). Estimates of change in chronic disability and institutional incidence and prevalence rates in the U.S. elderly population from the 1982, 1984, and 1989 National Long Term Care Survey. *Journal of Gerontology: Social Sciences* 48:S153–S166.

certified would be filled. In fact, the proportion of nursing home beds to the population over 65 has remained relatively stable at about 5% nationwide for years, but with a threefold or fourfold difference between high-supply and low-supply states. The population over 85, which truly is at greater risk of nursing home use, has increased dramatically over this 30-year period, and nursing home occupancy rates have generally gone up. However, as noted earlier, recent reports suggest for the first time declines in occupancy and evidence of excess nursing home capacity. Whether this phenomenon resulted from greater use of community-based care is not yet clear. Chapter 4 discusses state variation in nursing home supply and utilization in detail.

How did Medicare and Medicaid influence the nature of nursing homes? Because both these new financing programs intended to expend public money to purchase care from nongovernment, often proprietary enterprises, governments felt an immediate need to define and circumscribe providers eligible for funding. With accelerating concern as the programs matured, governments became preoccupied with assuring that they were getting their money's worth, that they were purchasing only necessary and appropriate care, and that the care purchased was of adequate quality. To be allowed to receive reimbursement from Medicare or Medicaid, all institutional or organizational providers needed to meet specific standards—known as Conditions of Participation. Such federal standards shaped nursing homes and home health programs for the next three decades.

Initially, standards for federally funded long-term care programs were set under time pressures and later governed by ever-present fears of or reactions to catastrophes (such as fires). Faced with the task of creating standards quickly for a modality of care that was largely unfamiliar, federal and state bureaucracies turned to available models. One of the models was the small hospital. A federal program to support the construction of rural hospitals in the 1950s, the Hill-Burton program, had created blueprints and standards for construction and staffing. Hence, the temptation to envision nursing homes as miniature hospitals was irresistible, and, indeed, was compatible with the view of the program's framers. At the same time, the strategy of using gigantic amounts of public money to pay private entrepreneurs under Medicare and Medicaid was accompanied by fears of headline-grabbing catastrophes, especially nursing home fires. Thus, the initial regulations placed strong emphasis on issues of life safety (for example, building construction, fire doors, and sprinkler systems). These elements were already incorporated into the hospital plans that were used as templates. Likewise, staffing requirements were designed to provide an environment akin to that of a small hospital with a complement of trained nurses, who might be expected to care for recuperating hospital patients.

In the earliest years, few facilities could meet the standards set even when older nursing homes were "grandfathered" into the program. Federal and state officials were threatened with an embarrassing situation in which they promised coverage of care in nursing homes, but excluded under their rules most of the places available to provide it. By 1971, bureaucratic ingenuity found a way out of the dilemma by creating a new class of facilities, called intermediate care facilities (ICFs), which would not have to meet such stringent requirements, especially for staffing. Nonetheless, the strong emphasis on structural elements, especially life-safety features, meant that many of the original nursing homes which had emerged out of boarding houses, could no longer continue operation. The costs of coming up to standards were too high. The modern nursing home thus came to look and function much more like a miniature hospital than a home. Many of the more homelike facilities went out of business.

Although federal certification rules govern minimum standards for nursing homes, states, which administer the federal regulations, are free to impose their own higher standards and are also required to inspect the appropriateness and quality of care received by Medicaid clients. Over the years, nursing home regulations have been revisited, modified, and strengthened. A thoroughgoing examination of nursing-home standards was conducted in the 1980s,[7] culminating in a revised federal statute in 1987. This legislation is known colloquially as OBRA '87 because it was part of the Omnibus Budget Reconciliation Act of 1987. The changes introduced conditions of participation for quality of life, residents' rights, and resident assessment; OBRA '87 also mandated an inspection process that included getting information directly from residents. Two important by-products of this nursing home reform initiative were the implementation of a federally mandated resident assessment instrument (RAI) and a concerted attempt to reduce the use of physical and chemical restraints in nursing homes. The quality assurance approaches developed under OBRA '87 are further discussed in Chapter 7.

Although the disadvantages of hospital-like accommodations with their crowding, shared space, and rigid routines in a dwelling place were well understood early on, states were reluctant to impose different regulations for the nursing home environments, both because of the lobbying power of the nursing home industry and because they would have been left paying for the presumed higher cost of doing business for their Medicaid residents. As Medicaid nursing home care became a major item in state budgets, efforts to control its costs became a political goal in most states.

How can we now characterize the nursing home industry? As Figure 2.5 shows, about two-thirds of nursing homes are operated for profit, and 52% of nursing homes are part of chain operations, most of which are for-profit chains. The independent nonprofit nursing home has a shrinking share of the market at 19%, and only 8% of nursing homes are government-owned. The for-profit homes are highly likely to be comprised of nursing home beds only, with 91% of them following that pattern, 7% having some independent living or assisted living units attached, and 2% hospital based. In contrast, 26% of nonprofit nursing homes and 42% of government nursing homes are hospital based, and 21% of nonprofit nursing homes and 14% of government nursing homes include independent living or assisted living units.[8]

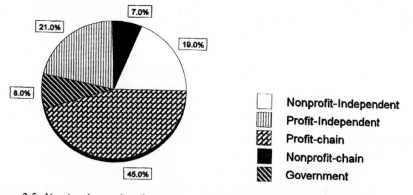

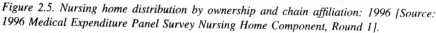

Figure 2.5. Nursing home distribution by ownership and chain affiliation: 1996 [Source: 1996 Medical Expenditure Panel Survey Nursing Home Component, Round 1].

Demonstrating Alternatives to Nursing Homes

Throughout the 1970s, nursing homes were the main publicly funded modality for long-term care. Medicare home health care, as described earlier, generally served the rehabilitation and recuperative function intended by the framers of Medicare. Medicaid home care tended to mirror Medicaid home health, thus filling mostly acute-care needs. Early in Medicaid's history, Oklahoma successfully lobbied for a personal care program under Medicaid, and several states used this optional program to fund personal-attendant programs. For many years, one state, New York, accounted for the majority of Medicaid's national home care expenditures.

Aside from Medicaid, some states purchased homemaking and other socially oriented home care programs with state-appropriated funds. Sometimes states used their Social Service Block Grant funds (under Title 20 of the Social Security Act for such expenditures). These programs tended to be relatively small. Although some states, notably Massachusetts and Pennsylvania, initiated a statewide network of socially oriented home care in the 1970s, even those programs were dwarfed by growing state expenditures on nursing home care under Medicaid.

By the early 1970s, funds for services to the elderly were also available to states under the Older Americans Act (a statute enacted the same year as Medicare and Medicaid). Among other things, the Older Americans Act promulgated rights for seniors, created the Administration on Aging (AoA) at the federal level to coordinate aging-related programs and to advocate for elderly citizens; established a network of State Offices on Aging and more than 600 Area Agencies on Aging (AAAs) to manage a largely contracted program of social services for the elderly in their geographic areas; encouraged volunteer and work programs for seniors; and established ombudsman and legal assistance programs to protect the rights of older citizens.

Initially, Older Americans Act service funds were largely used for Senior Centers and congregate meal programs, as well as a variety of social services, and the programs were targeted to the well elderly. Over the years, however, AoA has increasingly emphasized long-term care issues and encouraged redirection of service programs to the frail elderly, thus, Older Americans Act funds have often played a meaningful though supporting, role in community-based long-term care. The programs under this Act (sometimes known as "aging network" programs) vary in their involvement in long-term care. At their most effective, the State Units on Aging and the AAAs have provided leadership and a single point of entry for a coherent set of community services, managing other money besides grants under the Older Americans Act. For instance, the previously statewide state-funded programs developed in Massachusetts and Pennsylvania are largely managed by AAAs. About a third of the State Units on Aging (usually through the AAAs in the state) also manage Medicaid funds for alternative care. In only one state, Oregon, do the local case managers also manage the nursing home program, a feature we describe in subsequent chapters.

Beginning in the 1970s and continuing with increased intensity during the 1980s, federal and state authorities developed demonstration projects to reduce the reliance on nursing homes for long-term care.[9] These projects were inspired by the twin goals of improving the lot of older people with disabilities and saving money. For old people and their families, nursing homes were dreaded destinations because of the compromised quality of daily life in an institution and the impoverishment needed before public funds were available. For federal and state governments, the high cost of paying for about 50% of the growing nursing home bill was a budgetary headache. Both humanistic reformers and cost cutters resonated to the claims of theorists that care could be provided more desirably and less expensively in the home setting.

Thus, several waves of alternative programs were launched as demonstration projects (some with experimental designs) to test the potential substitution of home-and-community-based care services (HCBS) for nursing home care. These demonstrations used waivers of the Medicare rules, the Medicaid rules, or both to permit offering the demonstration clientele a fuller range of HCBS; often the financial eligibility rules under Medicaid were waived to permit coverage of a less poor clientele at risk of becoming eligible for Medicaid nursing home care once in a nursing home. Typically, too, Medicaid's requirements for statewide programs were waived to permit local demonstrations. (These demonstration waivers are known as 222 Waivers Under Medicare and 1115 Waivers Under Medicaid, not to be confused with programmatic HCBS waivers discussed in the next sections.) Services developed under demonstration authorities varied widely but tended to emphasize socially oriented homemaker and personal-care services (as opposed to home health services), and adult care.

Almost invariably, long-term care programs funded under demonstration waivers offered case management services to assess client needs, develop appropriate care plans, authorize purchase of services, arrange and coordinate services not in the care plans, and monitor quality of services. As time went on, case managers' functions became increasingly directed at targeting the waiver program to those whose functional status was similar to nursing home residents and monitoring the costs of care to ensure that the programs (for individuals and in the aggregate) did not cost more than nursing home care. One enduring legacy of the era of HCBS demonstration projects was the evolution of a technology for care coordination and case management at state and local levels.

The demonstration projects largely generated disappointing findings. With few exceptions, the outcomes for the demonstration group clients (in terms of functional status, illness rates, death rates, psychological well-being, and relocation to nursing homes) were no better than for control-group clients who did not receive expanded HCBS services and case management. And, since the main vehicle for cost-effectiveness was meant to be reduced use of nursing homes, the costs tended to be higher for the demonstration clients when the costs of case management and HCBS under the waiver were factored in. (This was not true of the Oregon FIG Waiver project, an HCBS demonstration conducted in several counties. However, Oregon ended the demonstration and decided to move immediately into statewide system change rather than continuing to conduct a narrow experiment.)

Why were the demonstrations of the cost-effectiveness of the "alternatives approach" a failure? First, some projects, especially early ones, had difficulty targeting services to people with high levels of disability and high likelihood of nursing home admission. Second, even when such targeting was done well, the projects inadequately reckoned with the general disinclination of people to use nursing homes as other than a last resort. In most of the programs, the control group members rarely used nursing homes, leaving little room for the demonstration clients to show an effect. Yes, the programs were reaching people with high levels of disability and frailty (the death rates demonstrated this), and yes, the consumers really "needed" the services. However, the clients tended to be people who never went into nursing homes at all or who went into nursing homes for a short time before their deaths. If a year of HCBS services prevents only a month of nursing home care, the cost-effectiveness of the former is unlikely.

In their increasingly energetic quest for clientele who were "eligible" for nursing homes, the demonstrations reinforced the home truth that many people are eligible for many services they never use. For something perceived as inherently negative, like the nursing home, many of those whose level of dependency qualifies them for such care will go to great lengths to stay in the community, even given the risk to their own best interests and the stress on their families. Thus it is correct to say that dependency (or disability) is a good predictor of nursing home use, but its predictive accuracy is still quite low. Dependency or disability is a necessary but not a sufficient condition for nursing home admission. The difficulty of identifying precisely who will enter a nursing home has made it difficult to target community services to those who might most readily be deflected from such care.

The more people who would otherwise not enter a nursing home receive care in the community, the less efficient is the alternatives approach, at least in the short run. However, if a state perseveres with efforts to change systems, eventually widespread use of HCBS can be associated with reductions in nursing home use. In its operational programs Oregon found that 2.6 people needed to be served in the community to eliminate a single nursing home slot and that eventually the strategy of community "placement" led to more people served for fewer total dollars. However, the studies of the 1980s were not designed to test a system's effect nor were the interviews rigorous enough, consistent enough, or targeted enough to displace nursing homes.

Other reasons can be cited for the unimpressive showing of the HCBS demonstrations. First, the price of the HCBS services (a function of how much service and what type of services the case managers ordered and how much the program was willing to pay for units of service) may have been higher than necessary. The social workers and nurses at the helm of the HCBS programs tended to order services from organized agencies, and they tended to be risk-averse and somewhat traditional in their views about the kind of professional care and oversight needed. Also, at least initially, some agencies successfully imposed minimum blocks of service hours—e.g., 4-hour, 3-hour, or 2-hour minimums, which drove up the price of HCBS. Some demonstration programs operated with complex procurement rules that required using a single contractor in a geographic area for each service and prevented case managers from getting the most value for the dollar.

Perhaps even more important, the price of nursing home care under Medicaid was rather low in many states, especially considering the full range of services (e.g., shelter, board, nursing care, personal care, recreation) that nursing homes are expected to provide. The demonstrations showed that the original premise was somewhat naive. Rather than being an expensive approach compared to the state-of-the-art in-home services at the time, nursing homes were inexpensive because of economies of scale and their ability to provide small increments of service on an unscheduled, as-needed basis. The care provided in a nursing home is extremely difficult to replicate at home at a comparable price for comparable people. For any individual, a break-even point can occur when the cost of home care equals and is in danger of exceeding the cost of nursing home care; that break-even point will be hastened if the person's needs are great, if the person has little family care, if the price of the in-home services are high, and if the price of the nursing home care is relatively low.

These were not easy or painless lessons. Indeed, some practitioners have failed utterly to internalize the message and still make claims that modest service programs (e.g., meal delivery, family support groups, volunteer friendly visiting) are saving money by preventing nursing home care. At the same time, state officials, having studied the lessons of the demonstration projects all too well, tend to be leery about undertaking any initiatives in long-term care, lest they add to, rather than substitute for, the state's nursing home bill.

The HCBS Service Spectrum

HCBS Waivers

The HCBS demonstrations can be criticized because they were just that—demonstration projects, which by definition have a limited ability to influence a marketplace. Most of the programs were evaluated after a period of no more than a year or 18 months of activity, and all were limited in enrollment. Thus, they were poorly positioned to influence the delivery system in the cities where they were located, or to change behavior of consumers and providers.

Fortunately for progress in long-term care (but unfortunately for the credibility of health services research), in late 1982 before the last results of the demonstration projects were in, Congress initiated an operational home-and-community-based services Medicaid waiver program. Known as "2176 waivers" (after the section of the authorizing legislation), they allow states to apply to receive federal matching Medicaid funds to provide a much wider range of HCBS services under Medicaid to a broader population under more flexible conditions. To obtain such a waiver, the state needed to prove that it would spend no more total Medicaid dollars on long-term care (including both nursing homes and HCBS) than the state would project to spend without the waiver. (Later, these waivers became known as "1914(c) waivers," again after a section of the law that authorized them.) Essentially, these operational Medicaid waivers opened the door for states to develop long-range plans for HCBS services. States also were able to build on the positive lessons of the HCBS demonstrations (some of which were still ongoing); whatever their results in terms of cost-effective alternatives to nursing homes, the demonstrations allowed states to develop capabilities for assessment, case management, and delivery of HCBS services.

States could include populations other than the elderly under HCBS waivers. Many 2176 waivers are targeted to children, people with developmental disabilities, people with physical disabilities, and, more recently, people with AIDS. Some HCBS waiver programs are tiny (the need for a program to be statewide could be waived) and targeted to a specific group; other waivers are broad and cover both seniors and persons with disabilities in the same waiver.

Some states have used their 2176 waiver programs effectively to develop or expand HCBS services, often integrating the program with other statewide programs funded from different sources (for example, state revenues or social service block grants) and with personal assistant services (PAS) programs under the regular Medicaid program. Typically, some form of in-home care is the central service offered; such home care may be medical in nature (such as home health care), but more often it is comprised of more socially oriented services such as personal care, homemaking, chore services, and companions. Usually the care is provided by nongovernment organizations, but some states also fund self-employed or client-employed workers under their waivers or their regular Medicaid PAS programs. As already mentioned, in some states, younger Medicaid recipients may receive services from individually employed personal assistants, whereas elderly clients cannot. We see great promise in these more individualized, nonagency approaches to long-term care, and discuss such programs in greater detail in Chapter 5.

In addition to a range of home care services, a wide variety of other services may be available to long-term care consumers. These include day health care, social day care, home modifications, home equipment, home-delivered meals, emergency alert systems, telephone reassurance systems, transportation, and a variety of services designed for family members (e.g., respite care, family support groups, and family education programs). Respite care is an odd category, because it is actually comprised of home care, day care, or short-term institutional care, and is distinguished from other kinds of care only because its clear purpose is to relieve a family caregiver. (Family caregivers are also often involved in the care of those receiving home care in general and presumably gain relief from this help, leading us to wonder if the designation of respite care has any use beyond its political utility.) Finally, case management is usually present and construed as both a service in itself (because of the assessments, care planning, counseling, monitoring, and referrals done by case managers) and as an administrative function to rationalize the program and allocate the resources. The availability of all the services described above varies considerably within as well as across states.

HCBS Providers

Describing the nursing home industry in terms of its ownership and size is much easier than describing the home care industry. Because home care agencies vary so markedly in the number of clients served and because, moreover, they can expand and contract to meet market demands and payment sources, the actual number of agencies per elderly person is hardly meaningful. Furthermore, information about Medicare-certified home health agencies, many of which also do Medicaid and private-pay business, is easier to amass than information about other agencies that are licensed by their respective states. The number of Medicare-certified home health agencies grew from 1,753 in 1967 to 8,747 in 1995. In 1997 for the first time in many years, the actual number of agencies declined somewhat, largely because of mergers and acquisitions.

Over the years the ownership of home health agencies has changed to reflect more hospital based agencies, more proprietary home health agencies, and more chain ownership.[10] The most recent information on home health agencies and hospice from the National Center for Health Statistics identifies 10,900 home health and home hospice agencies operating in 1994. That year there were 8,100 Medicare-certified home health agencies, 8,000 Medicaid-certified home health agencies (obviously many of the agencies held dual certifications), and 1,900 Medicare-certified hospices. Of all 10,900 agencies, 43% were part of chains and 23% were operated by hospitals.[11] A study based on 1992 data showed that for-profit, large, and new agencies generate more Medicare visits and higher Medicare costs per case and that hospital-based agencies generate higher costs per visit.[12]

Information about certified home health agencies tells only part of the story; the rest is more difficult to detail. According to a 1993 study, almost half the home care agencies in the country are *not* certified for Medicare, and about half of these are not licensed by the state.[13] Whether they are licensed is a matter of the policy in the particular states as to which kinds of home care agencies, if any, are required to be licensed. Medicare certification is more discretionary. Some agencies are not certified because they intend to serve a different segment of the market; moreover, they may not meet the technical requirements for certification. Most uncertified home care agencies are in the low-tech category, offering personal care and home-making. The exception are highly technical home-infusion agencies. Medicare does not ordinarily cover these services and thus agencies specializing only in infusion often do not become certified.

Spectrum of Residential Services

This chapter began with a discussion of nursing homes, and indeed the nursing home remains the major residential long-term care provider. Also, nursing homes are the only residential service covered by Medicaid as a package with a daily rate. But people who need long-term care often move into specialized residential settings where at a minimum they can be relieved of housekeeping and meal preparation and, in some programs, where they can receive some personal care and routine nursing services. Except in nursing homes or hospitals, the Medicaid program is prohibited from paying for room and board and, therefore, the earliest manifestation of new arrangements of housing with services developed in the private sector and were marketed to relatively well-to-do people who sought a more appealing living situation than a nursing home. However, some states do incorporate alternative housing arrangements into their Medicaid and Medicaid waiver programs by paying for the *services* received in the setting. In such instances, the client may well be able to afford the room and board out of income, especially if the state subsidizes the room and board for low-income recipients of Supplemental Security Income.

Thus, long-term care may be provided in, and sometimes by, staff of board and care homes, small group homes, adult foster homes, and assisted living programs. As with nonagency personal assistant services, we view the trend to new residential settings as a positive development and discuss the phenomenon in much more detail in Chapter 6.

Veterans Administration

The United States Veterans Administration (VA) has a substantial capability for directly providing and purchasing long-term care for veterans who are eligible based on their service history. The direct services are largely provided in long-stay

VA hospital units and nursing homes on the campuses of the VA hospitals. Some home care services are also provided by teams centered at the VA hospitals. In addition, the VA purchases nursing home care from community facilities and monitors its adequacy; in much smaller amounts, it also purchases day care, assisted living, and other HCBS. Because the veteran population is aging more rapidly than the general population, the VA system has led in training geriatric specialists in medicine, nursing, and social work and has pioneered in developing geriatric evaluation and management programs (such as described in Chapter 8), and interdisciplinary team models. Besides the capacity of federal VA programs, one or more state Veterans Homes operate in 42 states.

Like its civilian counterparts, the VA is challenged to shift its long-term care resources from nursing homes to HCBS, while simultaneously achieving a better articulation between acute care and long-term care. In 1995, the VA restructured itself into 22 geographically distinct Veterans Integrated Service Networks (VISNs), each with responsibility and accountability for managing its resources and constituted the primary care team as the focal point for service delivery. Care coordination and case management for long-term care will need to be achieved through the VISN system and the primary care teams.

At present the VA and the state Veterans Home Program are separate systems, not reimbursed by Medicare or Medicaid. Excluding any cost-sharing by the veterans, the VA spent 1.7 billion for long-term care in 1996, and 93% of these outlays were for nursing home or long-stay hospitals. Given that these public expenditures are substantial, any changed long-term care policies in the United States should be planned in tandem with the planning for the future of the VA system.

Issues in Service Provision

Health Care or Welfare?

In long-term care, form follows financing. Long-term care in the United States is largely viewed as a welfare program and is financed in large part by the Medicaid program, which is designed to cover health care for the poor. The growth in nursing home expenditures per se from 1960 to 1995, shown earlier in Figure 2.3, reflects a dramatic pattern of growth. The effects on Medicaid can be seen in the change from 1960, when total expenditures were only $0.8 billion, to $4.2 billion in 1970 soon after the program was launched, to $17.2 billion in 1980, and almost doubling in the next 5 years. By 1995 the costs had risen to $76.1 billion but the rate of growth had slowed. To underscore that this growth was not predominately a function of the aging of the population, the total per-capita expenditure on nursing homes in 1960 was $4, by 1970 it was $20, by 1985 it was $124, and in 1995 the per-capita expenditure on nursing homes was $285. The proportion of costs covered by Medicaid remains dominant but has actually diminished slightly since the program was well established in 1970, whereas Medicare expenditures have increased substantially in the last several years. In 1995 Medicaid paid 46.5% of the nursing home bill and Medicare another 9.4%. Out-of-pocket costs represented 36.7%. Because the major pipers are state governments, the tunes have been driven largely by government regulations, by striving to control costs, and by a desire to avoid major catastrophes during the terms of elected and appointed officials.

As a welfare program, the American notion is that long-term care is primarily a private expenditure, with governments playing a residual secondary role. Much of the discussion about how to pay for this care has been confused by an American version of double-entry bookkeeping, which somehow has created the belief that maximizing private funding and minimizing public funding were goals in themselves. The debate has been more about who should pay than what should be bought. Efforts have been directed at proposing various schemes to shift the responsibility from one sector to the other. This penchant for partners has led to recommendations for different approaches to public cost-sharing. Some have favored front-end loading and some back-end loading of the public money, but either approach continues to place heavy responsibility on the consumer. Front-loading allows coverage for the initial period of use, which then declines or ends over time. Back-end loading offers just the opposite, a period of little or no coverage (which may be thought of as a large deductible), after which coverage would begin. The latter responds to the high-cost, long-stay patients who face financial ruin. The former addresses more people but provides less coverage. These options were discussed in the early 1990s by the United States Commission on the Comprehensive Health Care (known as the Pepper Commission), which recommended the front-end variety coverage for nursing home care but provided broader coverage for home care in an effort to shift coverage in that direction.

The 1993 Clinton Health Care Task Force recommended a universal HCBS benefit that would be limited to people with quite severe disabilities (but would have no age limits) and which introduced modest cost-sharing for people whose incomes exceeded an established threshold. The Task Force's long-term care recommendations went down in flames with the rest of the health reform package, but the exercise highlighted the great ambivalence of policy makers about long-term care. Side by side with recommendations for expanded HCBS services were recommendations that would have provided incentives for insurance to finance nursing home care and other forms of long-term care. As a society, we have not quite determined where the responsibility for long-term care expenditures resides. Another intriguing side of the Clinton Health Care Task Force proposals is that they would have incorporated many services for people with chronic mental illnesses and developmental disabilities (currently part of state budgets) into the new long-term care entitlement, which would have been mainly federal money. This would have brought an infusion of much needed revenue into programs with training and vocational rehabilitation missions, but again raises the question about the proper boundaries for long-term care.

A sticking point in the United States has been societal reluctance to use public funds to subsidize care for older people while the beneficiaries of those subsidies are permitted to leave an inheritance after their deaths. This kind of intergenerational transfer is widely viewed as inappropriate. The tendency to expect Americans to first do all they can for themselves before rendering assistance culminates in a strong distaste for supporting older persons to permit them to leave a legacy. Even proposals for higher inheritance taxes fail to soothe the irate feelings over this issue; indeed, the American preference seems to be to reduce inheritance taxes. On the other hand, the public is responding with little enthusiasm to the opportunity to purchase long-term care insurance, a subject to which we now turn.

Private Long-Term Care Insurance

The zeal for private long-term care has been fostered by governmental concerns about the growing costs of long-term care and especially the governmental share. Under the belief that greater use of private insurance would reduce ultimate Medicaid obligations, several states have created incentive programs to encourage the purchase of private long-term care insurance. These usually take the form of promising asset protection equal to the insurance coverage to quality for Medicaid eligibility. For every dollar of coverage, the purchaser gets an additional dollar of asset allowance. In addition, federal policies in the mid 1990s have offered tax incentives to encourage employers and individuals to buy long-term care insurance.

The rationale for purchasing private long-term care insurance depends on several factors: costs, expected benefits, other expenses, and predictions about the future. For very wealthy people, who have little likelihood of spending down their assets to qualify for Medicaid, it is essentially a means of protecting their assets to allow them to be inherited. (On this basis one might perhaps expect their heirs to buy the insurance.) For those who anticipate they might qualify for Medicaid in stringent circumstances, the purchase of private insurance is driven by: (1) a desire to avoid the prerequisite poverty necessary for Medicaid eligibility and (2) a hope that they could purchase better care or more flexible care privately than would be available under Medicaid. In effect, for this group, especially as the welfare stigma of Medicaid seems to be giving way to a feeling of middle-class entitlement, the strongest incentive to buy private coverage is the poor quality of care under Medicaid. Such a situation can lead to perverse policy incentives. Those with limited incomes have neither the cash to pay the premiums nor the expectation that they will preserve enough assets to make the purchase worthwhile.

Analysts point to several unknown factors in purchasing long-term care insurance. Getting good rates depends on buying a policy many years in advance of likely use. The actuarial and economic assumptions are difficult. Would one be better off to simply invest a similar amount in a rapidly appreciating investment, especially since the near-term risk of needing coverage is very small? Then, too, there are concerns about the role of inflation. The value of a fixed policy benefit will be dramatically reduced over time, but policies with a inflation adjusters are very expensive. The biggest questions surround the future public policy. By buying private insurance one is effectively predicting that the government will not cover long-term care costs, but trends, albeit subtle ones, point in the opposite direction.

Efforts to estimate the potential market for long-term care insurance have been fairly bleak,[14] but activity in purchases has increased in the last decade. Between 1987 and 1995 the numbers of individual policies increased from about 815,000 to 4.3 million. In 1995, 125 companies offered LTC insurance policies. From 1987 to 1983 the number of employer-sponsored plans grew from two to 462; but employer sponsorship does not mean that the insurance is offered as a no-cost employee benefit.[15] For example, one large employer, the California Public Employees Retirement Plan, has agreed to offer a long-term care insurance policy through its auspices to allow public service workers an opportunity to obtain such coverage at much lower group rates, although the employees pay the full cost of the premium.

Unlike health insurance, which is offered as a fringe benefit by many employers, few companies offer to pay for long-term care insurance, except as part of a "cafeteria" plan for benefits where employees can choose any set of benefits up to a certain cash value. In such a case, the employee would have to choose long-term care coverage over another perk such as dental coverage or retirement. Some private-sector employers have been willing to use their group status as a marketing device to allow employees to purchase long-term care insurance out of their own pockets at a lower group rate. (This is analogous to the California Public Employees example just described.)

The actuarial payoff from this long-term coverage is still too early to estimate. Most companies selling the policies have had few claims to date. Many policies are designed to provide cash payments or broad coverage for a wide variety of care, but they also require substantial copayments (up to 33%). Thus, eligibility, which is usually predicated on some level of disability, but can also include cognitive impairment per se, can be generous as long as the clients must spend their own money first.

Opinions about the situation depend on one's perspective. Enthusiasts talk about the rapid growth in sales. Since it was first offered in the early 1980s, thousand of people have bought private LTC policies. But skeptics point out that this represents a market penetration of less than 3%. Legislation in 1996 permitting the payment of benefits to be received tax-free may further stimulate the private long-term care insurance market.

Another strategy to tap into the resources of older persons needing long-term care recognizes the high rate of home ownership in this country. Often a home is an older person's primary asset, and it is typically exempted from asset calculations for purposes of determining Medicaid eligibility. A proposal to use this asset was cast in the form of a reverse mortgage.[16] In essence, older persons could borrow against the value of their home. Instead of getting the payment in a lump sum and paying back the loan over time, they would receive a regular payment and continue to live in the home until death or serious disability that required nursing home admission. They would then get the remainder of their money, but the home would revert to the mortgage holder. Despite substantial efforts to promote the concept, it has not been well received. Seemingly, almost everyone likes this idea except elderly widows who own homes and need long-term care.

Federal or State Levels?

Another way that form follows funding lies in the way programs are encouraged to shift costs to other units of government. Most notably, a prudent state tries to maximize the use of federal dollars from the Medicare program (which is entirely federal) or to use federal matching dollars in Medicaid and Medicaid waiver programs.

The Medicare home health program is an interesting case in point. Although Medicare is not a major source of revenue for long-term care and although the home health benefit was designed for short-term use, changes since 1990 have led to an enormous expansion in the cost of the Medicare home health program, much of which can be attributed to cases where home health aides provide the major service. From 1987 to 1992, the percentage of Medicare beneficiaries using home health rose from 4.8% to 7.2%, while the average number of visits among users went from 23 to 54.[17] Some (82.2% of home health users) received fewer than 50 visits. The group receiving fewer than 150 visits had an average of 31 visits in 1992,[18] whereas the group receiving more than 150 visits (10.8% of home health users) had an average of 250 visits. The heavy home health users did not differ greatly from the lighter users in terms of living alone or disability levels. Heavier users were more likely to suffer from diabetes, osteoporosis, partial paralysis, and stroke. In general, the probability of using home health care increases with more dependencies in ADLs and IADLs. Greater disability is also associated with using more home health care, as is being on Medicaid. It seems clear that some proportion of Medicare beneficiaries use the Medicare home health benefit as a long-term care program even though the high levels of nurse supervision required render Medicare a peculiarly expensive way to deliver routine in-home services.

Reacting to Acute-Care Policy

Long-term care funding is, in part, a fallout from acute care financing. For example, when changes were made in the way that Medicare paid hospitals in 1984, the response was earlier discharge to nursing homes for short-term stays for convalescence, rehabilitation, or dying. In acknowledgment of new roles, some nursing homes have anointed themselves as subacute care providers to reflect their provision of a mix of services that were formerly provided in hospitals. Home health care providers have also geared up to serve people with higher levels of acuity, including even children on ventilators who might previously have been in intensive care units.

Long-term care consumers depend on high quality acute care, and the working arrangements between acute-care and long-term care programs are often less than ideal. Chapter 8 discusses models for geriatric care that better integrate and coordinate acute care and long-term care. The major change in funding of acute care on the horizon since the mid-1990s is the use of capitated payments under both Medicare and Medicaid. These funding changes will certainly alter the form of long-term care, even if long-term care services are not covered under the capitations. Chapter 9 discusses this emerging trend in considerable detail.

Unified Disability Agenda

Largely for political reasons, spurred by charges that older people receive disproportionate social benefits compared to children, long-term care became less a segregated program for older people from the 1980s on. Policy discussions now take great pains to describe long-term care programs as age-irrelevant. Instead, the clientele are defined on the basis of disability or other measures of need and disability. Thus, younger and older people with disabilities have become political allies, if not codependents. Old habits die hard, however, and, although every person getting long-term care has a disability, state literature often refers to programs in language such as "seniors and people with disabilities" or "disabled people and the elderly." Perhaps this is because older people needing long-term care do not identify themselves as "disabled." The negative repercussions of older persons' failure to embrace the term *disability* means that older people with disabilities seldom have access to the experience and resources that have been established for younger people, nor have they joined the political movement for the rights of people with disabilities. The common agenda for people with all disabilities of all ages has been largely at the level of policy discussion and general advocacy.

This uneasy merger resulted in part from a growing perception that the elderly population was receiving a disproportionate share of the health and social services dollar and in part from the perception that younger people had access to more generous and flexible per-person community benefits for long-term care. In fact, as we point out in Chapter 4, long-term care consumers under age 65 receive a disproportionately greater share of the HCBS long-term care dollar in relation to their presence in the population. This fact has been obscured because the sheer numbers of older people are so much greater and consume the lion's share of the total costs.

The unified agenda joins groups with quite different needs and expectations, and it may catalyze positive developments for long-term care in general. Spokespersons for younger people with disabilities have often been vocal about their insistence on being in charge of their own cases. Essentially, they advocate for money to purchase services that will allow them to function as normally as possible. They reject the concept of home care because it implies they should stay at home; they want attendants who can provide whatever assistance is needed to enable them to participate in a full range of social activities. They believe they can best choose their attendants and decide what these attendants should do. This is particularly true among people with spinal cord injuries, people with cerebral palsy, and even people with developmental disabilities accompanied by mental retardation; one of the ironies of long-term care is that some younger people with limited intellectual abilities demand (or their families demand on their behalf) and experience greater self-determination than many older people with unimpaired cognitive abilities.

Older clients have collectively been more passive. They have tended to accept professionally oriented case management and external definitions of what types and amounts of services would be provided. Indeed, their level of protest has been generally limited to refusing services when they are offered. Some of this difference in attitude may be generational and some may be situational. The generational argument is that people now entering old age will be more oriented to consumer rights and less stoical about making do with what they are offered than the Depression-influenced older people of the 1990s. The situational argument takes into account that the disabilities of older people are often due to a combination of diseases and ailments rather than a condition to rally around, and that older people themselves may be more sick, more subject to fatigue, and less needful of developing services for a lifetime than healthy younger people with disabilities. Despite these differences, however, some younger people with disabilities argue that their older counterparts simply need to be educated in the art of the possibilities for them to become active consumers.

The differences among the constituency groups needing long-term care are not limited to their expectations to control services. The type and style of services needed and the relevant cooperating organizations differ among target groups as well. When people with developmental disabilities are added to the disabled mix, the range of services becomes even more varied. Everyone would be disadvantaged if the results of the merger of target groups led to some expectation for a single approach to services. There may be a social equity argument for some type of equal basis of eligibility across groups. (It is to be hoped that eligibility will be more than a threshold determination; it should offer a titrated amount of service depending on the client's needs.) However, the nature of the service, and perhaps even the place and way it is provided, will surely differ among the groups. Just as there is individual variation in preferences for types of services, the variation across groups should be larger.

Although the unified approach has the advantage of increasing the voice of the long-term care consumer, difficulties occur even in creating a common agenda for all subgroups of younger people with disabilities. Part of the problem relates to historical categorical provisions for certain populations—for example, blind and deaf people, handicapped children, and more recently, people with Alzheimer's disease. The general rule of thumb is that each subgroup, regardless of age, tends to favor retaining any special funding streams for the particular group while sharing in any general long-term care revenues.

At the very least, and even without the latest merger of interests with the people with disabilities under age 65, long-term care for older people can be seen as serving five groups of older clients: *(1)* those who are in the terminal stages of disease (i.e., hospice care), *(2)* those who are severely impaired in cognition by virtue of dementia or brain damage to the point where they have no ability to appreciate their environment, *(3)* those who are primarily physically impaired, *(4)* those whose major problems are produced by cognitive failures (but can still appreciate their environment), and *(5)* those who have a strong expectation of significant improvement. These quite diverse groups of clients need very different types of care. The entities that have evolved under the banner of long-term care are ill-equipped to provide much of that care, certainly not under uniform auspices. We will elaborate on these subgroups as we discuss in-home HCBS in Chapter 5 and residentially based services, including nursing homes, in Chapter 6.

Summary

Long-term care is provided by a wide variety of programs, in a wide range of settings, and under a wide range of funding. The diversity in funding accentuates the fragmentation that exists in the service sector. Most notable, however, is that large sums of public (federal and state) and private money are expended on long-term care. Long-term care is also an enormous part of state budgets, and the bulk of the public expenditure is still spent on the program that consumers value least—the nursing home. The next chapter takes up what we consider the greatest public policy challenge—moving to systems that eliminate the nursing-home bias and make available a more balanced array of services for people who need long-term care.

Notes

1. Isaacs B, Livingston M, & Neville Y (1972). Survival of the unfittest. *A study of geriatric patients in Glasgow.* London: Routledge and Kegan Paul.
2. Dunlop BB (1979). *The Growth of Nursing Home Care.* Lexington, MA: Lexington Books. This book provides an excellent history of the nursing home industry.
3. See, for example, Mendelson MA (1974). *Tender Loving Greed: How the Incredibly Lucrative Nursing Home "Industry" Is Exploiting America's Old People and Defrauding Us All.* New York: Random House; Vladeck BC (1980) *Unloving Care : the Nursing Home Tragedy.* New York: Basic Books; Moss FE & Halamandaris VJ (1977). *Too Old, Too Sick, Too Bad: Nursing Homes in America.* Germantown, MD: Aspen Systems Corp.
4 Strahan GW (1997). *An Overview of Nursing Homes and Their Current Residents: Data From the 1995 National Nursing Home Survey.* (Advance data from Vital Statistics: No. 280). Hyattsville, MD: National Center for Health Statistics.
5. Levit KA, Lazenby HC, Sivarjan L, Stewart MW, Braden BR, Cowan CA, Dobham, CS, Long AM, McDonnell PA, Sensenig AL, Stiller JM & Won, DK (1996). Data view: health expenditures, 1994. *Health Care Financing Review* 17(3): 205-242.
6. Manton KG, Corder LS, & Stallard E (1993). Estimates of change in chronic disability and institutional incidence and prevalence rates in the U.S. elderly population from the 1982, 1984, and 1989 National Long Term Care Survey. *Journal of Gerontology: Social Sciences* 48:S153–S166.

7. Institute of Medicine (1986). *Improving the Quality of Care in Nursing Homes.* Washington, DC: National Academy Press.

8. Krauss NA, Freiman MP, Rhoades JA, Altman BM, Brown Jr, E, & Potter DEB (1997). *Nursing Home Update, 1996. MEPS Highlights*, July, Number 2. (Data drawn from the Medical Expenditure Panel Survey).

9. There are many separate and summary accounts of the demonstration projects in long-term care. One comparison of major studies leading up to and including a landmark study called the Long-Term Channeling Demonstration is found in Kane RA & Kane RL (1987). *Long-Term Care Principles, Programs and Policies* (pp. 313–340). New York: Springer. For another summary of a larger group of studies, see Weissert WG, Cready CM, Pawelak JE (1989). Home and community care: three decades of findings. In MD Peterson & DL White (Eds.), *Health Care of the Elderly: An Information Source Book* (pp. 39–126). Newbury Park, CA: Sage; Weissert WG & Hedrick SC (1994). Lessons learned from research on effects of community-based long-term care. *Journal of the American Geriatrics Society* 42:348–353.

10. Vital and Health Statistics (1997). *National Home and Hospice Care Survey: 1994. Summary.* (Series 13, DHHS Publication No. PHS 97-1787). Bethesda, MD: National Center for Health Statistics.

11. See note 10.

12. Goldberg HB & Schmitz RJ (1994). Contemplating home health PPS: current patterns of medicare service use. *Health Care Financing Review* 16 (1):109–130.

13. Silberberg M, Estes CL, & Harrington C (1994). Political perspectives on uncertified home care agencies. *Health Care Financing Review* 16 (1):223–246.

14. Wiener JM, Illston LH, and Hanley RJ (1994). *Sharing the Burden: Strategies for Public and Private Long-Term Care Insurance.* Washington, DC: The Brookings Institution.

15. Cunningham R (1997). Perspectives. In Faulkner and Gray's *Medicine and Health* 51(39), October 6. ERBI Issue Brief No. 163, July 1997.

16. Jacob B & Weissert WG (1987). Using home equity to finance long-term care. *Journal of Health Politics, Policy and Law* 12(1):77–95.

17. Mauser E & Miller NA (1994). A profile of home health users in 1992. *Health Care Financing Review* 16(1):17–34.

18. Vladeck BC & Miller NA (1994). The Medicare home health initiative. *Health Care Financing Review* 16(1):7–16.

3.

Obstacles to Balanced State Long-Term Systems

As we have seen, long-term care policy is largely forged at the state level of government, albeit with substantial federal money and some federal oversight. And state long-term care systems, in our view, require fundamental redirection. This chapter explores why fundamental change in state long-term care systems is so difficult to achieve.

We suspect that most state officials would readily assert that they intend their long-term care programs to make high-quality, user-friendly long-term care available in their state at a price the state and its citizens can afford. By this, they would mean that a long-term care system should pay attention to both the "quality of life" and the "quality of service"; that residential services should be designed not only to be safe, but also to be liveable; and that home-based services should not only be technically competent but be delivered in ways and at times that the consumer approves. Users of long-term care should not have to give up too much in the way they live in order to receive long-term care services. Though this hypothetical state official may not fully articulate it, achievement of this high-quality, user-friendly system would also mean that no provider group should dominate in the delivery of services, as nursing homes currently do in most states. A balanced long-term care system should allow a choice of services for each potential user whenever possible. Finally, to be practical the long-term care costs must be within the means of the citizens who pay for it privately and through their tax dollars.

States have two general mechanisms to achieve these goals—financing and management, on the one hand, and regulation, on the other. In the first instance, states shape the Medicaid, Medicaid waiver, Older Americans Act, and state-funded programs that subsidize long-term care, particularly for low-income people, in the state. For example, they decide on eligibility levels (based both on income and functional and health status), program characteristics, payment levels, and payment mechanisms. They design the systems to allocate this care and monitor its quality—either through case managers who are public employees at state or county levels or through contracts with community case-management providers. Second, the state can use the full range of its regulatory authority to influence the care that *all* citizens receive, regardless of payment sources. It does this through licensing and inspection programs, through legislatively derived standards that define various industries, through certificate-of-need programs designed to manage the supply of various services in the state, and through various adult protection programs. These and other state policies are discussed in more detail in Chapter 7. Here we simply stress that state policies have a much broader reach than to the low-income people who receive subsidies. They can determine, for better or worse, what will be available for anyone to purchase and, to some extent, what it will cost.

Achieving these user-friendly, balanced long-term care systems is challenging. No state has fully reached the goal. For that matter, it is likely that this goal is never attainable but rather something to be continuously sought as systems adapt to social, economic, demographic, and technological changes. Oregon seems to have come closest; at least it has demonstrated that it is possible over a 15-year period to make radical changes in the landscape of long-term care and reduce the dominance of the nursing home.[1] But Oregon's developmental efforts took 15 years, and every innovation and new service was fought by various interests that preferred the status quo. Any state that undertakes the task of reforming its long-term care system must expect opposition, at times intense opposition. For every two steps taken forward toward that goal, a step and a half will be taken backward. The key to achieving long-term care reform is clarity about the objective and tenacity in working toward it.

Long-term care is expensive: The average state spends 30% of its Medicaid budget on long-term care (excluding institutional services for people with developmental disabilities).[2] Because of the high amount of state general revenue spent to support long-term care (both in the match for Medicaid and other state efforts to round out the program), each state is keen to keep its costs as low as possible. This cost concern makes long-term care reform even more difficult. Simply adding more long-term care services can be very expensive, especially if these services fail to replace expensive nursing home services at lower costs. At the very least, for an interim period states will pay for both the old and the new services.

Long-term care is mainly a program for the elderly, and the elderly are the fastest-growing segment of the population. Leaders in each state know that unless they decide to take care of a smaller proportion of the population needing long-term care services (e.g., by making eligibility more stringent or capping clientele and creating waiting lists), their expenditures will increase each year. Current demographic projections indicate that these increases will continue until after the year 2030. Thus, states seek the least expensive method of caring for the long-term care population. Unfortunately, providers of each type of long-term care services claim that their particular service is the least expensive. Sorting out the valid claims is perplexing for state decision makers.

The key state decision makers are the governors and the state legislators. Generally, the occupants of these roles have only a limited understanding of long-term care and must depend on others to advise them. Since the research on the costs of long-term care services is ambiguous and often contradictory, advice proffered to elected officials is typically based on how the advisor perceives long-term care, and not on how best to achieve a viable, improved long-term care system overall.

Running for public office is expensive, and elected officials depend heavily on contributions to fund their reelection campaigns. Although contributions do not buy votes, they buy access, which allows contributors to advise elected officials. Nursing homes are more likely contributors than other long-term care providers, and accordingly they have the most access and provide the most advice to elected officials. Indeed, nursing homes contribute handsomely to state candidates in absolute terms, as well as in proportion to other long-term care providers.[3]

All states have made a large investment in nursing home care. In 1992 nursing homes accounted for over 78% of all long-term care expenditures (excluding both HCBS waivers explicitly for people with developmental disabilities and institutional services dedicated to developmental disability or mental retardation institutional services for the developmentally disabled). New York, which has about 7.5% of the nation's elderly population, spent about 43% of the home-and-community-based service care dollars in the United States in 1992, and this tends to skew the cost data. Indeed, only one state, Oregon, spent more on HCBS than it did on nursing homes, only four states (Oregon, New York, California, and Delaware) spent less than 75% of their long-term budget on nursing homes, and only eight states (adding Washington, West Virginia, Idaho, and Texas) spent less than 80% on nursing homes.

Most states have attempted to diversify their long-term care systems over the last 20 years. In fact, as of 1997, forty-nine states operate 192 home-and-community-based waivers which allow Medicaid funds to be spent on long-term care services outside of a nursing home.[4] Despite this effort, it remains true today that nursing homes are the dominant providers of long-term care services in the United States.

Obstacles to Change

If any real change, beyond minor tinkering, is to be achieved, three different, though related, types of obstacles must be overcome: political obstacles, logistical obstacles, and philosophical obstacles. In the final analysis, the real success of any long-term care reform will require that all three be addressed.

Political Obstacles

As previously stated, the United States has developed a nursing-home-dominated long-term care system. This occurred primarily because of favorable funding available to nursing homes through the Medicaid program (described in Chapter 2) and because of favorable federal and state regulations. States that attempt to balance their long-term care systems by providing more HCBS care and less nursing home care will find a plethora of opposition.

Nursing homes now form an enormous industry that is dependent on Medicaid for about half its revenue. Since Medicaid reimbursement levels are ultimately the responsibility of each state legislature, in order to protect their interest, nursing homes have become a powerful political influence in each state. They have used this influence quite successfully to retain their position as the dominate long-term care provider. Any state that attempts to reform its long-term care system by providing enhanced and expanded HCBS will encounter political opposition. Only a few states have been able to overcome this opposition to any degree.

States have also encountered political opposition from other provider groups when attempting to expand their HCBS system. State home-health associations object when states try to institute personal assistance programs that use nonagency personnel or embody the concept of the client as employer. They also may launch opposition to a meaningful role for case managers from outside their agency, claiming it is redundant but also concerned about abridgment of their autonomy and possible interference with their markets.[5] Professional associations advocate full and expanded use of their respective disciplines out of a combination of a genuine belief in their vital importance and guild-like self-interest. For example, state nursing associations and state boards of nursing object when states try to institute procedures by which nurses can delegate services to unlicensed paid personnel in home care settings. The organized board-and-care industry objects when states try to introduce standards of privacy and autonomy-enhancing amenities into the rules that certify residential settings other than nursing home for payment under Medicaid waivers.[6]

Though less often recognized, potent opposition to change comes from other quarters besides care providers. If the proposed change requires modifying the administrative structure at the state and county levels, state and local employees whose jobs are threatened (or perceived to be threatened) by such reforms will raise objections to the proposals. Any rationalization or reorganization of the service system or the state's system for case management in long-term care is bound to raise such concerns. Finally, groups representing seniors and people with physical disabilities can also mount opposition if they feel that long-term care reform will result in a loss of services or a loss of safeguards.

It is simply impossible to reform a long-term care system and keep all of the interested parties—care providers of all kinds, professionals, public employees, consumer advocates—happy at all times. Certainly, it is important to anticipate opposition and skepticism and to involve all stakeholders as much as possible in developmental steps. Furthermore, true expertise is reflected in the many constituencies that will rally around to object to innovation. The challenge is to achieve some consensus on the overall goals for long-term care, to take into account legitimate interests as much as possible, and try to develop broad public support for the changes. (For example, given the broad public support for welfare reform in 1997, the objections of other stakeholders, such as providers who might have supported the status quo, got little attention.)

Each special interest group has become adept at forming arguments against changing the long-term care system. Many have developed strong influences in the legislative process and have been successful in preventing or delaying changes. Without some outside leverage, such as a major state revenue shortfall or changes in federal laws and regulations, it is usually extremely hard to attempt to overcome political barriers. An important strategy to achieve change is to organize groups of people with disabilities and older people at risk of incurring disabilities into a clear constituency that may become a counterpoint to provider interests. This strategy has the compelling added advantage of providing a litmus test for whether proposed policies are really user-friendly. Unfortunately, however, consumers cannot advocate for change in a vacuum, and without education, reflection, and discussion many have no alternative vision for long-term care other than to improve care in nursing homes and reform the financing system so that families need not expend huge personal resources on them.[7]

Logistical Obstacles

The logistical barriers to long-term care reform begin with financing issues. This includes determining how to raise the money, maximizing federal dollars in the system, and finding start-up funds for alternative care systems. Once money is found, a wide range of logistical problems arise related to designing and managing the service system, some of which are quite technical. Scattered within state bureaucracies, often at lower tiers and lesser visibility than key department heads and program planners, are people who have acquired substantial expertise in tailoring solutions in their own states.

Maximizing federal money. Almost all long-term care reforms include an expansion of HCBS. Federal funding support, at present, is more certain for nursing homes than it is for HCBS. Since 1981, the HCBS Medicaid waiver mechanism has been available, and many states have capitalized on it, though some state legislatures were slow in deciding to appropriate the money needed for the state share. Any state long-term care reform that expands HCBS must obtain and retain as much federal Medicaid funding as possible. Failing to do so has the effect of raising the cost of such reforms, since the federal Medicaid program pays at least half (and in most states more than half) of these costs. Thus, the first logistical problem that must be faced in any long-term care reform that expands HCBS is how to retain as much federal funding as possible. This will become more difficult if a federal spending cap is placed on Medicaid. In general, going after the federal dollar is more difficult when the federal policies themselves are in flux.

Finding start-up funds. States must also undertake these reforms and the expansion of HCBS in the face of limited state government funding. Certainly, most all successful long-term care reforms implemented by states in the last 15 years have done so, at least partially, on the premise that they would eventually save that state long-term care dollars. A successful state long-term care reform should, indeed, save dollars over time, and most states that have implemented successful reforms report cost savings. Some of the savings represent the results of real diversions from nursing homes. Others are political fabrications derived from naive or disingenuous assumptions that every one receiving HCBS would otherwise be in a nursing home. These real savings come from diverting people needing long-term care services away from the more expensive nursing home services toward the usually less expensive HCBS. But, perhaps the greatest logistical problem facing states bent on long-term care reform is finding the money to start the program.

Start-up costs can be considerable because, until the HCBS program is operating with enough success to have an impact on the long-term care system, states must continue to support the existing (usually over-bedded) nursing home program. Indeed, most states start the expansion of their HCBS in a limited fashion: They usually allot a set number of HCBS placements and form waiting lists once this number of people is reached. Of course, once HCBS waiting lists are formed, any person needing immediate, formal long-term care services must go to a nursing home, thereby negating the impact of the expanded HCBS.

Some sources of start-up have included state lottery monies (notably in Pennsylvania) and foundation grants, but typically legislatures need to make appropriations from general revenues. Until recently, Pennsylvania used ear-marked lottery money for its LTC program and did not have an HCBS waiver at all. In some states, substantial funding comes from county and municipal levels from required or optional cost-sharing. In Ohio, various counties have developed levies that raise substantial funds for long-term care for older people; however, these funds are designed to supplement and enrich the state program rather than provide the basic service.

Defining the services. States can design service systems by providing selective incentives for some providers to develop, and disincentives for growth in other sectors. They have leverage because they determine what services will be subsidized for low-income people through state-run programs. They also shape the service system by developing regulations that define each service component. When the state has determined licensure categories for doing business (which may relate to staff qualifications, staffing ratios, building features and equipment, and even the allowable disability levels of the clientele), then that state has influenced what people paying privately can buy and what it is likely to cost. At present, states tend not to deliver services directly through state employees, but there are some exceptions to the preference to contract out services to private nonprofit or for-profit agencies. Sometimes, contracts are let to county government agencies such as public health departments, human service departments, and AAAs run by city and county governments. In such cases, additional logistical problems arise, especially in states with a tradition of strong, independent counties.

States need to determine the array and amount of HCBS that should be subsidized for low-income people through Medicaid, Medicaid waivers, and state dollars. Most states have programs subsidizing in-home assistance and case management services of some type. Some states subsidize adult day care programs, and many states offer housing options such as adult foster homes and assisted living facilities. Most states and many localities subsidize transportation programs for people with disabilities, but these are often underfunded and a weak link in the ability of older people with disabilities to live independently. Some states have made specific investments—for example, developing respite care programs or day centers, sometimes earmarked for Alzheimer's disease. But, despite the large number of long-term care programs at the state level (sometimes dozens of different programs), these programs are seldom available on a statewide basis; and they are often not subsidized in enough quantity (because of caps on clientele) to have a practical effect on the dominant role of nursing homes. When a need for long-term care arises that cannot be met solely by family, one can usually eventually find a nursing home, whereas the likelihood of finding other arrangements is less predictable.

Managing the program. A myriad of logistical problems arise in determining how to best manage the program, including how to organize state governmental agencies and determining roles for county and voluntary agencies. At both state and local levels, change will be strategically advanced if the same organization controls public expenditures in the nursing home sector and in the HCBS sector and can make trade-offs between these budgets. Other logistical issues include determining eligibility, designing a system for case management and deciding how much it should cost, developing some kind of assessment tool and management information system that helps the state target its programs and evaluate its successes, and creating a quality assurance program.

Philosophical Obstacles

Philosophical obstacles to the development and implementation of long-term care reforms are usually subtle, but may be the most difficult to overcome. The success of any long-term care reform depends more than anything else on the people who operate the long-term care system at state and local levels and who provide the services "on the ground." Generally speaking and despite vested interests, most parties to the issue are well motivated and have in mind doing something good and appropriate for old people. The prototypic older person evokes everyone's parents and grandparents and, in contrast to public attitudes about other disadvantaged or dependent groups, there is a widespread collective desire to "do right" by senior citizens. Nonetheless, deep-seated beliefs about what is right to do or what will work in practical terms interfere with meaningful change.

Philosophical obstacles are especially apparent among case managers at the local level who recommend and monitor placements and service plans. Most case managers were trained and worked in an era when nursing home placements were justified as being the best possible placement for most individuals. They, like most people, developed a philosophical outlook that coincided with the work they were required to perform. Changing this philosophy to one that entails substantially increased use of HCBS can be very difficult. This is usually compounded by the fact that there is always more work (for the usually overworked case manager) connected with an HCBS arrangement than there is with a nursing home placement.

Hospital discharge workers, physicians, and family members are similarly affected by entrenched attitudes. Placements in nursing homes after hospitalization are influenced by two sources: hospital discharge workers and family members. Historical relationships facilitate transfers to nursing homes. For families, nursing homes are known commodities, which are expected to provide all necessary services. Physicians are involved in both instances: They advise hospital personnel about the discharge needs and certify the "medical necessity" of the nursing home, and they also advise family members. Physicians typically lack familiarity with the HCBS services in their community and often assume that a nursing home is the only viable placement. This is often particularly true if the alternative service is not a medically based service.

The Medicare prospective hospital reimbursement system based on DRGs was implemented in 1984. As discussed earlier, this system limits the amount of money a hospital can receive for a Medicare patient based on the diagnosis at discharge. The resultant pressure on hospital personnel to foster quick exits has been enormous. These workers often have less than 24 hours to make placements, and they have found that it is usually much easier to make a nursing home placement than a home-and-community-based care placement. Moreover, the patients being discharged are often actively ill at the time, requiring plans to be based on a predicted course rather than a relatively stable situation at hospital discharge.

The circumstances for adequate discharge planning are far from ideal. According to a study analyzing model programs in discharge planning,[8] conceptually, a good discharge plan should include five steps:

1. The people most in need of discharge planning should be identified, preferably as early as possible. Immediate and eventual candidates for long-term care would likely need such attention.

2. The risks, costs, and benefits of alternative post-hospital modalities of care (such as rehabilitation, nursing home care, home health care) should be discussed. Once apprised of the facts, patients and their families should make the decision about where the patient will go. Discharge planners and medical experts should supply information and offer opinions, but not make the final determination. Unfortunately, the database to support such advice is weak and further compromised by early discharges which require crude predictions about a patient's future course. In some cases not only may the discharge planners disagree with the patient, but there may be discord within the family or among the various health professionals involved. Several conflicting opinions may be held. Resolution requires time and discussion.

3. Once a general modality of long-term care has been selected, the specific provider should be chosen. The choice of the actual nursing home, assisted living program, home care vendor, and so on should be a deliberate one based on what is known about the capacity and other characteristics of each. The criteria for this choice may depend on such factors as convenience and compatibility with personal preferences (e.g., religion) as well as quality.

4. Information needs to be transmitted promptly to assure continuity of care. Both the next level of caregivers as well as the patient and family need information about treatments and prognosis.

5. Some form of feedback about the outcomes is needed to learn from the experience and thereby improve the database for future estimates. In practice, many patients discharged to some form of post-hospital care will require more than one type of care. Hospital discharge planners are poorly positioned to oversee the entire episode. Some other type of case management may be needed.

In truth, few hospital discharges come even close to this idealized model. The pressures for rapid action tend to promote availability as a primary criterion. Because it may take more time and effort to organize a discharge to the community, an available nursing home bed may appear attractive. With a destination in mind, the alternatives are packaged to achieve patient compliance with the foreordained decisions. Under those circumstances, the dice are loaded against developing a new philosophy for discharge planning that gives much greater consideration to HCBS arrangements.

Attitudes of family caregivers are also important. When family caregivers reach a point where they can no longer continue to provide informal care, this often results in a catastrophic situation for the family, usually accompanied by a great deal of guilt. By placing the family member in a nursing home (which is most often seen as providing a level of care above what the family can provide), they can view their decision as inevitable and the guilt can be alleviated. If a community alternative is selected (e.g., a home-care provider, a live-in attendant, or placement in a foster home arrangement in the community), family members may view the success of these arrangements as a reproof. Even more important, family members often embody a protective philosophy, especially toward a widowed elderly parent who lives alone. They understandably want to protect their relatives. Finally, family members, just like professionals, are more familiar with nursing homes than the alternatives. Like them or not, they are the known commodity.

The philosophical barriers to meaningful change in long-term care policy are fueled by some persistent beliefs about long-term care. The following nine beliefs may be deeply embedded in the philosophies of all the key actors, from public officials to policy-makers to long-term care consumers and their families.

Belief 1. HCBS is more expensive than institutional care. This statement is often given as justification by nursing homes to rationalize their own prices. It has been incorporated into the thinking of many policy-makers. If believed, it becomes a self-fulfilling prophecy, immobilizing any real investment in making home care and other HCBS programs work as genuine alternatives to nursing homes. As indicated in Chapter 2, state officials noted the results of the Long-Term Care Channeling Demonstration, completed in about 1985. The study concluded that many people who used HCBS would never have never ended up on the state payroll for nursing home care. Since HCBS did not substantially reduce nursing home usage, they constituted add-on costs for a new population.[9]

Criticism of the Channeling projects has come from several quarters. Many have suggested that the projects did not target services well and tested a rather low intensity of case management or a costly model of service. Some suggested that the intervention was too limited in time and number of people served to truly change the incentives for program stakeholders. Both providers and consumers were hesitant to count on a small program expected to be of 18 months' duration. Moreover, those who did not like its thrust could wait it out, especially because it affected only a few hundred clients in then market areas.

One of the earlier demonstrations, which was a precursor to Channeling, done in three areas of South Carolina, showed that the new services were cost-effective. Persons receiving HCBS had 38% fewer nursing homes days, compared to a control group.[10] This South Carolina program was particularly effective because it targeted the intervention to low-income people who were clearly eligible for nursing homes by dint of functional status and, in many instances, were actually on the way toward admission. The program interrupted the trajectory toward the nursing home for the experimental group. Similar efforts have been made to alter the course of the consumer's destiny in operational programs; for example, Oregon's HCBS waiver program, described in Chapter 5, made enormous efforts to help Medicaid clients move out of nursing homes, even though this often meant reconstructing some kind of living and support system because the original housing of the nursing home resident had been given up.

Every state that has offered HCBS as a large-scale operational program has found that it is less expensive than nursing homes. A recent study found that in two states this was pronounced. In Oregon in 1994 the cost per day for HCBS care was $13.52, while the cost per day for nursing home care was $57.97. Texas had similar numbers at $12.27 for HCBS and $46.55 for nursing home care.[11]

The argument that some people would use HCBS programs who would never enter a nursing home is known as "the woodwork effect." That is, people will come out of the woodwork to take advantage of desirable programs, and this added use will more than offset any reductions in the use of established programs. Undoubtedly, there is validity to the concerns about a woodwork effect, but Oregon and other states that have heavily invested in alternatives found this effect was not overwhelming and could be offset by efficiencies in the HCBS programs. The woodwork effect could be a greater problem in states with a low level of current provision and high poverty rates, thus creating a pent-up demand for service—for example, Alabama and Georgia, but even then a carefully targeted and managed program with available and well-priced services should, in the long run, reduce overall long-term care costs while serving more people.

By 1980 an influential analysis by William Weissert and colleagues[12] argued that socially oriented home care—specifically homemaker services—will not reduce nursing home care enough to save money. Although actively urged, this argument that a real investment in HCBS will not reduce nursing home care is simply untrue. The provision of increased HCBS does not result in a one-to-one replacement of nursing home care, but it does substantially reduce this care over time. For example, Wisconsin increased the use of its Community Options Program in the 1980s, resulting in a 12% reduction in nursing home use.[13] Indeed, eight states had negative nursing home utilization growth rates during the 1980s, and twenty states were able to keep the nursing home utilization growth rate during this decade to less than 10%. Each of those states expanded its HCBS during this same period.

Belief 2. If HCBS is subsidized, long-term care caseloads will rise drastically. The reasoning here is that many people will use HCBS who would delay or refuse nursing home care, and that families giving free care to help their relatives avoid nursing homes will stop helping once an HCBS benefit is more available. Though this belief is widely held by many decision makers in state government, there is little or no evidence that family withdrawal will occur. Summarizing the evidence to date, in 1994 researchers from the Brookings Institution asserted: "Most studies suggest that when the disabled elderly receive paid home care, such as adult day care, skilled nursing services, personal care, and homemaker services, the unpaid care given by family members does not change significantly."[14] The experience from other countries with more expansive public support for LTC shows little or no reduction in the efforts of informal caregivers. In the United States, William Weissert compared twenty-seven controlled demonstrations of home-and-community-based-care. He identified fifty-three findings that related to the effects of paid home care on unpaid family care; forty-one were findings of no statistically significant differences, seven suggested a significant *increase* in unpaid support with the addition of paid help, only four suggested a significant decrease of family care, and one was indeterminate.[15]

Belief 3. Most people in nursing homes "need" nursing home care specifically rather than care in general. This argument is often voiced by nursing homes as a means to justify their existence. For example, the Wisconsin Health Care Association (a nursing home trade association) recently distributed a letter that stated that the long-term care populations that use home-and-community-based care were entirely different from the populations that use (or need) nursing home care.[16]

Several studies, including a classic study by the U.S. General Accounting Office[17] have shown that fully two-thirds of all people needing long-term care services are cared for at home by family or friends. Indeed, many of these people have very high care needs and would easily qualify for nursing home care. Ironically, some people are judged to be too sick for nursing homes and can get sufficient nursing personnel at home. Oregon has shown that, although nursing homes tend to care for a higher percentage of people with heavy long-term care needs, people with similar levels of disability can be found in significant numbers in every other long-term care setting.

Nursing homes often attempt to convince the public that all of their residents require nursing home care. Two recent studies show that this is not the case. A study of Texas nursing homes showed that 27.3% of the residents had no deficiencies in the activities of daily living and low medical needs.[18] A second multistate study estimated that up to 35% of people residing in nursing homes could be candidates for other long-term care settings.[19]

Belief 4. It is feasible and desirable to develop a continuum of care based on measured needs, and to move consumers "appropriately" within that continuum. A wide range of service options for long-term care should exist in local areas. This is the only way consumers have choices. The options should ideally include a range of in-home services and personal assistance, transportation assistance, home-delivered meals, adult day care, adult foster homes, assisted living facilities, and nursing homes. This array should be a balanced system so that the numbers of any particular type of provider do not heavily dominate the system.

The myth of the continuum is that it is feasible and desirable for professionals to pinpoint exactly what long-term care setting should "appropriately" be used to serve a particular person. This belief fuels efforts to design scoring systems so that case managers can assign people to settings and gives rise to studies on how many people are in nursing homes who "do not need to be there."

We reject as a harmful myth the premise that one can and should design a continuum of services and optimize each person's care through scientific assignment. It is overly restrictive to maintain that there is a "right" place for each person to live and get care. People's preferences differ, and many different service packages and settings are capable of serving a given individual appropriately. Perhaps few people "need" nursing home care literally in the sense that a nursing home is the only place where their needs could be met, but, conversely, there are few people in nursing homes today with zero need for care. Also, people's levels of need change over time, and the concept of moving people to different residential settings with different service levels to precisely titrate their "needs" is both unworkable and inhumane. We are on record with a recommendation that the continuum of care be abandoned as an ideal because of its connotations of conveyor belt decline and pigeon-hole classifications. Instead, we suggest that states aspire to a repertoire of services from which consumers, with the help of professionals as needed, can choose.[20]

Belief 5. Many routine procedures needed in the daily lives of people with disabilities must be performed with close supervision of a nurse. Most people needing long-term care who have physical illnesses and disabilities are on medication regimens. Administration of medications of all types (oral, topical, suppository or injections) can be the Achilles' heel that makes long-term care plans in the community prohibitively costly if the client cannot manage the regimen independently and no family members are present to help. Other nursing tasks that are often part of the plan include catheter care, ostomy care, tracheotomy care, wound care, and respirator care.

It is simply untrue that laypeople cannot be taught to perform routine nursing tasks competently. Many of these tasks are performed daily by family members. Only when they become paid services do rules about professional oversight come into force. Several states have shown great success with nurse delegation laws that allow nonprofessional people to perform these tasks. Also, state programs providing personal assistant services to younger people with disabilities have sometimes waived requirements for a nurse to do certain procedures without deleterious repercussions. One of the Medicare-reimbursed functions of nurses and therapists in home health agencies is teaching family or friends how to perform a wide range of health procedures. Yet, the idea that nurses can and should also teach nursing tasks to unlicensed paid personnel such as those working in the home and in socially oriented group residential settings is controversial. Once the assumed protection of a family relationship is removed, professionals are concerned about safety issues. However, most of the tasks done by nurses (as opposed to the nursing assessment) are concrete and capable of communication to others.

For many long-term care clients, paid helpers are present doing personal care and homemaking tasks; surely they could be drawn upon for nursing tasks as well. They could also be taught to perform nursing tasks in socially oriented home-like residential settings too small to afford the regular presence of a nurse. The unthinking acceptance that certain tasks *must* be done by licensed nursing has dramatically increased the price of long-term care outside of large facilities that can afford to hire full-time nurses.

Belief 6. The physical safety of older persons should guide policy and programs above all other values, concerns, and goals. Federal and state regulations are rife with rules and procedures regarding safety of clients and residents. Advocates for the disabled and elderly often cite safety as their leading concern. This is a natural concern and part of the human condition: We all want people to be safe from harm, especially those that we care dearly about. Unfortunately, we are often forced to trade other, equally important, values like independence, privacy, and choice for safety.

Over the years, the passage of so many state and federal laws and regulations concerning safety has not been as successful in yielding desired results. Abuse still exists in long-term care settings despite all of the additional laws, and the cost of implementing these laws and regulations has been very great. In fact, every time a new law or regulation was passed, it had the effect of removing a little bit of the personal freedoms that long-term care clients desire. In nursing homes, for example, the facility is totally responsible for its residents, and unfortunately, total responsibility often leads to total control.

When safety is viewed as paramount, personal preferences tend to be trumped by professional judgments about safety. In turn, this has often led to more expensive care than necessary. The success that Alaska and New York have enjoyed in their long-term care services for persons with developmental disabilities proves this case. Alaska and New York provide these services based on the preferences of the client, even though these preferences often contradict professional judgment, and they found that these plans cost less than nursing homes in the same states. Alaska and New York have shown than the cost of these "wraparound" services are substantially less than institutional care. (New York and Alaska are two states at the higher end of the price spectrum for all forms of care.) A small-scale demonstration in New Hampshire dramatically showed the same thing: The plans preferred and designed by the person with the developmental disability were much less expensive than professionally designed plans, and problem rates were not greater because of the compromise with safety entailed in the plans.[21]

One of the most insidious features of the safety myth is that it leads professionals to take protective actions without ever learning the results. People are "placed" in nursing homes or legal procedures are implemented to arrange guardianship for a person. Yet, little is known about whether people thus protected are better off even in terms of their physical well-being and health, let alone their social and psychological well-being. One of the most dramatic examples is the case of physical restraints, once widely in use in nursing homes for protection of residents and now in disrepute.[22] As part of the movement to "untie the elderly," studies have been done showing serious injuries as a result of using restraints, including bedrails.[23] Thus, an orthodox practice justified on safety grounds has largely been discredited *even* in terms of safety itself. Another consequence of the way safety is enshrined as a goal means that home care providers and case management agencies sometimes withdraw from serving clients whom they believe they cannot adequately protect within the available resources for services. Paradoxically, if the withdrawal does not have the intended effect of precipitating relocation to a more protected setting, this may result in the person having no service at all and being less safe.

Belief 7. Frail elderly people cannot live alone, especially if they have cognitive deficits. This is a widely held belief by many individuals involved in long-term care services. It is most often stated by providers who operate congregate care facilities like assisted living facilities or nursing homes. Study after study has shown that it simply is not true. Thousands of frail elderly people and people with cognitive impairments continue to live alone in their homes and apartments. Many of these people receive intermittent care from home health and home care agencies and from family and friends without having live-in providers. Innovative programs in other countries have demonstrated the feasibility of managing the care of people with dementia, even if they live alone. One such program has been implemented widely in Adelaide, Australia, a city of about one million people.[24] A specially trained group of paraprofessional workers, under nurse leadership, provide a range of practical services, going in and out of the home at brief intervals during the day. The care is interspersed with help from family members, and a chart kept in the consumer's home allows for communication and documentation of who has done what. Program leaders comment that many of the very disturbing behavior problems exhibited by people with dementia cease to be problems when nobody is there to be bothered by them. In other words, they were more a problem for the family members because of the sadness, anxiety, or annoyance they evoked than for the consumer.

Belief 8. It will do them no harm and may benefit older people to be placed involuntarily in the same room as other older people. Nothing in federal law or regulation requires that older (or younger) people should involuntarily share their space with others. The myth that such sharing is acceptable is commonly generated by providers of institutional long-term care services, who believe they can increase their profits (or lower their costs) by placing more than one person in a room. It is sustained by people who assume that older people with diminishing capacities to move about independently will be lonely if they have private rooms in nursing homes or other residential settings. It is also sustained by those who believe older people easily adjust to the necessity of shared accommodations.

Providing private rooms does not substantially increase the cost of care, especially in nursing homes where the facility costs tend to be a minor part of the total costs. Assisted living facilities with only private rooms and private baths are being constructed in several states and construction costs have been affordable. More important, older people express a very strong preference for privacy in their bedrooms and bathrooms. A recent study by Michelle Teitelbaum showed this clearly for nursing home residents; the sample surveyed had not wanted shared rooms to begin with and did not get accustomed to the lack of privacy and the lack of space.[25] A telephone survey of a representative sample of 694 citizens over age 50 indicated their strong preference for private rooms in assisted living, which respondents preferred to larger apartments.[26] A focus-group study done by Rosalie Kane and colleagues found the same results.[27] Therefore, we believe that an important plank in long-term care reform is to offer normal, privately occupied small apartments as a minimum provision for people who cannot practically get long-term care in their own homes, a topic discussed in detail in Chapter 6. Here we just note that the persistent and deeply entrenched belief that it is good for older residents to be spared the isolation of a private room is as powerful a deterrent to change as the dubious assertion that private rooms are too expensive to be a standard expectation.

People are social animals, and meaningful social involvement is essential to most people's perception of a life worth living. But arbitrarily pairing people in their living quarters does not achieve such social involvement. Studies show that people in the close quarters of a nursing home tend to withdraw from communication with others, including roommates.[28] Space for privacy, for contemplation, personal planning, regrouping, and conducting a chosen social life is needed. We cannot exaggerate the human unhappiness that has arisen from the widespread acceptance of the idea that it is alright to assign roommates to older people needing care.

Belief 9. Good long-term care can prevent bad things from happening. The beliefs discussed here are interrelated. The emphasis on safety, professional presence, and "scientific" long-term care placements is related to keeping bad things from happening. The formulations that state that home care is more expensive than institutional care are predicated on costly personnel meant to keep people safer and to promote the best results. At the heart of many of these tenets is the view that somehow good long-term care will mean that the consumers remain alive, and suffer no accident or injury. In particular, a view prevails that long-term care should be organized in such a way that a negative event, such as a fall or a serious illness, be prevented or at least discovered instantly. "What if something should happen?" is a watchword for long-term care planners.

Some bad things that might happen are on a different plane from disease, accident, and natural death. The family might abuse, neglect, or exploit the patient, with long-term care programs "letting it happen." Worse, somebody employed in the long-term care labor force—either giving services in the client's home or in a residential facility—might exploit, neglect, injure, or otherwise abuse the patient. A client might perish in a fire. Not only do clinical personnel often feel responsible for such events and believe they should have prevented them, but public officials have a deep dread of a case of abuse or neglect on their watch.

Of course, we do not condone neglectful or abusive behavior and we are saddened by accidents and injuries, particularly if the client is alone and unable to summon help for hours afterward. Prudent long-term care plans should incorporate precautions to minimize accidents and the predicament of being unable to get help in an emergency (for example, safer homes, alarm systems, telephone checking systems). But the view that anything bad that happens is a caregiving failure defies common sense. The population getting long-term care—at least its elderly portion—is at risk for death and increasing disability. And do what one will, some pathological and destructive behavior will occur within our families and communities that cannot be predicted or prevented. Criminal checks of personnel is one useful and prudent approach to minimizing the potential problem of abusive behavior on the part of paid caregivers. But bad things will happen, and the larger the population receiving long-term care, the more incidents will occur. Unfortunately, the constant preoccupation with the bad things that might happen and many of the strategies undertaken to mitigate them create extensive present misery for the consumer. This nagging sense that good long-term care requires that nothing bad happen to the consumer has foreclosed needed discussion about the kind and volume of untoward events that might be tolerated and how to resolve the trade-offs between protection and freedom for long-term care consumers.

The corollary to the belief that we should prevent bad things from happening is: If bad things happen, program staff and public officials will be sued, and probably successfully. Attorneys have written a great deal about this persistent belief.[29] Long-term care providers can, it is suggested, remain relatively impervious to successful liability suits if they follow some straightforward practices, discussed further in Chapter 7 where we treat issues of accountability and quality assurance.

To summarize, the obstacles to achieving the goals of a more user-friendly, more balanced long-term care system are myriad, falling into political, logistical, and philosophical categories. To overcome those obstacles, as earlier stated, tenacity is the key word. The political situation in most states is constantly changing, and what may be infeasible at one point may be possible at another. States that have successfully changed their long-term care systems have found that well organized and focused senior and disabled advocate groups can offer enormous help in this effort.[30] Because these groups have little or no fiduciary interest in long-term care services, they have greater credibility, and, therefore, can sometimes convince key legislators that changing the long-term care system can improve the system. Not only that, but they and their family members are voters.

Federal Policies Favoring Nursing Homes

Even if they overcome the barriers described so far and summon the political will to act, states must contend with the barriers of federal laws and regulations that tend to favor nursing homes. In this section we describe some federal policies— seemingly rather technical—that taken together show that the federal government has definitely favored nursing homes over all other providers of Medicaid long-term care services. This has resulted in a nursing home–dominated long-term care system in the states, because long-term care is too expensive to operate without federal help.

Entitlement Status for Nursing Homes
Entitlement status means that any person who is eligible for nursing home services cannot be denied that service as long as a Medicaid-certified nursing home bed is available. States cannot deny nursing home services because of state revenue short-falls or budget considerations. Home-and-community-based care waiver services do not enjoy this entitlement protection status. Clients eligible for HCBS waivers can be denied services because of state budget considerations, and often are. Many states (like Wisconsin) have long waiting lists for HCBS, and these are mainly caused by the amount of money in the state budget appropriation for this service.

Personal care services and home health services that are part of the state's Medicaid state plan are also entitlement services. However, these services have lower income eligibility levels and therefore are not available to all those eligible for nursing home care.

Mandatory Nature of Medicaid Nursing Home Services
States must have a statewide nursing home program in order to qualify for any Medicaid funding. These services must be offered in the same amount, for the same duration, and have the same scope of services available. These federal laws mean that states must have a fairly extensive nursing home program that is also fairly uniform.

HCBS programs are an optional service under Medicaid, and states can choose whether to have such services available. In addition, most HCBS waivers have exceptions to both the need to have the program statewide, and the amount, duration, and scope requirements.

Higher Income Eligibility for Nursing Home Coverage Under Medicaid

Medicaid allows a higher income status for covering nursing homes than for covering HCBS in many states. To be eligible for nursing home care under Medicaid a resident must not have an income above 300% of the Supplemental Security Income (SSI) standard. As of January 1994, this federal payment was set to ensure an income of $494 a month for disabled and elderly people. The 300% standard permits an income of $1,432 dollars a month. In addition, a spouse of a nursing home resident living at home is able to reserve a large portion of the available income and assets, under the "spousal impoverishment laws." Many states allow even higher incomes for covering nursing home care under the Medically Needy option in Medicaid. If a person's income is above 300% of the SSI standard (about $1,410 a month), but below the Medicaid nursing homes charges, Medicaid will pay the difference if a state has added this option to the Medically Needy program.

Although all of these eligibility options are also available to states under the HCBS waiver program, they are not available under other Medicaid services like personal care and home health services. In reality most states have adopted an income limitation of 300% of the SSI standard for home-and-community-based waivers, but few have extended the spousal impoverishment provisions or medically needy eligibility to these clients. The income limitation for personal care and home health services is 100% of the SSI standard ($494 a month), and in about five states, which opted for lower eligibility levels in 1972 when SSI was enacted, it is even lower than this. Spousal impoverishment provisions do not apply to these services. Medically needy provisions can apply to these services, but few states have implemented this option.

Guarantee of Inflationary Increases

Nursing homes are guaranteed inflationary increases by federal law, while home-and-community-based services are not. The Boren amendment, enacted in the late 1970s (and repealed in 1997), declared that states must pay the full costs of an efficient and economic facility but, no specification was given by either federal law or federal regulation. Because of the law's vagueness, most states paid little attention to it until the late 1980s when a lawsuit in Virginia (*Virginia Hospital Association vs Wilder*) ruled against that state and required that it raise its reimbursement of nursing homes.

Since then almost every state has been sued by either hospitals (which also were governed by the Boren Amendment) or nursing homes, and often by both. The states tended to lose most of these suits, and a large body of court law resulted.

States were then required to do cost finding on nursing homes and hospitals, define the costs of an efficient and economic facility, and pay all costs up to this amount. This type of reimbursement is inflationary, because it most often means that the more one spends in the current year the higher the reimbursement will be the following year.

HCBS had no such protection under federal law or regulation. States are not required to grant any inflationary increase to these services, and often do not. Indeed, several states have even reduced the reimbursement rates to HCBS when there has been a shortfall in state revenues.

Over the years, this discrepancy in federal law and regulations has resulted in nursing homes receiving much higher annual inflation increases than HCBS providers. States are often required to pay hospitals and nursing homes higher annual increases than the annual increases in state general revenue. This has meant that a higher and higher percentage of the state general revenue must be used to support hospitals and nursing homes. Under these conditions it becomes even more difficult to obtain dollars for HCBS programs.

The effects of repealing the Boren amendment remain to be seen. A new state of equity with HCBS could ensue, or nursing homes may find other political bases for maintaining their inflationary advantage. The emerging managed care phenomenon, discussed in Chapter 9, may offer prepaid organizations a financial incentive to use HCBS instead of nursing homes, though managed care organizations would need to overcome their own habits and philosophical biases to deal comfortably with purchasing very complex and possibly informal community arrangements for very sick people.

Ease of Increasing Bed Supply

Nursing homes can increase the bed supply without prior federal approval, while most HCBS programs cannot expand their capacity without such approval. Most states have prior approval processes through their Certificate of Need (CON) programs, a state process that requires approval of all medical facilities and expensive equipment. These processes are rather loose in many states, and some states have eliminated CONs altogether. Many states have placed a moratorium on any new nursing home construction, and this has tended to lower the bed supply over time.

The federal government, however, has no limitation on the number of nursing home beds a state may certify for Medicaid funding. This led some states to add substantial numbers of nursing home beds during the decade of the 1980s. At the extreme, for example, Indiana saw a 247% increase in nursing home beds between 1981 and 1991.

Although there is also no federal prior approval process for personal care and home health, this is not true for HCBS waivers. All of these services must have prior approval from the federal government before they are eligible for Medicaid funding. A lengthy and complicated request for approval must be submitted by the states in order to obtain waivers, or to add to the number of waiver slots available for Medicaid funding. While obtaining federal approval for HCBS waivers is much easier today than it was in the 1980s, it still requires much more additional effort by the states, and has tended to limit the number of waiver requests.

State Laws and Regulations

States must also make changes to their own laws and regulations that often protect particular providers of long-term care services and embody philosophical beliefs about what is necessary for vulnerable elderly people. Although it is easier for state officials to critique federal regulations, sometimes they will need to conclude, with Pogo, that the enemy is us.

All states have enacted laws and regulations concerning long-term care services. These laws and regulations tend to vary greatly from state to state, and they also tend to define any particular state's long-term care system. They describe who is eligible for long-term care services, which providers can provide these services, and under what conditions these services will be provided. Many of these state laws and regulation present barriers to the development of more user friendly, more balanced long-term care systems. States must also modify any state laws and regulations that unduly protect particular providers of long-term care services.

Eligibility Issues

States have some flexibility in defining financial eligibility for Medicaid long-term care services but are mostly required to use federal standards. For example, states could use anywhere from 100% to 300% of the SSI standard for nursing home and HCBS waiver income eligibility levels, though most adopted the 300% level. Asset limits are $2,000 for single people, and $3,000 for a couple, except that qualified Medicare beneficiaries have assets at $4,000 for single people, and $6,000 for couples. In addition, spousal impoverishment allows states higher levels of income and asset requirements, and states have responded with a variety of levels in their adoption of these regulations.

Although financial eligibility for long-term care services is mostly defined by the federal government, impairment eligibility is largely defined by the states. The only federal requirement is that a physician must certify medical necessity. Many states, especially southern states, have adopted this federal requirement as the only impairment requirement for entering a nursing home or HCBS. Most other states have added additional requirements that compell potential state and Medicaid-funded long-term care clients to meet minimum levels of functional impairment.

These additional impairments requirements vary from state to state, but they are usually defined as needing assistance in at least two or three activities of daily living. (Activities of daily living are usually defined as eating, toileting, ambulating, dressing, grooming, and bathing.) Several existing assessment instruments exist that can measure these activities of daily living, but most states have created their own instrument. Thus, some potential clients will be eligible for long-term care services in one state but not in another. Texas, for example, has no impairment requirements for entering a nursing home and has about 25,000 Medicaid nursing home residents (27%), who have no functional impairments and low medical needs.[31] Most of these clients would not be eligible for any long-term care services in states like Oregon, Washington, and Wisconsin.

Long-term care programs that do not use Medicaid funding are free to define both financial and impairment eligibility levels. Although these requirements vary from state to state, eligibility requirements for state-funded programs are usually more permissive than the Medicaid requirements. Long-term care programs that are not Medicaid funded usually attempt to fill the gap between those who are eligible for Medicaid and those who can afford to pay privately for long-term care services. Alaska, for example, probably has the most developed long-term care programs that are not funded by Medicaid. Alaska spends more state general revenue on Pioneer homes (a state-funded program) than on the state share of nursing homes. These Pioneer homes have a residency requirement of 1 year, making them ineligible for Medicaid funding, and they provide care mostly for residents with Alzheimer's disease and related disorders, who are not eligible for nursing home services in Alaska. In addition, Alaska pays each elderly resident a longevity bonus of $250 a month if they lived in Alaska for 1 year and were age 65 before January 1, 1994. This makes many older Alaskans ineligible for SSI and Medicaid. Alaska has instituted an Alaska Longevity Bonus-Hold Harmless program which allows such people to receive the same services as Medicaid clients, but the payment is made entirely through state general revenue funds.[32]

Coverage Issues

All states have a nursing home program and all state have a HCBS program. The amounts and types of services offered in the nursing home program are fairly standard between states, but the amounts and types of services offered in the HCBS programs vary greatly between states. Every state has implemented some kind of home care program, several states have implemented adult day care programs, and some states have implemented housing options that also provide personal assistance, like adult foster homes and assisted living facilities.

Each state has laws and regulations that define what HCBS can be offered, who can provide these services, and under what conditions they may be offered. These laws and regulations are often the result of strong lobbying efforts by particular providers, and can often be termed "protective regulations." For example, most states have laws that limit the number of days a provider, other than a nursing home or home health agency, can retain a client who needs skilled nursing care. These laws most often apply even if the provider employs skilled medical professionals and is fully equipped to handle the client's condition. In addition, the number of days allowed varies greatly from state to state (e.g.,10 days in Oregon and 45 days in Alaska).

Other examples of protective regulations include the provision in many states that only home health agencies can provide home care and the provision that only licensed medical professionals can provide personal care services. Both of these provisions raise the cost of HCBS substantially, and several states have now instituted "nurse delegation" regulations that allow nonlicensed persons to provide personal care services, often including dispensing injectable medicines, under the supervision of a nurse.

In addition, many states have regulations that prevent the normalization of congregate living situations. Some states, having recognized that a nursing home is not a normal living situation, are attempting to develop alternate housing options (usually assisted living facilities) to provide more homelike environments. These housing options usually include private apartments with locking doors, private bathrooms, living and sleeping areas, and small kitchenettes. In some states where these housing options have been developed (e.g., Oregon, Washington, Texas, and New Jersey) regulations found on the books have delayed the implementation of these options, such as provisions against locking doors and having stove-top burners or microwave ovens.

States, of course, are free to change any of their own laws or regulations as long as they do not create a conflict with federal laws and regulations. But this is usually much easier said than done. Each state has built up a history of tradition over the years that helps to define long-term care. This history is often based on myths about long-term care that were espoused by particular special interest groups that wanted long-term care to take a specific form. These myths tend to persist and are often very hard to overcome.

Concluding Comment

The picture painted in this chapter suggests formidable obstacles to redressing the imbalance between nursing homes and HCBS. But, we do not want to end on a bleak note. The next chapter describes remarkable variation in states' abilities to shift resources from nursing home care to other forms of care. Then, in the Part II we discuss substantive approaches that hold enormous promise to improve the American way of doing long-term care.

Notes

1. Oregon has made sustained efforts to develop a range of alternative long-term care programs, design them for efficiency and to conform with consumer preferences, and target them to people with substantial disability. The system has been described in several reports, including Kutza EA, Neal MB, Peterson M, Lansing J, Carder P, & Shell D. (1991). *Independent Assessment of 1915(d) Waiver: Home and Community-Based Waiver for the Elderly* (Technical Report). Portland, OR: Portland State Univer-

sity Institute on Aging; Kutza EA (1995). *Long Term Care in Oregon.* (Paper prepared for the 1995 White House Conference on Aging and distributed by the National Association of State Units on Aging). Portland, OR: Portland State University Institute on Aging; Ladd RC (1996). *Oregon's LTC System: A Case Study by the National LTC Mentoring Program.* (Wendy J. Nielsen, Series Editor, Case Report Number 1). MN: Minneapolis, Institute for Health Services Research, University of Minnesota School of Public Health.

2. The comparative state figures cited in this and the next chapter come from work that the authors did to develop benchmarks of progress toward more balanced state long-term care investments. Using existing 1992 data, we compared all fifty states and the District of Columbia on a number of expenditure and utilization parameters. Unless specified, the state statistics cited in this chapter are found in Ladd RC, Kane RL, Kane RA, & Nielsen WJ (1995). *State Long-Term Care Profiles.* (Report of the National LTC Mentoring Program). Minneapolis, MN: University of Minnesota School of Public Health.

3. According to a *New York Times* article, "while money often buys access to power in Washington, the efforts of the nursing home industry are particularly well documented." The article goes on to identify large gifts to the Democratic party directly from the American Health Care Association, and key fund-raising roles of nursing home executives. See Pear R (1997). Big donors from nursing homes had access. *New York Times,* Wednesday, April 23, p.A16.

4. United States General Accounting Office (1994). *Medicaid Long-Term Care. Successful State Efforts to Expand Home Services While Limiting Costs. (GAO/HEHS-94-167, August 1994).* Washington, DC: Government Printing Office.

5. Kane RA & Frytak J (1994). *Models for Case Management in Long-Term Care: Interactions of Case Managers and Home Care Providers.* (A report submitted to the U.S. Office of Technology Assessment in October 1993 and disseminated by the National LTC Resource Center, University of Minnesota). Minneapolis, MN: National LTC Resource Center, University of Minnesota School of Public Health; Williams JK (1992). *Case Management: Opportunities for Service Providers.* (Prepared for the Home Care Association of New York State, February 12, 1992). Mimeo.

6. Kane RA & Wilson KB (1993). *Assisted Living in the United States: A New Paradigm for Residential Care for Frail Older Persons?* Washington, DC: National Association of Retired Persons.

7. In 1996, the Pew Charitable Trusts began an exploratory process to examine the presence of genuine advocacy groups in long-term care at the state level and to consider ways to stimulate their development See Ladd RC (1997). *State Strategies and Methods Used To Balance Long-Term Care Systems.* (A paper commissioned by Pew Charitable Trust). Austin, TX: Ladd, Mimeo. Unfortunately the foundation's board aborted its plans for a national program to strengthen consumer groups in long-term care.

8. Potffhoff SJ, Kane RL, & Franco SJ (1995). *Hospital Discharge Planning for Elderly Patients: Improving Decisions, Aligning Incentives.* (Final report to the Health Care Financing Administration under Master Contract 500-92-0048, September, 1995). Minneapolis, MN: University of Minnesota School of Public Health, memo.

9. See the entire issue of the *Journal of Health Services Research,* Volume 23 (1), 1988 for a group of articles that succinctly summarize the methods and results of the Long-Term Care Channeling Demonstration.

10. Nocks BC, Learner M, Blackman D, & Brown TE (1986). The effects of a community based long-term care program on nursing home utilization. *The Gerontologist* 26:150–157.

11. Ladd, RC. (1995). *Long-Term Care in Texas: Recommendations for Reform.* Austin, TX: Lyndon B. Johnson School of Public Affairs.

12. Weissert WG, Wan TTH, Livieratos BB, & Pellegrino J (1980). Cost-effectiveness of homemaker services for the chronically ill. *Inquiry* 17:236–240.
13. Wisconsin Bureau of Long-term Care (1994). *Using the HCFA 2082*. Annual Medicaid Program Statistics Report. (Available from Department of Health and Human Resources, Health Care Financing Administration). Baltimore, MD: Division of Information Distribution.
14. Wiener JM & Harris KM (1990).Myths and realities: why most of what everybody knows about long-term care is wrong. *The Brookings Review* Fall: 30.
15. Weissert WG, Cready CM, & Pawelak JE (1989). Home and community care: three decades of findings. In MD Petersen & DL White (Eds.), *Health Care of the Elderly: An Information Sourcebook*. Newbury Park, CA: Sage.
16. Personal Communication. Letter from Tom Moore, of the Wisconsin Health Care Association, to the legislator.
17. U.S. General Accounting Office (1979). *Entering A Nursing Home—Costly Implications for Medicaid and the Elderly*. (Report No. PAD-80-12). Washington, DC.
18. Ladd RC. See note 11.
19. Newcomer R & Lee P (1994). *State Innovations in Residential Care for the Elderly: A Profile of Best Practices in Range of Care, Placement Control, and Financing*. San Francisco: University of California at San Francisco, Institute for Health and Aging.
20. Kane RA (1993). Dangers lurking in the "continuum of care:" A repertoire of services is a better goal. *Journal of Aging and Social Policy* 5(4):1–7.
21. Nerney T & Shumway D (1996). *Beyond Managed Care: Self Determination For People With Disabilities*. Concord, NH: Institute on Disability, University of New Hampshire.
22. Kane RL, Williams CC, Williams TF, & Kane RA (1993). Restraining restraints: changes in a standard of care. *Annual Review of Public Health* 14:545–584.
23. Miles S & Irving P (1992). Deaths caused by physical restraints. *The Gerontologist,* 32: 762–766; Parker K & Miles S (1997). Deaths Caused by Bedrails. *Journal of American Geriatrics Society* 45:797–802.
24. Mykyta LJ & Lovell G (1989). Community care for dementia sufferers. *Australia Journal of Aging* 8(3):17.
25. Teitelbaum M (1996). *Evaluation of the LTC Survey Process*. (Report to the Health Care Financing Administrator). Boston: Abt.
26. Jenkens R (1997). *Assisted Living and Private Rooms; What People Say They Want*. Washington, DC: American Association of Retired Persons.
27. Kane RA, Baker MO, Salmon J, & Veazie WJ (1998) *Consumer Perspectives on Private Versus Shared Accommodations in Assisted Living Settings*. Washington, DC: American Association of Retired Persons.
28. Kaakinen JR (1992). Living with silence. *The Gerontologist* 32(2):258–264. For a discussion of perceived isolation in nursing homes. Also see Sheilds RR (1988). *Uneasy Endings*. Ithaca, NY: Cornell University Press.
29. See Kapp MB (1997). Who is responsible for this? Assigning rights and consequences in elder care. *Journal of Aging and Social Policy* 9:51-65; Kapp MB (1991). Malpractice liability in long-term care. *Creighton Law Review* 24:1235–1260.
30. Ladd (1997). See note 7.
31. Ladd (1995). See note 11.
32. Ladd (1996). *Long-term Care in Alaska: Recommendations for Reform*. (Report submitted to the Alaska Department on Aging, November 1995). Austin, TX: Ladd & Associates.

4.

Progress Toward Balanced Long-Term Care Systems

We have repeatedly stressed that long-term care policies are invented and implemented at state and local levels. Thus, state governments are the entities that have been handed, and in various ways have risen to, the challenge of developing operational long-term care programs. Although many state officials and health and human service providers are dedicated to the mission of fashioning long-term care services that conform to the evident human need and administering those services fairly, they have been hampered by the barriers described in Chapter 3. They all contend with financial pressures on state governments, rigid federal program definitions, and limits to their own ability to imagine an entirely new philosophy that could transform long-term care.

Perhaps because of those barriers, few states have made serious efforts to reverse the dominance of nursing home expenditures over HCBS expenditures, although excellent models for promising HCBS approaches can be found scattered across the country. On the other hand, states vary enormously on the crucial matter of how they balance expenditures for their HCBS and nursing home programs. No ready markers have been available to examine how far states have come and how far they need to go. Therefore, in states that have devoted considerable creative and imaginative energy to HCBS programs, legislators, state officials, HCBS providers, and the general public may believe that those state efforts have actually achieved more reshaping of the entire system of care delivery than is actually the case.

This chapter provides one answer to the question, How well are states doing regarding long-term care? For this purpose, we assembled statistical markers of progress for the fifty states and the District of Columbia to examine how well each state has controlled the growth of nursing home expenditures (which we argue must proceed simultaneously with investment in HCBS) and how much it has invested in HCBS programs. Recognizing that the hands dealt to states are uneven, we also created indicators of the demand for long-term care and, specifically, for publicly financed long-term care in each state.

In this chapter we present broad-based information, largely using 1992 data.[1] (We are updating our analyses based on 1996 data. Undoubtedly, small changes will be found, but we expect the message conveyed by these figures will remain unchanged.) We also recognize that data about state resources expended in broad categories of nursing home and HCBS programs say nothing about the nature and quality of those programs. These caveats aside, the statistics presented in this chapter tell a useful and compelling story. First, they show how far we need to go as a nation to balance our long-term care systems. Second, and more encouragingly, they present a story of great variety in patterns of state expenditure and provide evidence that some states have made transitions in emphasis, despite extraordinary demographic demands on their systems. What some states have accomplished in shifting priorities of expenditures, all states can accomplish.

Federal Matches

All states have implemented Medicaid programs, and this provides some consistency across states. Medicaid differs from Medicare in two major respects. First, it is a program for poor people, including poor elderly people, and second, it is a state-administered program with the states and the federal government sharing the costs. The state share of Medicaid ranges from 22% to 50% depending on the state's per capita income compared to the national average. This formula has led to substantial variation in the contribution states must make. When Medicaid waivers became available for HCBS services, the same matching formulas applied.

Table 4.1 shows the state match rate or share of the Medicaid program for 1996. In 1996, Mississippi paid the lowest share at 21.9%, twelve states were at the maximum of a 50% share, and the average state share in the Medicaid program was 39.9%. However, wealthier states that pay a larger share in Medicaid also tend to purchase more long-term care services than those states receiving less federal money. Therefore, taken together, states pay an average of about 43% of total long-term care costs under Medicaid, with the federal government paying 57%.

The Medicaid matching formula attempts to equalize the ability of poorer states to acquire funds by requiring lower match rates. It accomplishes this to some extent, but it is probably not the fairest formula for achieving equity among states. If the 50% upper limit for state expenditures were removed, the match rates for the twelve states matched at the maximum 50% would change dramatically.[2] Connecticut, for example, would be required to pay 88.6% of its Medicaid long-term care bill, New Jersey 84.2%, the District of Columbia 74.5%, Massachusetts 74.6%, New York 69.4%, Maryland 67.3%, Alaska 66.6%, New Hampshire 61%, California 60.4%, and Illinois almost 60%. The farther a particular state's average per-capita income

Table 4.1. State Medicaid Percentage Share in 1996

State	State match %	State	State match %
Alaska	50.00%	Ohio	39.83
California	50.00	Vermont	39.13
Connecticut	50.00	Oregon	38.99
District of Columbia	50.00	Georgia	38.10
Hawaii	50.00	Texas	37.70
Illinois	50.00	Indiana	37.43
Maryland	50.00	Maine	36.68
Massachusetts	50.00	Iowa	35.78
New Hampshire	50.00	North Carolina	35.41
New Jersey	50.00	Tennessee	34.36
New York	50.00	Arizona	34.15
Nevada	50.00	South Dakota	33.34
Washington	49.81	Idaho	31.22
Delaware	49.67	North Dakota	30.94
Virginia	48.63	Montana	30.62
Colorado	47.56	Alabama	30.15
Pennsylvania	47.07	Oklahoma	30.11
Rhode Island	46.14	Kentucky	29.70
Minnesota	46.07	South Carolina	29.23
Florida	44.24	Louisiana	28.11
Michigan	43.23	New Mexico	27.13
Kansas	40.96	Utah	26.79
Nebraska	40.51	West Virginia	26.74
Wisconsin	40.33	Arkansas	26.39
Wyoming	40.31	Mississippi	21.93
Missouri	39.94	United States	39.89

is above or below the national average per-capita income, the better deal the state receives on a Medicaid match rate. Table 4.2 makes this concept more clear by using a couple of assumptions. First, Table 4.2 assumes that the national average per capita income in $10,000, and second, it assumes that all states have a 1% tax on personal income for use in Medicaid long-term care programs.

Table 4.2 shows that having a personal income close to the national average (as in Michigan, Pennsylvania, Florida, Washington, Minnesota, Colorado, Rhode Island, Nevada, and Hawaii) is disadvantageous. Both wealthier and poorer states are better able to make their tax dollars generate more Medicaid funding. Since Medicaid is a program designed to serve poor people, we would argue that the

Table 4.2. Relative Effect of the Medicaid Match Rate Assuming a National
Per-Capita Income of $10,000, and a 1% Tax on Personal Income for
Long-Term Care

Per-capita income as % of national average	State share match rate (%)	Amount of per-capita state tax available for Medicaid LTC ($)	Total available per capita with Medicaid match ($)
130	50	130	260
120	50	120	240
110	50	110	220
100	50	100	200
90	40	90	225
80	30	80	267
70	20	70	350

percentage of a state's population living under the poverty level compared to the
national average is probably a better base to use in affixing a state's contributions.
Some states like Florida, Georgia, and Texas have near-average per-capita income
levels, but very large percentages of their populations live in poverty.

State Variations in Nursing Home Care

Nursing Home Use

If states are to reset the balance of their long-term care systems toward HCBS,
then they must simultaneously curtail their expenditures on nursing homes. Using
several statistics to assess the states' progress in controlling both nursing home
utilization and expenditures, we found substantial variation among the states on
both fronts.

Although nursing home supply is conventionally described according to the population age 65+, the average age for nursing home residents is well over age 80.
Using the population age 85+ as a denominator provides a more realistic indicator
of the relative bed supply in the state. Indeed, substantial differences emerge when
the different denominators are used. For example, Alaska is ranked third highest
on the number of beds per 1,000 persons age 85+, but it is ranked eleventh lowest
when the base is persons age 65+. (Alaska has the smallest age 85+ population
in the nation at only 0.25% of the total Alaska population.) States with higher
percentages of age 85+ elderly, such as Kansas, Iowa, and South Dakota, are
ranked lower in supply when the age 85+ statistic is used, whereas some sun-belt
states with lower percentages of people over age 85 (for example, Alabama, North
Carolina, and Mississippi) appear to be better supplied with beds when the more

realistic 85+ figure is used for the ratio. States will have a more accurate perception of their challenge if they use the age 85+ figures rather than the more often cited, but less meaningful, statistics about people over age 65.

Table 4.3 shows the number of nursing home beds per 1,000 persons age 85+ by state in 1992. Louisiana had the highest bed supply at 834 beds per 1,000 persons age 85+, and Florida had the lowest at 306.3 beds per 1,000 persons age 85+, whereas the national average was 527 beds.

Table 4.4 shows the number of nursing home residents on Medicaid in 1994 per 1,000 people age 85+ in 1992 by state. This proportion ranged from 15% in Arizona to 59% in Louisiana, with a national average of 31%. The ratio of nursing

Table 4.3. Nursing Home Beds per 1,000 Age 85+ in 1992

State	Beds per 1,000 85+	State	Beds per 1,000 85+
Louisiana	834	Maine	539
Indiana	787	Utah	536
Alaska	757	New Hampshire	498
Oklahoma	721	Pennsylvania	497
Missouri	720	Washington	487
Wyoming	711	South Carolina	475
Texas	682	Mississippi	472
Illinois	657	North Carolina	463
Nebraska	650	Kentucky	463
Georgia	644	Virginia	459
Arkansas	643	Vermont	456
Rhode Island	639	Michigan	451
Wisconsin	638	New Jersey	447
Minnesota	635	Idaho	447
Kansas	628	Alabama	443
Ohio	628	New Mexico	424
Iowa	621	New York	421
Connecticut	614	California	418
Delaware	609	Nevada	396
North Dakota	591	District of Columbia	391
Montana	590	Arizona	389
South Dakota	590	West Virginia	379
Colorado	574	Oregon	351
Tennessee	563	Hawaii	311
Massachusetts	556	Florida	306
Maryland	552	United States	525

Table 4.4. Number of Nursing Home Residents Receiving Medicaid in 1994 per 1,000 Persons Aged 85+ in 1992

State	NH residents 85+ per 1,000	State	NH residents 85+ per 1,000
Louisiana	590	Virginia	310
Arkansas	540	New York	310
Georgia	470	Colorado	300
Rhode Island	440	Alabama	300
Tennessee	410	New Jersey	300
Maine	400	Kansas	300
Connecticut	390	Vermont	290
Minnesota	390	Pennsylvania	290
Wisconsin	390	Missouri	290
Ohio	390	Nebraska	290
Alaska	380	Washington	280
Indiana	380	District of Columbia	270
Mississippi	370	Iowa	270
Oklahoma	370	Michigan	260
Massachusetts	370	New Mexico	260
New Hampshire	370	West Virginia	260
Texas	360	Utah	250
Montana	360	Delaware	240
Illinois	340	Idaho	230
Wyoming	340	Nevada	220
North Carolina	330	California	220
North Dakota	330	Hawaii	210
Maryland	330	Oregon	180
Kentucky	320	Florida	170
South Dakota	310	Arizona	150
South Carolina	310	United States	310

home residents on Medicaid and the ratio of nursing home beds per person age 85+ are highly correlated in a positive direction. The few exceptions include Kansas, Iowa, and Nebraska, which are ranked on the high end as far as supply of beds and the low end as far as proportion of Medicaid residents, and Mississippi, which has a relatively low supply of beds and a high proportion of Medicaid residents. The number of Medicaid nursing home residents per 1,000 age 85+ population is also positively correlated with the following: the percentage of persons age 65+ living below poverty level, the percentage of persons age 65+ on Medicaid, the number of persons with severe disabilities per 1,000 persons age 65+, and the percentage of nursing home residents on Medicaid.

The ratio of Medicaid nursing home residents to the 85+ population and the amount of state and local expenditures on nursing homes are not significantly correlated. However, the population of all nursing home residents on Medicaid may be thought of as a fairly reliable predictor of how many resources a state will invest in the nursing home program. As seen in Table 4.5, this percentage varies from a low of 50% in Iowa to a high of 89% in the District of Columbia, with a national average of 69%. States with relatively high poverty levels tend to have higher percentages of nursing home residents on Medicaid. The proportion of nursing home residents on Medicaid is also linked to the Medicaid reimbursement rates.

Table 4.5. Percentage of Nursing Home Residents on Medicaid in 1994

State	% NH residents on Medicaid	State	% NH residents on Medicaid
District of Columbia	89%	Vermont	67%
Alaska	88	Maryland	67
Mississippi	83	Indiana	67
Louisiana	83	Washington	67
Georgia	82	California	66
Maine	78	Oklahoma	66
New York	78	Wyoming	65
Arkansas	78	Nevada	65
Tennessee	77	Missouri	65
North Carolina	77	Utah	65
Kentucky	76	Illinois	64
West Virginia	75	Minnesota	64
Rhode Island	75	Pennsylvania	64
Texas	75	Florida	63
Hawaii	74	Colorado	62
South Carolina	74	Idaho	61
New Hampshire	73	Montana	61
Massachusetts	73	Oregon	61
Alabama	73	North Dakota	57
New Mexico	71	Arizona	57
New Jersey	70	South Dakota	55
Virginia	70	Delaware	54
Ohio	70	Nebraska	53
Connecticut	68	Kansas	51
Michigan	68	Iowa	50
Wisconsin	68	United States	69

Source: Health Data Associates (1994). Rounded to the nearest whole percentage.

The higher the state rates, the more Medicaid residents. (Alaska, with the highest Medicaid reimbursement rate, has 88% of its nursing home residents on Medicaid.) It would appear that the higher the nursing home utilization rate, the fewer the residents who can afford to be privately paying clients. The percentage of nursing home residents on Medicaid is also significantly correlated with several other variables: state and local nursing home expenditures per person 85+, the severity of impairment in nursing homes as measured by the Propac Acuity Index,[3] the proportion of persons 65+ per 1,000 who are severely disabled, Medicaid nursing home residents as a percentage of the age 85+ population, and the percentage of the age 65+ population on Medicaid.

Nursing Home Expenditures

Authorities commonly believe that the more nursing home beds that are available, the harder it will be to change the long-term care system. The often-stated reason for this is that a state with a high bed supply relative to the elderly population has invested more per person in nursing homes and would have a greater difficulty in reallocating funds for HCBS. Our analyses challenge this contention.[4] State and local Medicaid nursing home expenditures per person age 85+ are only loosely correlated with the number of nursing home beds per 1,000 persons in this age group. Since the number of nursing home beds per 1,000 persons age 85+ had little to do with the amount of state and local nursing home expenditures, presumably some states could control nursing home expenditures without reducing the number of beds. However, those states may not opt to invest the difference in HCBS.

State and local general revenue spending for Medicaid nursing home residents per person 85+ ranges from $14,254 in Alaska (an outlier) and $7, 813 in the District of Columbia (the second highest spender) to a low of $1,020 in Utah, with a national average of $3,152. Generally, states with higher per-capita incomes spend more state and local money on Medicaid nursing home matches per person 85+. There is a significant correlation between the state and local Medicaid nursing home expenditures and the state per-capita income. Indeed, of the thirteen states that have state Medicaid match rates of 50%, all but two (California and Virginia) have above average Medicaid nursing home spending per person age 85+. One of the exceptions, Virginia, has a relatively low Medicaid cost-per-day nursing home rate ($51.96).

The Medicaid cost per day in nursing homes in 1992 ranged from highs of $223.61 in Alaska and $177.83 in the District of Columbia to lows of $36.44 in Oklahoma and $40.24 in Iowa, with the national average being $71.03 per day. The Medicaid cost per day in nursing homes is positively and strongly correlated with the state and local nursing home expenditures; that is, when states spend more on nursing homes, part of that expenditure is accounted for by more generous reimbursement rates under Medicaid. States with above-average per-capita taxes also have above-average state and local spending on Medicaid nursing homes per person age 85+, which is also correlated with higher reimbursement. Only three states are exceptions to this pattern: New Hampshire, Maine, and Ohio all have above-average nursing home costs per person age 85+ and below-average per-capita taxes. Seemingly, state and local nursing home expenditures are highly dependent on the percentage of nursing home residents who are Medicaid clients, the average Medicaid cost per day in nursing homes, the state per-capita income, and the state and local taxes per capita.

Table 4.6 shows that in 1992 the amount of state and local general revenue that each state spent on Medicaid nursing home care varied substantially. Although these are small percentages, the dollar amounts are large. Collectively, state and local governments spent $10.3 billion dollars on Medicaid nursing home care in 1992 and raised about $514.5 billion dollars in state and local taxes. All seven states with state and local Medicaid nursing home costs above 3% of the total state and local taxes collected also had very high nursing home costs per person age 85+. All of these states, except Maine, also had state Medicaid match rates above 45%, indicating fairly high per-capita incomes. Maine's Medicaid match rate was 38%, but it had a high average Medicaid nursing home cost per day ($82.00 in 1992) Thirty-nine states had state and local Medicaid nursing home expenditures that fell between 1% and 3% of state and local tax revenues. Of the five states with state and local Medicaid nursing home costs below 1% of the total state and local taxes collected, only Alaska has a state Medicaid match rate above 40%.

Table 4.6. State and Local Nursing Home Expenditures as a Percentage of State and Local Taxes in 1992

>3%	2% to 3%	1.5% to 2%	1% to 1.5%	<1%
Rhode Island	Dist. of Col.	Arkansas	Iowa	Oregon
New Hampshire	Ohio	Tennessee	Colorado	New Mexico
Massachusetts	Pennsylvania	Missouri	N. Carolina	Alaska
Connecticut	North Dakota	Kansas	Virginia	Arizona
New York	Indiana	Maryland	Montana	Utah
Maine	Wisconsin	Florida	Michigan	
Minnesota	Illinois	Alabama	Oklahoma	
	New Jersey	Louisiana	California	
	Nebraska	Washington	Mississippi	
	Vermont	Hawaii	W. Virginia	
	South Dakota	Georgia	Texas	
	Delaware	Kentucky	Idaho	
			S. Carolina	
			Wyoming	
			Nevada	

Alaska has a Medicaid match rate of 50%, but it also has the highest state and local taxes per capita in the country at $4,069 in 1992. Beyond the state variation illustrated in Table 4.6 is another message: Despite the large dollar amounts that states expend on long-term care, these outlays still represent only minute fractions of state and local tax revenues. Education, for example, garners a much larger share of the state and local tax dollar.

Generally, the nineteen states with state and local Medicaid nursing home costs above 2% of the total state and local taxes collected had higher per-capita incomes. All of these nineteen states except North and South Dakota had state Medicaid match rates of over 36%. Both North and South Dakota had a fairly low state and local taxes per capita ($1,562 and $1,447, respectively, in 1992).

State Variation in HCBS Programs

States not only use different amounts of HCBS, they also use widely different services. Although all states have some sort of program for in-home services and many have adult day care programs, relatively few have services in nonmedical residential settings that serve as viable alternatives to nursing homes. These settings are licensed under widely different names from state to state: for example, residential care facilities, homes for the aged, adult family homes, personal care homes, domiciliary homes, adult foster homes, and assisted living facilities. In some states these facilities are used mainly for people with chronic mental illness and are nothing more than a housing option, providing few, if any, long-term care services. Increasingly, states are evolving service programs for elderly persons with functional disabilities in residential settings other than nursing homes. Our tabulation of expenditures on HCBS services counts any home-based or residentially based HCBS programs that the particular state funds (either from Medicaid, Medicaid waiver programs, or state-funded programs); therefore, we can present only a crude estimate of commitment to HCBS services. Closer inspection may reveal that some of the residentially based services counted under HCBS may be more institutional than home-like in nature even though they are not defined as nursing homes.

Although we assume that states vary widely on the percentages of their populations using HCBS, no good data exist to compare states on that dimension. No standard method of counting HCBS clients exists comparable to the measure of resident days in the nursing home sector. Left on their own, states have evolved several different methods. Some states attempt to develop unduplicated counts of HCBS clientele and others do not. States with unduplicated counts use varied time periods (e.g., weekly, monthly, semiannually).

States also vary widely in the extent to which state and local tax revenues are spent on HCBS. The amount of money spent on HCBS is more standardized and can be used for making cross-state comparisons. Table 4.7 shows the nonfederal dollar amounts spent by each state in HCBS programs per person age 85+. The

Table 4.7. State and Local HCBS Expenditures per Person Age 85+ in 1992

State	Amount per 85+	State	Amount 85+
New York	5,779	Florida	634
Alaska*	5,692	Kentucky	620
Delaware	1,940	Rhode Island	619
California	1,931	Louisiana	613
North Carolina	1,619	Utah	610
Oregon	1,588	Nevada	608
Massachusetts	1,449	Vermont	580
Washington	1,394	Oklahoma	538
Maryland	1,263	Georgia	517
Hawaii	1,117	Colorado	512
Wisconsin	1,107	South Carolina	509
Texas	1,050	Arizona	500
Connecticut	1,013	Montana	461
Minnesota	1,006	Nebraska	452
New Hampshire	978	Ohio	447
New Jersey	911	Michigan	444
Illinois	874	Missouri	408
Wyoming	842	Pennsylvania	397
Indiana	840	Iowa	388
Maine	819	North Dakota	367
Idaho	808	Tennessee	346
District of Columbia	805	Kansas	275
Virginia	743	South Dakota	259
New Mexico	656	Alabama	240
West Virginia	641	Mississippi	234
Arkansas	636	United States	1,251

* Includes Pioneer Homes: Alaska facilities that are not licensed as nursing homes. Numbers are rounded to the nearest dollar.

national average expenditure figure is skewed by the state of New York, which, with about 7.5% of the nation's elderly, spends about 35.8% of the total state and local HCBS dollars in the country. (Here we would wish for accurate utilization figures. Lacking these, we can only speculate that New York serves many fewer people in HCBS for its large investment than do other states with lower prices and less rich patterns of service allocation.) Of the sixteen states with HCBS spending above $900 per person age 85+, exactly half have nursing home beds per 1,000 persons age 85+ that are below the national average, and half are above the national average on that dimension. Indeed, there is virtually no correlation between the number of nursing home beds per 1,000 persons 85+ and the state and local home-and-community-based care expenditures.

Combining data on state and local nursing home expenditures and state and local HCBS expenditures, Table 4.8 presents a ratio of the types of expenditures in the first column. In the second column, federal money has been included to create a ratio of all public HCBS expenditures in the state to all public nursing home expenditures in the state. Once again, widespread variation is revealed. Looking at

Table 4.8. Ratio of Public Spending on Nursing Homes to Spending on HCBS in 1992*

State	State + local	Federal + state + local	State	State + local	Federal + state + local
Dist. of Columbia	**9.71**	**12.25**	Hawaii	3.90	7.22
Rhode Island	**8.65**	**12.19**	Virginia	3.57	5.39
Ohio	**8.39**	**13.17**	Indiana	3.56	6.56
Pennsylvania	**7.76**	**17.61**	Iowa	3.51	8.45
Alabama	**7.22**	7.31	South Carolina	3.37	6.76
Connecticut	**6.89**	9.81	Maryland	2.99	4.70
Kansas	**6.57**	**11.28**	Wisconsin	2.85	5.05
Tennessee	**6.30**	**18.29**	Kentucky	2.67	6.24
Georgia	**5.99**	7.66	Oklahoma	2.67	**4.56**
South Dakota	**5.85**	**14.90**	Florida	2.63	4.84
New Hampshire	5.59	9.71	Arizona	2.56	4.79
Maine	5.45	6.93	Arkansas	2.55	4.58
North Dakota	5.43	**17.26**	Wyoming	2.55	7.74
Mississippi	5.42	**21.53**	Alaska	2.50	4.99
Colorado	5.40	9.29	New Mexico	2.33	4.61
Michigan	5.36	7.70	Washington	**2.11**	**3.10**
Vermont	5.11	10.48	West Virginia	**2.05**	**3.44**
Nevada	4.80	8.09	Delaware	**1.85**	**2.99**
New Jersey	4.79	6.54	Texas	**1.85**	**3.79**
Nebraska	4.57	9.06	Idaho	**1.76**	**3.75**
Minnesota	4.43	8.08	Utah	**1.67**	5.42
Missouri	4.23	7.29	California	**1.50**	**2.33**
Illinois	4.14	7.16	North Carolina	**1.34**	**3.01**
Massachusetts	4.07	6.89	New York	**1.26**	**1.31**
Montana	4.06	6.53	Oregon	**0.84**	**0.98**
Louisiana	3.93	**11.72**	United States	2.52	3.69

*Note. Boldface and underlined numbers show the states most unbalanced toward nursing home expenditures. Bold and double-underlined figures show the states with the most balanced long-term care expenditures.

state and local dollars only, the District of Columbia spends nearly ten times more on nursing home care than it does on HCBS, whereas Oregon is the only state to spend more state and local money on HCBS than it does on nursing home care. The table shows the dominance of nursing homes, with only eight states spending less than twice as much on nursing home care as on HCBS. When federal expenditures are added, the imbalances become even more pronounced, suggesting that some states use their solely state-funded discretionary programs for HCBS while directing Medicaid funds to institutional care. More than twenty times as much public money is spent on nursing homes in Mississippi than on HCBS; in five states at least fifteen times as much is spent on nursing homes; and in eleven states, at least ten times as much is spent on nursing homes as on HCBS.

By and large, the rankings of states with the greatest imbalance and those with the greatest balance in their systems are similar whether state and local dollars only are counted or federal money is added (see Table 4.8). When federal dollars are included, however, the rank order does differ somewhat. A few states figure in the ten most or least balanced with one indicator and not the other. The differences are most distinctive at the upper end of the table. In state long-term care expenditures alone, Mississippi, North Dakota, and Louisiana do not figure in the ten states with the greatest bias toward spending public money on nursing homes. Yet, when all dollars are counted, these states respectively use more than 21 times, 17 times, and 11 times as many resources on nursing homes as on HCBS. In all states, the imbalance toward spending on nursing homes is more pronounced when the federal money is counted, but in states with more balanced state and local expenditures (e.g., Oregon, New York, California, North Carolina, Delaware, and Idaho), the states have seemed to use federal contributions more effectively to maintain a thrust toward HCBS.

Simple ratios can be misleading, however. For example, in terms of state and local expenditures, New York, California, and Delaware all have ratios of nursing home care to HCBS under 2.0, but all three of these states spend relatively *high* amounts on *both* nursing homes and HCBS per person age 85+. In contrast, Idaho and Utah also have ratios under 2.00, but both of these states spend relatively low amounts on *both* nursing homes and HCBS per person age 85+. Only Texas, North Carolina, and Oregon spend relatively low amounts on nursing home care per person age 85+ and relatively high amounts on HCBS per person age 85+.

Table 4.9 shows the proportion of state and local general revenue each state spends on HCBS as estimated for 1992. No state, except New York, spends more than 1% of its state and local tax collections on HCBS programs. In fact, only thirteen states spend more than one-half of 1% of their tax collections on HCBS. A wide gulf exists between New York, which spends 2.3% of its state and local taxes on home-and-community-based care, and Mississippi, which spends only 0.009%. Most states are spending between 0.1 and 0.4% of their state and local tax collection on HCBS.

The amount of state and local expenditures on HCBS is not significantly cor-

Table 4.9. State and Local General Revenue HCBS Expenditures as a
Percentage of Estimated 1992 State and Local Taxes

State	Percent	State	Percent
New York	2.341	California	0.259
Alaska	0.990	North Dakota	0.231
Oregon	0.961	Alabama	0.227
Massachusetts	0.883	Hawaii	0.227
North Carolina	0.863	New Hampshire	0.213
Wisconsin	0.734	Pennsylvania	0.212
Delaware	0.711	District of Columbia	0.211
Maine	0.584	Iowa	0.210
Idaho	0.574	Arizona	0.193
Arkansas	0.541	Louisiana	0.188
Connecticut	0.522	Georgia	0.182
Washington	0.509	Vermont	0.178
Indiana	0.505	Utah	0.176
Kentucky	0.469	Colorado	0.175
Florida	0.447	Michigan	0.175
Illinois	0.427	New Mexico	0.174
Minnesota	0.406	Tennessee	0.170
Oklahoma	0.372	Ohio	0.161
Rhode Island	0.361	Nebraska	0.159
West Virginia	0.357	South Dakota	0.151
New Jersey	0.330	Virginia	0.127
Wyoming	0.329	Kansas	0.111
Montana	0.278	South Carolina	0.110
Maryland	0.277	Nevada	0.090
Texas	0.271	Mississippi	0.009
Missouri	0.265	United States	0.568

related with the percentage of nursing home clients on Medicaid. However, the
other three variables that were highly correlated with state and local nursing home
expenditures are also correlated with state and local HCBS expenditures: These
were the Medicaid cost per day in nursing homes, the state Medicaid match rate,
and the state and local taxes per capita. One of the best predictors of how much a
state will spend on HCBS is the state and local expenditures on nursing homes.
On average, the more a state spent on nursing home care in 1992, the more it was
likely to spend on HCBS.

State Variation in Total Long-Term Care

If New York State is eliminated as an outlier from the national averages on state nursing home expenditures and state HCBS expenditures, the results are intriguing. Eliminating New York, the average state and local revenues spent in 1992 on Medicaid nursing home care per person 85+ was $2,809.77, and the national average for HCBS expenditures for persons 85+ was $870.96.

Using these figures, we divided states into the four categories in Table 4.10: based on expenditures on nursing homes and HCBS, each divided into above and below the average.

Nine states had above-average nursing home costs and below-average HCBS costs. Table 4.11 shows some interesting comparisons for these nine states. Note that:

- The District of Columbia had the highest percentage of Medicaid nursing home clients in the United States and the second highest nursing home rate. This combined with below-average spending on HCBS made the District of

Table 4.10. Classification of State Spending Patterns on Nursing Homes and on HCBS in 1992

		Nursing Home Expenditures			
		Below Average		Above Average	
HCBS Expenditures	Above Average	Connecticut New Hampshire New Jersey Minnesota Illinois Massachusetts Hawaii	Maryland Wisconsin Alaska Washington Delaware California New York	Texas North Carolina Oregon	
	Below Average	Rhode Island Ohio Pennsylvania Georgia District of Columbia	Maine Vermont Nevada Indiana	Alabama Kansas Tennessee South Dakota North Dakota Mississippi Colorado Michigan Nebraska Missouri Montana Louisiana Virginia	Iowa South Carolina Kentucky Oklahoma Florida Arizona Arkansas Wyoming New Mexico West Virginia Idaho Utah

Table 4.11. Comparisons of the Nine States with Above-Average State and Local Nursing Home Expenditures and Below-Average State and Local HCBS Expenditures

State	Ratio of nursing home expense to HCBS expense	HCBS percent of per-capita taxes spent on nursing homes	Medicaid per-day rates for nursing homes ($)	Percent of nursing home residents on Medicaid	Percent of per-capita taxes spent on HCBS
District of Columbia	9.71	2.79	177.83	89.4	0.211
Rhode Island	8.65	4.18	78.47	74.8	0.361
Ohio	8.39	2.74	72.43	69.7	0.161
Pennsylvania	7.76	2.50	79.23	63.5	0.212
Georgia	5.99	1.58	49.86	82.3	0.182
Maine	5.45	3.48	81.75	78.3	0.584
Vermont	5.11	2.07	76.65	67.3	0.178
Nevada	4.80	1.03	101.92	65.1	0.090
Indiana	3.56	2.43	68.94	66.6	0.505
National Average	2.52	2.00	72.42	68.7	0.568

Columbia the most nursing home–dominated long-term care system in the country.

- Rhode Island had the highest percentage of state and local taxes spent on nursing homes in the nation (4.2%). Rhode Island has so much invested in nursing homes that it faces difficulty investing more in HCBS. However, New Hampshire, which also spent over 4% of its state and local taxes on nursing homes (4.1%), invested 58% more than Rhode Island in HCBS programs per person age 85+.
- Ohio had the eighth lowest percentage of state and local taxes invested in HCBS in the nation and the ninth highest percentage of state and local taxes invested in nursing home care in the country. This resulted in Ohio spending 8.39 times as much on nursing home care per capita as on HCBS, the third highest such comparison in the nation.
- Pennsylvania was similar to Ohio, but spent slightly less of state and local taxes per capita on nursing homes and a little more of state and local taxes per capita on HCBS. Even so, nursing homes still dominated in Pennsylvania, receiving 7.76 times more spending per capita than HCBS (the fourth highest ratio in the nation).
- Georgia had the fifth highest percentage of nursing home residents on Medicaid (82.3%) in the country. This statistic, combined with a fairly low HCBS expenditures as a percentage of state and local taxes, produces six times more spending on nursing homes than on HCBS.
- Maine had the sixth highest percentage of state and local taxes spent on nursing homes in the country. Even though Maine spent only slightly less than the national average on HCBS per person age 85+, the high nursing home expenditures produced a differential of 5.45 times more spending per person 85+ on nursing homes than on HCBS.
- Vermont was similar to Georgia, but spent slightly less on both nursing homes and HCBS as a percentage of state and local taxes. Vermont also differed from Georgia in having higher nursing home rates but a lower percentage of nursing home residents who were on Medicaid.
- Nevada had the sixth highest nursing home rate and the second lowest percentage of state and local taxes spent on HCBS in the nation. Nevada had relatively few Medicaid nursing home residents as a percentage of the age 85+ population (22.0%). However, the high nursing home rates combined with the low spending on HCBS produced a differential of 4.8 times more spending per person 85+ on nursing homes than on HCBS.
- Indiana was only slightly above the national average on nursing home spending per capita age 85+ and slightly below the national average on home and community care spending per capita age 85+. Indiana, however, appeared to be moving in the wrong direction. Medicaid nursing home utilization increased 246.7% in the 1980s (the highest in the nation), and nursing home expenditures increased 86.0% in the 1980s (the eleventh highest in the nation).

Table 4.12. Comparisons of the Three States with Below-Average State and Local Nursing Home Expenditures and Above-Average State and Local HCBS Expenditures

State	Ratio of nursing home expense to HCBS	Percent of per-capita taxes spent on nursing homes	Medicaid nursing home resident rates ($)	Percent of per-capita taxes spent on HCBS
Texas	1.85	1.19	44.69	0.271
North Carolina	1.35	1.44	63.74	0.863
Oregon	.84	0.97	59.23	.961
National Average	2.51	2	72.42	0.568

Table 4.12 shows similar comparisons for the three states that have below-average nursing home expenditures and above-average HCBS expenditures per person age 85+. Note the following:

- Texas did not spend a great deal of state and local taxes on *either* nursing home care or HCBS. Texas had the eighth lowest percentage of state and local taxes spent on long-term care services, but a large part of what it spent went to HCBS: the amount spent per person 85+ was above the national average. Texas has been working, with much success, for at least 20 years to expand its HCBS program. Also, Texas nursing home rates are substantially below the national average, and if these rates were above the national average, Texas would probably fall into the category of spending above the national average on both nursing homes and HCBS per person age 85+.

- Like all southern states, except Georgia, North Carolina spent less than the national average on nursing home care per person age 85+, but it had the fifth highest spending per person age 85+ on HCBS. However, a high percentage of state and local HCBS expenditures in North Carolina (63.4%) goes to domiciliary homes which, for the most part, appear to lack the privacy and home-like lifestyle that we would associate with user-friendly services. Without its high expenditure on domiciliary homes, North Carolina would be ranked with the states that spend below average on both nursing homes and HCBS per person age 85+.

- Oregon had the fifth lowest state and local expenditures on nursing homes per person age 85+ and the sixth highest expenditure on HCBS care per person age 85+. Like Texas, but more pronounced, Oregon has been working for the last 20 years to expand HCBS. It is the only state to spend more state and local tax dollars on HCBS than on nursing home care. Oregon enacted state policies on aging and disabilities in the 1980s, both of which stated that persons needing long-term care services should be placed in the least restrictive setting whenever possible.

Among the fourteen states with above-average nursing home costs and above-average HCBS costs, all except Minnesota, Wisconsin, and Washington, had higher than average per-capita incomes, and Medicaid match rates of 50%. Indeed, all of the thirteen states with Medicaid match rates at 50%, except the District of Columbia and Virginia, are included in these fourteen states. All of these fourteen states, except New Hampshire, also collected above-average amounts of state and local taxes per capita and have decided to spend relatively high amounts of state and local taxes on both home-and-community-based care and nursing home care. These fourteen states tend to disprove the generalization that the more a given state spends on nursing home care, the less it will have available for home-and-community-based care.

The twenty-five remaining states had below-average nursing home expenditures and below-average HCBS expenditures. All of these states, except Wyoming and Michigan, collected below-average amounts of state and local taxes per capita. All of them, except Virginia, had state Medicaid match rates of less than 50% and relatively low per-capita incomes.

With a few exceptions, states with high per-capita incomes and high state and local tax collections spent more on nursing homes. Many of these states, however, did not spend a great deal on HCBS. Also, with very few exceptions, states with low per-capita incomes and low state and local tax collections spent less on both nursing homes and HCBS. From this, one might generalize that those states that have the money spend it on long-term care, and that those that don't, don't.

As noted earlier, the Medicaid match formula does not redress the imbalance. Indeed, it favors the rich states. Thus, the same generalization appears to apply to total (both state and local taxes, and federal funds) nursing home expenditures and total home-and-community-based care expenditures. Some poorer states with favorable federal match rates (notably Alabama and, to a lesser extent, Oklahoma and Arkansas) improve their relative position compared to other states on the balance between HCBS and nursing home expenditures when federal contributions are added. But the federal contributions could also tip the balance in the opposite direction toward a greater relative spending on nursing homes (notably in Mississippi, and to a lesser extent, in Louisiana and Utah). In other states with favorable federal match rates, such as West Virginia, New Mexico, South Carolina, and Kentucky, federal funding did not change their relative ranking. It is true that public expenditures on nursing homes are completely cost-shared with the federal government, whereas HCBS programs are not. However, our analyses suggest that, consciously or not, states chose whether to use their federally matched funds in the service of more HCBS or more nursing home care. The match rates do not predict how much the state will spend in either sector in relationship to the other.

Varying Demand for State-Supported Services

So far we have looked at relative public expenditures on HCBS and nursing homes at the state level. But, what about the need for such expenditures? That, too, can vary markedly by state. Long-term care services directly provided by or purchased by state governments are designed to serve people needing long-term care services who cannot afford to purchase them on their own. Although many states make some long-term care services available without regard to a person's income, most state long-term care programs are designed for persons with low income. Once again using primarily 1992 data, we compared the demand for state-supported long-term care services by state. Table 4.13 lists the demographic factors believed to be related to demand for LTC.

As proportions of people over age 85 increase, and as proportions of older people over 65 living alone (who, therefore, have less access to family care) increase, the demand for formal long-term care services also rises. Given that minorities are less likely to use formal services than others of similar age and income, the demand for formal services varies inversely with the proportion of minorities in the population. Trends in these indicators, especially the increase in population over age 85, suggest to states what they can anticipate in terms of demand for formal long-term care.

The demand for publicly funded long-term care will be particularly sensitive to disability rates and poverty rates. Disability rates of both older people and adults under 65 are pertinent here; we constructed an indicator based on the rates of adults with severe disabilities per 1,000 in the population. The proportion of Medicaid recipients over age 65 in the state, while obviously correlated with the state's poverty rates, indicates even more directly the demand on publicly subsidized long-term care programs. We used both indicators of poverty to compare this demand across states.

Table 4.13. Predictors of High Demand and High Public Demand for LTC

Factors predicting high general demand for long-term care services	Factors predicting high demand for publicly funded long-term care services
Greater population age 85+	Greater population age 85+
Greater growth rate in population age 85+	Greater growth in population age 85+
More people living alone age 65+	More people living alone age 65+
Fewer minorities of color age 65+	Fewer minorities of color age 65+
	Higher poverty rates age 65+
	Higher disability rates in adults of all ages
	Higher percent Medicaid recipients age 65+

Table 4.14. Relative Demand on State Supported Long-Term Care Services

Highest	Very high	High	Average	Low	Very low	Lowest
Mississippi	Louisiana	North Carolina	New York	Iowa	Maryland	Utah
	Arkansas	Oklahoma	Maine	Nebraska	Nevada	
	Alabama	District of Columbia	Vermont	Minnesota	Delaware	
	Tennessee	Texas	Virginia	Massachusetts	New Jersey	
	South Carolina	Rhode Island	Montana	Pennsylvania	Washington	
	Kentucky	North Dakota	Florida	Idaho	Connecticut	
	West Virginia	South Dakota	Ohio	California	Hawaii	
	Georgia	New Mexico		Michigan	Colorado	
		Missouri		Illinois		
				Indiana		
				Kanasa		
				Alaska		
				Arizona		
				Wisconsin		
				Wyoming		
				New Hampshire		
				Oregon		

Table 4.14 compares the relative demand for state-supported long-term care in the fifty states and the District of Columbia based on the three demographic factors—rates of severely disabled persons, poverty rates, and Medicaid rates (posited to affect public demand). For comparison purposes, we divided the states into quintiles from very high demand to very low demand based on the distribution of the composite scores. All southern states have a high or very high potential demand on state coffers for long-term care services, whereas the West Coast states have low or very low demands. No other regional patterns seem to exist; however, a strong inverse relationship between the demand for long-term care services and a state's relative wealth does seem to exist. A strong positive correlation exists between the proportion of people age 65+ who are severely disabled and the proportion of people over age 65 who live below the poverty line. In addition, the first thirteen states listed in Table 4.14 (that is, Mississippi through Texas) all have very high or high poverty levels for the age 65+ population.

It would appear that poverty is associated with an increase in severe disabilities among the elderly and that this increases the demand for long-term care services. In general, the relative wealth of a state influences the demand for state-supported long-term care services, with higher demand being evident in poorer states. Unfortunately, the states with the highest potential demand for long-term care services tend to be the states that can least afford them. In 1990, per-capita income in the

United States averaged $17,539, ranging from $24,318 in Connecticut to $12,038 in Mississippi. State and local per-capita tax revenues in 1990 averaged $2,017 nationally, ranging from $4,069 in Alaska and $3,806 in the District of Columbia to $1,262 in Mississippi. Nearly all of the states with high or very high demand for long-term care services had per-capita incomes below the national average (the exceptions being Rhode Island and the District of Columbia). Significant negative correlations exist between the proportion of people age 65+ who live below the poverty line, and both state and local per-capita taxes and state per-capita income. No other regional patterns seem to exist; however, the demand for long-term care services and a state's relative wealth are highly related. A strong positive correlation exists between the proportion of people age 65+ who were severely disabled and the proportion of people over age 65 who lived below the poverty line. The first thirteen states listed in Table 4.14 with the greatest demand for long-term care (that is, Mississippi through Texas) had very high or high poverty levels for the age 65+ population.

Almost all of the nine states with very high or high demand on state-supported long-term care services had below-average per-capita incomes, the exceptions being Rhode Island and the District of Columbia. It follows that all of the states with very high demand on state-supported long-term care services also had low state Medicaid match rates; indeed, all are under 30%, except Tennessee (at 34.36%), Alabama at (30.15%), and Georgia (at 38.10%). Thus, these poorer states are advantaged by needing less from state and local tax dollars to match federal Medicaid dollars, but as stated earlier, they sometimes have difficulty convincing legislators to appropriate the state dollars. In part, this hesitation may be due to the lack of familiarity with HCBS services in comparison to the much better understood nursing home program. It may also be due to the differing tax policies of states and their varying abilities to raise revenues.

To a great degree the differences among states reflect each state's wealth. Indeed, a significant correlation exists between state and local taxes per capita and the per-capita income. Poor states tax their citizens less, but not necessarily less relative to their personal incomes. For example, in 1990 New Jersey's per-capita tax of $2,519 represented 10.8% of personal income, while Mississippi's per-capita tax of $1,264 represented 10.5% of personal income. Although most states tend to tax their citizens between 10% and 12% of personal income, in 1990 the tax rates ranged from a high of 19.9% in Alaska to a low of 8.3% in New Hampshire.

The amount of state and local tax dollars spent on HCBS programs per person 85+ is highly correlated with the state and local taxes per capita. States with more tax dollars per capita tend to spend more on home-and-community-based care, and states with less tax dollars tend to spend less. An even stronger correlation exists between state and local spending on nursing homes per person 85+ and state and local taxes per capita.

These relationships will have significant consequences if the country moves toward requiring states to absorb more of the costs of Medicaid long-term care services. High per-capita tax states, with their higher demands on the long-term care system, will be able to respond much better than low per-capita tax states. Indeed, one could reasonably expect these low per-capita tax states to provide even less long-term care services in the future.

Generally, the higher the demand on state-supported long-term care services, the harder it is to change the long-term care system. This is especially true if that change entails adding HCBS. Most states have added HCBS programs to their long-term care repertoire for two reasons: the potential users of long-term care prefer these services, and unit-for-unit, HCBS services cost states less than nursing home services. The investment in HCBS is much more likely to happen in states where the demand for state-supported services is low or very low. An encouraging exception is Arkansas, a very high-demand state that has been able to control nursing home growth fairly well by adding HCBS. (Arkansas saw a Medicaid nursing home utilization growth rate of 5.9% in the 1980s, compared to the national average of 33.3%).

Program Variations

So far, we have emphasized that almost all states invest in long-term care programs that are heavily weighted to nursing home care, despite the preference of the consumers, but that the extent of this imbalance differs substantially from state to state. We have also shown that some states have a greater challenge than others in shifting the balance or making any changes because of the sheer force of expected demand for publicly subsidized services. In the remainder of the chapter, we examine some of the more qualitative variations in state long-term care programs.

Medicaid Programs

Medicaid has been the driving force in determining how states have developed their long-term care systems. In 1992, the year for which we assembled the statistics in this chapter, Medicaid provided 94% of all state and local government expenditures for long-term care in the United States. The Medicaid program's basic provisions give some common shape to state long-term care programs. At the same time, the substantial flexibility of the Medicaid program , especially as it has evolved, has made possible some distinctive program departures in the various states.

When Medicaid was enacted in 1965, it was conceived as a medical program for poor people who were unable to gain coverage for health care through private health insurance. The only long-term care programs available under Medicaid were skilled nursing-home care and home health care, both of which were considered more acute care programs than long-term care programs. As described in Chapter 2, the first three decades of Medicare and Medicaid altered that vision until Medicaid has now become an enormous long-term care program.

Medicaid is an open-ended funding source for states. Although there have been many proposals to cap the federal funding contribution, at this writing there is no limit on the amount of Medicaid dollars a state can receive. Because of this, and the way the federal match is calculated, Medicaid has been a boon to the states, and they have used it as the main funding source for long-term care programs. Under Medicaid, a state can purchase a dollar's worth of long-term care service for an average of 39 cents. In contrast, states must pay the full dollar if they purchase these services with state general revenue funds. In actual practice, some wealthier states have spent more money on long-term care in their Medicaid programs because it is easier for them to appropriate the state match to stimulate more generous programs. Although Medicaid could serve as a basis for economic development for those relatively poor states that receive much higher federal shares, such states sometimes have difficulty raising the revenue for the state match in the first place and, therefore, tend to have less generous Medicaid programs.

Changes in Medicaid long-term care services over the years have resulted in changes in how states operate their long-term care programs. The following major changes in the Medicaid program have occurred since 1965:

- In 1967 amendments, Intermediate Care Facilities (ICFs) were added to the list of services eligible for Medicaid funding. Prior to that, only Skilled Nursing Facilities were covered.
- In 1972, income eligibility levels went up to 300% of the Supplemental Security Income (SSI) standard for residents receiving institutional long-term care (nursing home care). Although meant to address the problem that many low-income people could not afford nursing homes, this provision meant that it was easier to qualify by income for nursing homes than the HCBS alternatives. (By 1997, this difference amounted to the difference between an income of $494 for a single person to qualify for Medicaid in general and $1,482 to qualify for nursing homes.)
- In 1975, institutional services for mentally retarded and developmentally disabled people were included in the Medicaid program. Over the years, partly because of strong advocacy on behalf of people with developmental disabilities, these groups have received larger and larger shares of the HCBS dollar and the services for those populations have broadened to include a range of training and "habilitation" programs that go beyond the usual definition of long-term care.
- In 1975, states were given the option to include a personal care program under their statewide Medicaid programs. This option, which not all states took up, allowed for less professionalized, less expensive, more flexible attendant-style services to be used in lieu of home health services for people needing long-term care services in their own homes. When a state incorporates personal care into its regular Medicaid program, the benefits are technically accessible statewide to all Medicaid target groups. However, in some states the Medicaid

personal care programs have become de facto benefits for younger people. By 1996, thirty-two states had personal care programs under Medicaid.

- In late 1981, the major waiver for HCBS care (described in Chapter 2) for individuals with functional impairment who would otherwise have been in nursing homes became available for people with incomes that go up to 300% of SSI eligibility level. States using the 300% of poverty for eligibility could reduce some of the perverse incentives to use nursing homes. Many of the innovations discussed in the next part of the book were stimulated by Medicaid waiver programs.
- In 1981, a waiver of freedom of choice was initiated, permitting states to limit who could provide Medicaid services. This encouraged some states to develop Medicaid managed care programs for acute care and, much later, for long-term care.
- In 1987, a major nursing home reform program was ushered in. One provision combined skilled nursing facilities and intermediate care facilities into one nursing facility program, and made this program a mandatory Medicaid service for persons over age 21 years. Other provisions mandated assessment and alternative planning for all Medicaid clientele in nursing homes who primarily had mental health disabilities.

The Balanced Budget Act of 1997 made it easier for states to set up managed care plans that include long-term care. As mentioned in Chapter 2, this law also deleted the Boren amendment, which governed reimbursement for costs in nursing homes and hospitals. At the same time, however, it substantially reduced federal funding to the states, primarily by reducing the federal portion of the Disproportionate Share program. (This is the Medicaid provision that allows hospitals that serve a disproportionally high percentage of Medicaid patients to receive higher reimbursement than other hospitals.) Although the cumulative effects of these changes are uncertain, it seems likely that the future will bring more Medicaid managed care plans, a tightening of dollars available for long-term care, and lower nursing facility payments for Medicaid residents. The combined effect could actually eliminate some of the incentives favoring nursing home use over HCBS.

Although Medicaid constrains state variability, it also allows many optional methods of providing services. States have developed their long-term care systems differently by taking advantage of some options and not instituting others. Most of the variability in Medicaid long-term care programs is in the HCBS programs. Medicaid allows more flexibility in these programs than in nursing home programs, and states have responded with many different types of services in both their regular Medicaid program and their Medicaid waiver programs.

Other Funding Sources

In addition to developing HCBS programs under Medicaid and Medicaid waivers, states have developed HCBS programs with other federal sources (for example,

Older Americans Act, Social Service Block Grants, Community Service Block Grants) and they have used their own revenues (general tax dollars, earmarked taxes, and, in the case of Pennsylvania, lottery revenues) to develop such programs.

States have used all of these funding sources, sometimes in conjunction with each other, and sometimes by themselves, to develop their distinctive long-term care programs, resulting in a hodgepodge in the HCBS arena. HCBS programs are better organized and coordinated in some states than in others. The viability of these programs as genuine alternatives to nursing homes varies greatly. In addition to interstate variation, intrastate variation also occurs, especially when locally raised funds are used to strengthen long-term care programs.

Indeed, inconsistency seems to be the rule, instead of the exception. States call similar programs by different names. For example, domiciliary care, personal care homes, residential care facilities, and rest homes are all terms that states use generally to connote light care and nonmedical services in congregate living facilities.[5] At the same time, states also use the same names in different ways. For example, assisted living facilities in some states are really the same thing as residential care facilities offering light care. In other states, assisted living facilities have been designed to replace nursing homes. In some states, the term *assisted living* is reserved for residential programs that assure a modicum of privacy (either distinctive apartments or at least singly occupied rooms), whereas in others no such provision exists.[6] The term *adult foster care*, sometimes called "family home" or "small group home," although typically designated as a private home, is defined variably with regard to the kind of services allowed, the staff requirements, the admission and retention requirements, and size—sometimes three or fewer clients, often five or fewer clients, sometimes six or fewer. To illustrate an atypical extreme, Michigan recognizes four size-based categories of adult foster home, with the largest housing twenty-one or more people.[7]

States also have taken programs with similar names and functions and operated them differently. For example, all states have one or more case-management program. Although these programs may be named slightly differently (care coordination and care management are the current favorites), they perform similar functions and are widely recognized as the vehicle to assist long-term care clients in obtaining and maintaining services. In some states, these case-management programs are operated by state staff with local offices (e.g., South Carolina and Missouri). In others, case management is done by local public agencies, such as county welfare or health departments (e.g., Minnesota and Wisconsin). In yet other states, case management is done largely by Area Agencies on Aging (for example, Oregon, Massachusetts, Pennsylvania, and Arkansas). Finally, some states vest the case-management function with nonprofit agencies under contract (for example, Florida, New York, and California). When this last mechanism is used, many different kinds of agencies, such as hospitals, home care organizations, Area Agencies on Aging, or family service associations may serve as the lead in a geographic area. Furthermore, the state will have its own particular stipulations about the relationship of its case-management contractors to its service providers. In New York, the HCBS waiver program, called Nursing Home Without Walls, certifies a large number of case-management providers, which, in turn, usually provide most of the services, though they do contract out for some services as well. In contrast, in California, the HCBS program called the Multipurpose Senior Services Program requires its case-management contractors to have an arms-length relationship with service providers. Finally, it is more usual than not for a state to have major variations of its standard state model in one or more of its local regions, usually arising because of historic circumstances or the unique demands of rural areas.

The variation among and within state long-term care programs in the United States results in complex systems. In fact, it is partly because of this complexity that states have developed case-management programs. Potential clients and their families experience great difficulty in understanding the different long-term care programs in the United States, in knowing which might meet their needs, and in gaining access to the services.

Varying Organizational Structures

State governments have tended to be generally consistent in organizing some functions and inconsistent in organizing others. For example, states have highway or transportation departments that are organized in similar fashions, and most states have correction departments and departments of public safety that contain many similarities. This is not true of health and social service agencies.

Health and social services cover a broad array of services and usually make up about a third of state government expenditures. States have three basic methods of organizing these programs:

- Some states have organized health and social service programs along functional lines. For example, states have a mental health agency that usually serves people with mental health problems, despite their age, disability, or other demographic characteristics. These mental health agencies, which are often part of larger agencies, also use a variety of funding sources. However, no state has a similar single state agency for all long-term care programs.
- States can organize health and social service programs around different populations. For example, states usually have an agency for the elderly and one for children, though in many states these agencies are a part of a larger agency. No state has combined all long-term care functions and funding sources for all populations into a single agency.
- States can organize health and social service programs around funding sources. Vocational Rehabilitation is probably the best example of a state agency organized around a funding source. Indeed, it is the only health and human service program that is required to do so by federal law. Even in this example,

though, there is variability between states with some vocational rehabilitation programs split into two agencies: one for the blind, and one for all other disabilities. Many vocational rehabilitation agencies are also part of other larger agencies, and in some states they are in departments of education rather than in health and social services.

No state has been successful in organizing all, or even most, of the health and social service programs using only one of the three methods. Indeed, all states use a conglomerate of all three methods, thereby creating much confusion and many separate agencies. In addition, states seem to disagree about the nature of some functions. For instance, most states treat Medicaid not as a funding source but rather as a functional program and have placed all Medicaid-funded services into one agency. Other states, like Texas, Arkansas, Washington, and Oregon, have viewed Medicaid as a funding source and split Medicaid funding between the health care agency, the elderly agency, and the agency for mental disabilities.

In response to this situation, most states have created "umbrella" agencies that are usually charged with coordinating and supervising many different smaller health and social service agencies. In many states these "umbrella" agencies have direct line control over many smaller agencies, but no state has combined all health and social service agencies into one such larger agency. The many different functions, populations, and funding sources for health and social service programs have made these programs very difficult to organize and very difficult to manage. Added to this difficulty is the fact that three of the very large health and social service funding sources (namely, Medicaid; Aid to Families with Dependent Children, now Temporary Assistance to Needy Families; and the food stamp program) have been entitlement programs, meaning that states have had to serve all persons who applied for and qualified for these programs. This has made budgeting for and managing these programs extremely difficult.

Because of the nature of health and social service programs, it may be next to impossible to integrate these programs into one large agency. Many states have achieved a degree of integration in some health and social programs like mental health and vocational rehabilitation, but no state has done this for all of its health and social service programs. States have fragmented health and social service programs, which are very hard to manage, and create much confusion. This observation is especially true for long-term care programs.

No two states employ identical organizational structures to administer long-term care programs. States tend to view long-term care not as a program by itself but rather as a subpart of several other different programs. Only four states, specifically Washington, New Jersey, Kansas, and Oregon, have attempted to integrate long-term care programs. Both Washington and Oregon have integrated all long-term care services for the elderly and disabled into a single state agency, but neither of these states has integrated long-term care services for the developmentally disabled into these agencies. Indeed, no state has developed a structure that places all long-term care programs for all populations into one state agency. For example, no state has combined long-term care programs for the elderly with long-term care programs for the developmentally disabled. Many states have separated nursing home services and HCBS among different state agencies. In most states, nursing home services are the responsibility of the state agency that administers Medicaid, and HCBS programs are split among several different agencies, including the Medicaid agency, the aging services agency, the developmental disabilities agency, the health department, and the social service agency. This is further complicated in several states because of the different structures for the Medicaid agency itself. For example, in several states the Medicaid programs are part of the health department, in other states they are part of the social service agency, and in others, Medicaid comprises a stand-alone agency.

Further adding to this confusion, the administration of long-term care programs at the local level varies considerably. In some states, staff at local branch offices of state government are responsible, while in others the job falls to city or county government. Additionally, in some states local administration is contracted to local (usually not-for-profit) agencies. Mostly, but not always, these are Area Agencies on Aging. In addition, most states usually contract only part of the long-term care program to local government or agencies, and in most states there are two or more local agencies administrating different parts of the long-term care program.

Thus, the administration of long-term care programs is usually confusing, hard to coordinate between agencies, and difficult for potential users to negotiate. Indeed, almost every state has set up information and referral services and case management programs to help potential clients, but access to the long-term care system remains confusing and elusive. State and local level agencies administering parts of long-term care have added to much of the confusion surrounding these programs. Some of these agencies attempt to be all things to all people, and they often duplicate long-term care services provided by other agencies. Some of these agencies have concentrated on some particular long-term care program, and tend to think that all knowledge of this program lies with them. Turf battles between state agencies (and between state and local agencies) make administration even more difficult and result in some clients falling through the cracks in the long-term care service network. For example, not uncommonly people who are *both* elderly and mentally disabled find it difficult to gain access to long-term care services anywhere.

Integrating long-term care programs is difficult, and proposals to do so always have more detractors than supporters. Some of the obstacles resemble those standing in the way of balancing systems away from nursing home care, which were described in the previous chapter. For example, state and local employees of the agencies administering the current long-term care programs may fear that their jobs will be changed or eliminated or that their functions will be absorbed by a different agency with different philosophies and different working conditions. State and local employees frequently subscribe in theory to the goal of consolidating and integrating programs, but progress breaks down on specific technical points such as how to integrate bureaucracies with different pay scales and working conditions, or where and how to physically locate programs. Some states, have mounted task forces perennially, and have repeatedly received recommendations that they integrate their long-term care service structures, but it is far easier to create another task force to restudy the problem than to make structural change.

Advocacy groups may also object to changing the structure because they want a distinct agency for their constituents. Advocates for the elderly, for example, often want a department, and preferably one that is cabinet level. (This motivation led to the creation of Florida's Department of Elder Affairs in 1991; however, only some of the functions related to long-term care for the elderly were actually moved to the new department, so fragmentation continued.) Advocates for the elderly usually prefer that their programs, even when funded by Medicaid, not be operated at the local level by welfare departments, which are perceived as more stigmatizing than the Area Agencies on Aging or the county health departments. In many states, these advocates resist combining aging programs under the Older Americans Act with Medicaid programs. To reiterate from Chapter 3, advocates for persons with Alzheimer's disease, though their numbers and interests overlap enormously with elderly long-term care consumers, often pursue special state legislation for their constituency. Thus, special HCBS programs may exist for Alzheimer's respite care or family support, when clients with other diseases (for example, stroke or Parkinson's disease) could benefit equally from the services. Similarly, advocates for younger people with disabilities are zealous in guarding special programs (for example, for the blind or for people with cerebral palsy), while striving for a share in any state general programs.

From the perspective of many elected officials and upper-level state bureaucrats responsible for Medicaid, the Older Americans Act programs, Social Service Block Grant programs, Community Service Block Grant programs, and state funded home care programs are seen as social programs of doubtful consequence and are given less credibility than the Medicaid program. Most states also give low credibility to HCBS waiver programs. Because of the perceived dubious impact of these programs, they have remained minor long-term care programs compared to the nursing home program. State-level bureaucrats and elected officials have an inherent distrust of both the federal government and local governments. They usually see the federal government as being too prescriptive and local governments as being unsophisticated. As a result,the administration of the nursing home program remains under the direct control of state agencies in most states, even those with a strong county government presence in HCBS.

Concluding Comment

As this chapter has illustrated, state long-term care programs are complex and diverse. No two states have identical programs, and variation is the rule. Most state long-term care programs are fragmented into different programs administered by different agencies. From a consumer's perspective, gaining access to long-term care services can be very difficult, although all states have established information and referral units to assist potential clients. From a planning perspective, envisaging the entire system is exceedingly difficult. Getting beyond the welter of programs to consider how well their totality advances the purposes of long-term care is a daunting task.

More positively, progress has been made to break the stranglehold of nursing homes on the state long-term care dollar. Even in the states where nursing homes claim the lion's share of the available state money, model programs have been established that have substantial promise. In Part II of this book, we examine the building blocks for long-term care programs that have the best potential for meeting the common sense goals of long term care; namely, to provide people with functional limitations, mostly older people, with the kind of help that allows them to transcend their disabilities as much as possible and lead meaningful and satisfying lives.

Notes

1. The data presented in this chapter are based on work that the authors did under a grant from the Administration on Aging. An earlier version was published in Ladd RC, Kane RL, Kane RA, & Nielsen WJ (1995). *State LTC Profiles Report*. Minneapolis, MN: National LTC Mentoring Program, Institute for Health Services Research, University of Minnesota School of Public Health. When not otherwise cited, statistical indicators are derived from that report, where the method is also outlined in detail. In general, the figures used to create our indicators were derived from census data and from various reports that states make to the Health Care Financing Administration on expenditures under Medicaid and Medicaid waivers. For information on state expenditures long-term care expenditures outside the Medicaid program, our only source was a special intramural study of the Administration on Aging, which gathered 1992 data from the relevant state agencies; these results are published in *1992 Medicaid Home-and-community-based Care Expenditures: Infrastructure of Home-and-community-based Services for the Functionally Impaired Elderly: State Source Book*. Washington, DC: Administration on Aging, 1995.
2. All data that describe and compare state per-capita income and state taxation in this chapter are derived from Harlender S (1993). Assessing your state tax burden. *Consumers' Research Magazine* 76 (Feb): 32.
3. Harrington C (1995). *ProPac Acuity Index Average Facility Scores by State: Nursing Facilities, Staffing, Residents, and Facility Deficiencies, 1991–1993*. San Francisco: University of California at San Francisco, Center on Health and Aging. This index compares acuity differences in nursing facilities based on determining the proportion of residents with the following characteristics: being bedfast, needing assistance with ambulation; needing full eating assistance; needing some eating assistance; having an indwelling catheter; being incontinent; having a pressure ulcer; receiving bowel or bladder training; and receiving special skin care. Each of these characteristics is weighted by the average amount of nursing care it requires.
4. See Kane RL, Kane RA, Ladd RC, & Veazie WJ (1998). Variation in state spending for

long-term care: factors associated with more balanced systems. *Journal of Health Politics, Policy and Law*. 23(2):363–390.

5. Hawes C, Wildfire JB, & Lux LJ (1993). *The Regulation of Board and Care Homes: Results of a Survey in the 50 States and the District of Columbia*. Washington, DC: Research Triangle Institute, American Association of Retired Persons.

6. Mollica RL & Snow KI (1996). *State Assisted Living Policy: 1996*. Portland, ME: National Academy for State Health Policy, US Department of Health and Human Services.

7. Folkemer D, Jensen A, Lipson L, Stauffer M, & Fox-Grage W (1996). *Adult Foster Care for the Elderly: A Review of State Regulatory and Funding Strategies*, Volumes 1 and 2. Washington, DC. American Association for Retired Persons.

II
PRACTICE OF
LONG-TERM CARE

5.

Home Care and Personal Assistant Services

Home care and personal assistant services (PAS) are the most important building blocks in a user-friendly system of community-based long-term care. Flexible, reasonably priced services for people living at home are the key to people staying at home. If states are to achieve balance in their long-term care programs, they need to forge a range of home care and PAS services. Designing such services is challenging because of the wide range of needs to be met, the diversity of home environments and life circumstances of the consumers, the necessity of building upon the help of family members when possible, and the need to keep costs down by using generalist personnel while maintaining acceptable quality.

The very use of the term "home care" is controversial. A vociferous and growing constituency of long-term care consumers prefer terminology such as personal assistant services or, as embodied in the proposed 1997 Medicaid Community Attendant Services Act (CASA),[1] personal attendants. PAS or personal attendant care is not identical to home care because PAS provides services outside as well as within the consumer's home and is intended to allow the consumers to function in a variety of contexts consistent with "normal living." Also, home care, in some versions, incorporates more medical, rehabilitation, and health-related services than does most PAS. Finally, PAS is often (though not always) associated with a mode of service where the consumer directly hires and supervises the caregivers. The overlap in what the two models can achieve, however, is considerable.

The purview of this chapter includes a range of nonfacility HCBS services that could supplement home care and PAS, such as adult day care, home-delivered meals, emergency call systems, home-delivered equipment, home modifications, telephone reassurance systems, and transportation programs. It also includes case-management services, which may be used to organize and monitor an entire HCBS plan. We reserve for the next chapter a discussion of residential settings ranging from nursing homes to various forms of congregate housing with services. In contrast, this chapter is devoted to the entire potpourri of services that taken together support long-term care consumers in their own homes. Thus, when we use the general term *in-home care* or *home care*, we mean to include the full range of in-home, PAS, and community-based supportive services for people living in their own homes.

Goals of Home Care and PAS

We discussed the goals of long-term care in general in Chapter 1, pointing to a wide range of possible objectives, including maintaining or improving functioning, improving health status, minimizing pain and discomfort, meeting unmet needs, promoting psychological well-being, promoting social well-being, maintaining consumers in the "least restrictive setting," enhancing choice and autonomy, and promoting meaningful lives. These various and sometimes conflicting goals are pertinent to home care and PAS, to which is often added another almost tautological goal—allowing the consumer to remain at home and connected to his or her community. As Chapter 2 stressed, proving that provision of services to people in their own homes actually keeps them there is extraordinarily difficult.

Of all the goals of home care and PAS, perhaps the most important from a consumer perspective is allowing consumers to live meaningful lives and to preserve their own dignity and sense of self despite whatever disabilities they have. To the extent possible the services promote opportunities for 'normal'' experiences for people with disabilities serious enough to require care. By definition, the lives of people with severe disabling illnesses, or with Alzheimer's disease or any number of other conditions that require help from others, are not "normal"—that is, they do not fall within the normal distribution for the population. The activities that others take for granted—sleeping late or getting up early, hopping out of bed, throwing on clothes, deciding to have a late night out with friends, taking a shower—may require painstaking planning and substantial assistance for a person dependent on long-term care. The challenge for home care and PAS is to minimize the difficulties and, above all, not to exacerbate them through insensitive, inflexible programs of care and assistance.

The services people want and need will, of course, depend on their condition—its severity, recency, and prognosis. Generally speaking, the service categories of home care can be reduced to six kinds of help: *(1)* personal care (that is, ADL assistance with bathing, dressing, toileting, moving about, even eating); *(2)* housekeeping, cooking, laundry, and chore services, including driving and escort assistance (that is, IADL assistance); *(3)* routine nursing and health maintenance activities, which include assistance with medications, monitoring of physical illnesses and their recovery, and palliative assistance to relieve pain and suffering for people who are dying; *(4)* supervision and oversight for safety (particularly important when the consumer suffers from cognitive impairment); *(5)* rehabilitation services to increase functional abilities, including movement, speech, and bowel and bladder training, which may require the specialized help of physical, occupational, and speech therapists, as well as nurses and other experts; and *(6)* management help, such as assistance in arranging for specialized care and learning how to live with and take care of oneself with specific diseases and disabilities.

Services of home care agencies can be considered broadly according to five categories of activities: rehabilitation services, convalescent care, hospice care for the dying, ongoing care to meet recurrent and routine care needs, and respite care to give relief to family members who have primary responsibility for care. Payment programs, as we will show, tend to separate these various functions of home care, in turn requiring the consumer to piece together the services needed. In fact our six categories (personal care, housekeeping and chore services, nursing services, rehabilitation, supervision, and care management) are more accurately reflective of real needs than the broad types of care created by payment programs.

From the perspective of those providing the services, we can further reduce the goals of home care to two general types, *therapeutic* and *compensatory*, terms foreshadowed in Chapter 1. Therapeutic goals suggest an effort to achieve some sort of measurable improvement or to forestall some sort of measurable deterioration as a result of one's efforts. Compensatory goals involve striving to help consumers and their families pursue their own lives despite the consumer's disability. Those dedicated to a compensatory approach tend to emphasize consumer satisfaction and autonomy as evidence of their success. We return to this distinction in the next chapter on residential care, and again in Chapter 8 on providing acute care to those who need long-term care. We keep reverting to this dichotomy because therapeutic approaches and compensatory approaches seem to be like oil and water, even though long-term care consumers need both. Those emphasizing therapy sometimes use that as an excuse to run roughshod over consumer preferences. Those emphasizing compensatory care sometimes use that as an excuse for lack of attention to ways to improve the consumer's health and functional status. Those who manage care according to therapeutic models may adhere to overly narrow definitions of "benefit from care." Those in the compensatory model may rely too much on the initial assessment, failing to recognize arising needs for further health investigations or rehabilitation potential.

Issues in Home Care

Home care is different from other venues of health care and long-term care in several ways. First, it is personal and intimate, and it enmeshes the workers in the daily lives and routines of the consumer. Those who endeavor to help the consumer must enter into that person's territory, and they can do so only at the invitation of the person getting the help. Second, the unit of scale is narrow—generally, one person at a time receives home care or PAS. Efficiencies are difficult to achieve and the care is often labor-intensive. Some efforts have been made to get more care for the dollar, for example, through "cluster care," where teams of in-home workers are assigned simultaneously to multiple clients living in close proximity,[2] or through use of a variety of contracted services such as laundries and restaurants with delivery in lieu of having a worker in the home doing laundry and making meals.[3] But the usual way to keep services within a reasonable price range despite their individualized nature is to reduce their amount, perhaps reducing them to a level which consumers or, more likely, professionals feel is inadequate. Third, family members are often central providers of care as well as direct targets for efforts of home care providers—such as training, support groups, assistance with particular technical tasks, and respite care.[4] Although family members are important adjuncts to care even when the consumer resides in a residential care setting or a nursing home, family members are relied upon to help public home-care programs balance their books.

Important interrelated issues flow from this situation, all of which pose perennial problems for policy-makers.

1. Who should receive home care and PAS? An argument can be made to limit such care, at least in public subsidy programs, to people with substantial disabilities.

2. How much service should be provided? Notions of appropriate levels of service range from the ideal of 24-hour shift care that until recently characterized the Medicaid personal-assistance program in New York City to minimalist approaches that subsidize just enough care to support an acceptable threshold of safety and comfort. The optimal approach is somewhere in between. Care must be sufficient to really promote a meaningful lifestyle, yet at a level that is possible to replicate for the entire community that needs such care.

3. Who should be in control? This is perhaps the central question. There is a growing conviction that the consumers should be in control of their care and, therefore, their lives. In operational terms, this might mean that the consumer dictates the timing and nature of services, chooses particular tasks to be performed over others, and chooses or at least vetoes the actual care providers who assist him. Competing for this control are providers of home care, who have professional opinions about the kind of care that is necessary and how to perform it; case managers who arrange care; and public programs that attempt to develop an equitable way to distribute resources. We favor consumer control, but within a system where the allocation from public resources is distributed according to some objective criteria for need. The first two questions about who should receive service and how much service need to be translated into an allocation of hours or dollars. Cash payments constitute the approach to home care that offers maximum consumer control and, as this chapter describes, this approach is being cautiously tested in a variety of publicly subsidized programs.

4. What sorts of consumer protections need to be built in? Consumer protections

and consumer restrictions are two sides of the same coin. There is a sense that long-term care consumers are vulnerable, especially those who are frail, elderly, and live alone. Those with sensory impairment and memory loss are even more vulnerable and could be prey to unscrupulous people coming into their homes. Various regulatory protections have been established that limit even what services people may purchase privately in various jurisdictions, and the tendency is to develop even more protections in public programs. Yet, each protection tends to raise the cost of the service. Also in contention is whether family members should be viewed as a natural layer of protection or as part of the danger against which long-term care consumers need protection. Elder abuse has become an important topic nationally and internationally in the last few decades and, with the lens focused on how to prevent, identify, and counteract the abuses that occur within families, policy is often crafted as though family abuse were the norm rather than a pathological aberration. In our view, developing policy for programs for the elderly with the expectation of elder abuse is as sensible as building policies for parents with the expectation of child abuse. Child abuse exists, as does elder abuse, as a tragic exception, but programs should be developed with the assumption of normal family relationships. On the other hand, public policy should not force enormous sacrifices from family members against their will. This tension poses a paradox. We rely on family help and cannot afford in-home services without it, yet we cannot in good conscience require family assistance beyond the statutory obligations of parents of minor children and spouses to each other.

Funding Programs

For three decades in the United States, home care has largely been shaped by the financing programs described in Chapter 2. These principal payment sources, as for long-term care in general, are Medicare; Medicaid, including Medicaid waivers and other state programs; and private pay. Although ultimately it is necessary to think "out of the boxes" to construct a new hybrid service, it is useful to examine the boxes that have been created by existing funding programs. At present, the kind of service package the long-term care consumer receives is much more a function of the programs paying for the care than a careful examination of the kind of help the person wants and needs.

Medicare

The Medicare program pays for home health care from certified home health agencies; it covers nursing, physical therapy, occupational therapy, speech therapy, medical social work, and home health aide services when skilled services are deemed medically necessary. Medicare also covers home hospice under a different set of requirements for Medicare-certified hospices for terminally ill people who decide to forgo life-prolonging therapies. Hospice must, for example, provide skilled pain relief and symptom management, psychological and social services, pastoral care, and, for the survivors, bereavement counseling.

Home health care as defined under Medicare sits at the expensive end of in-home services. Originally it was designed for short-term treatments for post-hospital patients who were likely to need a high level of skills from a multidisci-plinary team to achieve rehabilitation or ward off complications during the recuperation. In that sense, it was designed more as acute care than long-term care. The one permissible paraprofessional provider, that is, the home health aide, is expected to perform personal care under the supervision of the nurse or therapists and is enjoined against providing housekeeping, cooking, and similar household help except under very limited circumstances. In theory, home health care is a service for people who have intermittent needs for skilled care. In theory, too, a physician makes a specific prescription for home health care and oversees each plan.

As pointed out in Chapter 2, the aggregate costs of Medicare home health have soared both because more people are being served and at greater intensity of serv-ice, and because home health care has been partly transformed into a chronic-care service. The trend toward more use of home health care was hastened by various programmatic changes and clarifications. Notably, the definitions of home-bound and parttime were liberalized, and also home health agencies were able to keep cases open when they could argue a need for skilled "evaluation and manage-ment," even when no specific skilled service was needed. The result is that sub-stantial numbers of consumers rack up long episodes of continuous home health care (lasting for many months) with hundreds of visits. Analyses by the Health Care Financing Administration show the extent of long-term use of Medicare home health varies greatly by state, and that home health consumers getting large num-bers of visits per year are more likely to be poor and also to be eligible for Med-icaid.[5]

Our own analyses suggest a trade-off between Medicare and Medicaid support for home care. We compared 1992 state expenditures on HCBS to Medicare home health expenditures in those states in 1994. Of the ten states that fell into the highest quintile of Medicare home health expenditures, six had the lowest state expendi-tures on HCBS per person over age 65. In general, above-average state expenditures on HCBS were associated with below-average billings to Medicare home health in the state.[6] State policy cannot, of course, directly control the use of Medicare home health, but it does seem that Medicare is picking up some of the shortfalls of other subsidized home care programs in the state.

The conclusion that Medicare home health has become, at least in part, a long-term care program is reinforced by analyses prepared from 1992 home health Med-icare claims data to guide a prospective payment demonstration where home health agencies would be paid a fixed amount per episode.[7] The researchers defined an episode as up to 120 days of care after the initial admission. They found that the average number of visits for the episodes that were contained in the 120 days was 42 days. In contrast, for the 25% of episodes that exceeded 120 days, the average duration of service was 264 days. For-profit agencies, new agencies, and large agencies generated more visits per episode and longer episodes. Facility-based home health agencies (largely hospital-based) had shorter episodes but higher billings per visit. Although nurses accounted for more than half the home health visits that year (as one would expect because a nursing visit triggers other home health providers), for those consumers with episodes that lasted more than 120 days, home health aides provided 48% of all visits in the episode and 62% of all visits after the 120-day mark.

Ordinarily, there is no outside care management function in Medicare home health to rationalize the use of those resources. Leaving aside Medicare managed care organizations (discussed in Chapter 9), once the Medicare beneficiary is referred for home health care, the home health providers themselves determine the intensity and duration of care needed (subject to reviews by payers and retrospective disallowing of reimbursement if the care is deemed inappropriate under the program rules). The home health program has been vulnerable to particularly flagrant abuses by unscrupulous providers billing for fictitious visits and even deceased patients.[8] In part as a response to such concerns, at the time this book went to press the Health Care Financing Administration (HCFA) had declared a moratorium on certifying any additional home health agencies for Medicare.

Medicaid

State Medicaid plans must include home health care as well as nursing home care. At state option, the Medicaid program may also have a personal care program, and that program may include PAS from independently employed vendors. Some Medicaid programs have narrowly defined their home care as home health care with services identical to those offered under Medicare-certified home health. Often, however, agencies that are not Medicare-certified are also reimbursed by state Medicaid plans. Such agencies may emphasize personal care services, homemaker chore services, or both. New York, for example, has separate licensure for Medicare-certified home health agencies and for a large number of home care agencies that are more socially oriented and do not provide the full range of home health services.

Many states include PAS as a Medicaid service, but the models for Medicaid PAS differ across and even within states. Because Medicaid does not pay for services in advance, the Medicaid program reimburses the provider after service has been delivered rather than paying the consumer directly, who would then pay the provider. Typically, the PAS worker is deemed to be employed by the client. The number of allowable hours is usually authorized by county social service agencies and, once the client certifies the time sheets for the hours expended, the worker receives payment directly from the Medicaid program. Sometimes the checks are cut by the state (as in Oregon), by the county, or by an agency that is designated as a fiscal intermediary (as in Wisconsin). In New York City, where Medicaid

PAS is an enormous program, a consumer cooperative called Concepts in Independent Living acts as a fiscal agent and also provides a variety of supports for consumers who are employing PAS workers under Medicaid. California also is a large user of Medicaid PAS. In 1997, almost 200,000 Californians received Medicaid PAS, about 55% of whom were over 65. In this program, counties could decide whether to use an independent provider model (the dominant model), an agency model, or a supportive independent provider model (where the county provides some training, backup, and other support to the consumer), or to have all three models.

Other states provide PAS under Medicaid to varying degrees, and Medicaid programs differ as to the extent to which relatives can be the PAS provider. Technically relatives cannot be paid to give services under Medicaid, but states are free to define "relative." In Michigan, the definition of a relative specifies only a spouse, making it possible to pay everyone else. In some states, relative is defined as a spouse or parent, so parents cannot be paid for the care of their minor children with disabilities, but a wide range of other relatives can be compensated.

Medicaid Waivers
Like Medicaid proper, Medicaid waivers can fund, at state option, the entire range of home care from home health, through services from personal care, homemaker, or chore agencies, to PAS. The key difference between the waiver and the regular state plan is that the waiver services may be targeted to specific groups. Not uncommonly, younger long-term care consumers are offered PAS, whereas older consumers are offered only agency-based services. As we pointed out already, Medicaid waivers may also be used to fund a full range of HCBS services, including case management and adult day care, as long as these services are enumerated in the state waiver plan.

Other Public Payers
The Social Services Block Grant authorized by Title 20 of the Social Security Act, the Older Americans Act, and the Veterans Administration also cover in-home services and PAS. Because Title 20 block grants have not kept up pace with inflation, it is even more to a state's advantage to use the Medicaid waiver program where the federal match is applied to each person served. The California Medicaid PAS program described above was, in fact, transferred from Title 20 to Medicaid in the early 1990s to reinfuse the program with funding. A major distinction between Title 20 and Medicaid is that services funded under Medicaid must be medically necessary (ordered by a physician) and supervised in some way by a nurse, whereas Title 20 funds can be used in numerous ways with few restrictions and many claims on the money. Home care funded under the Older Americans Act tends to be social in nature, emphasizing homemaking, chore, and companion services. Veterans Administration home care services, in contrast, tend to be medically oriented and involve an entire team of professionals, including physicians, who serve patients within a reasonable radius of the hospital.

Private Payment

A great deal of home care and PAS is paid for privately. Information about the nature of privately financed provisions is hard to come by. Some people pay privately for care provided by agencies, including home health agencies, other home care agencies, and employment registries. More often, however, privately purchased provision comes from self-employed people and is highly individualized. The person employed may be a private duty nurse, a licensed practical nurse, or a certified nursing assistant, or may have no formal credentials at all. Sometimes, the privately paying consumer receives a referral of a private duty worker from a physician or a social worker. In large urban areas, particularly those that are magnets for retirees, fee-for-service care coordinators or case managers may maintain rosters of individuals with experience in providing personal care or homemaking. Very often the private-pay consumer finds the worker through newspaper advertisements or recommendations from friends. Sometimes, the consumer expands the job description of someone who had previously provided house-cleaning and similar services before that consumer needed long-term care. A growing number of resource books are available to assist consumers in selecting personal caregivers,[9] some of which have been developed by Independent Living Centers (ILCs). ILCs have been established in many states by and as a resource for people with disabilities. Initially oriented toward encouraging maximum independence among working-age people with disabilities, ILCs have recently turned their attention to older people with disabilities, including those who first incur their disability in old age.

If home care is being paid for by private insurance, the service is more likely to come from home care agencies than from an independently contracted provider. The exception is if the long-term care insurance pays off in the form of an indemnity payment, where the consumer is essentially paying out of pocket and is likely to use the more informal methods to find a privately employed in-home worker.

In summary, it seems likely that privately purchased home care resembles the PAS model more than the home care agency model, but surprisingly little is known about the home care people buy with their own money. To further complicate matters, older people can and do combine home health care purchased by Medicare and small amounts of home health care that they purchase privately with personal-assistance services and homemaking that they purchase entirely privately. Under these circumstances, the point of accountability for in-home services is hard to identify.

PAS versus Agency Services

Much has been made of the contrasts between PAS and agency-based home care, and PAS is assumed to be more compatible with consumer direction. Table 5.1 contrasts these two forms of in-home service along broad parameters. The key

Table 5.1. Comparison of Agency-Based Home Care and Personal Assistant
Services (PAS)

Agency-Based Home Care	Personal Assistant Services (PAS)
Common terms: home health care, personal care, homemaker service, chore service	Common terms: personal assistant, attendant
Delivery models: certified agencies, licensed agencies, unlicensed agencies, employment agencies	Delivery models: self-employed workers; fiscal intermediaries
Providers: nurses, PTs, OTs, speech therapists, home health aides, personal care workers	Providers: attendants, personal care workers, live-in companions
Services: wide range of services with substantial division of labor	Services: emphasis on services to meet ADL and IADL needs either through direct hands-on care or cueing, reminding, and supervision of tasks; little division of labor
Medication administration and nursing procedures included	Medication administration and routine nursing procedures done only under specific delegation or waiver of nursing regulations
Supervision: hierarchical structure with paraprofessionals supervised by professionals	Workers supervised by consumer or consumer's agent
Location: services delivered in the consumer's home	Services delivered in consumer's home or the community—e.g., at a workplace, in a school, or while consumer is engaging in recreational or other activities in the community, such as shopping
Being homebound often required for service	Being homebound not required for service
Funding: Medicare, Medicaid, Medicaid waivers, other public programs, private pay	Funding: usually Medicaid or private pay

distinctions concern organizational structure and control over the services. In-home services from agencies may draw upon a range of professional and paraprofessional personnel with the latter supervised by the former. PAS tends to rely on one or more all-purpose workers who are hired and supervised by the consumer or the consumer's direct agent. In a manifesto called *Attending to America*, the World Institute on Disability advocated forcefully for a PAS model in which the person with the disability selects, trains, supervises, pays, and (if necessary) fires the attendant.[10] Although at least in theory consumers should be able to exercise choice and autonomy when services are provided by an agency, PAS has come to be equated with consumer control and social as opposed to medical models of care. As with so many aspects of long-term care, a sharp dichotomy has been drawn when a pragmatic blend of agency-based care and PAS would be useful for many people. Indeed, some older people prefer not to be faced with hiring and firing responsibilities or with the various tax-withholding and other legal tasks of an employer.[11] Furthermore, the legal requirements of an employer are rather complex, and long-term care consumers who use PAS help around the clock may find themselves in the unwanted role of managing a payroll similar to that of a small business.

Three practical issues must be solved for PAS to live up to its potential to help people with severe impairments and heavy needs. First, what to do about backup? Second, what to do about medications and other nursing services? And, third, are worker's rights consistent with independent models of PAS?

Backup Services

No matter how effective the PAS arrangements may be, consumers are still at risk of finding themselves without help at crucial times, perhaps because of illnesses or other unavoidable absences of the attendant. Some might say that the consumer who elects to use independent PAS providers must accept the negative consequences that come from lack of an agency backup along with the positive features of lower unit costs and more control over the services. A less extreme position would at least try to develop some well-publicized source of emergency backup assistance to which consumers could turn if their care arrangements were to fall through. In some jurisdictions—notably, Oakland–Berkeley in the San Francisco Bay area, the local government authority is attempting to develop a reliable and efficient backup service that Medicaid consumers who use PAS for personal care can draw upon.

Nursing Tasks

In every state, nursing is a licensed function. Its scope is defined by state statute and oversight is performed by the State Board of Nursing. If a service is defined as nursing, it may not be performed by anyone without the proper license. Some states formally exempt relatives who are unpaid and domestic servants from this prohibition, and others do not prosecute family members for practicing medicine when, for example, a mother hands a pill to her child or a wife administers an injection to her elderly husband. When money changes hands, the sensitivity about practicing nursing without a license increases. The legal and liability ramifications of delegating nursing and medical practices to unlicensed personnel is a new area of exploration.[12]

The indisputable fact is that many long-term care consumers do need regular assistance with nursing tasks. This will be particularly true for medications administration if, because of physical or cognitive impairment, the long-term care consumer cannot take the pills, put in the eyedrops, or administer the injection. Home health aides work under the regular supervision of a nurse and can, therefore, manage medications. The PAS worker, in all probability, is not a licensed nurse or, for that matter, a certified nursing assistant. If he or she cannot administer medications, the value of the service goes way down. Moreover, if medications are needed on a frequent basis, the sheer cost of having a licensed professional nurse come to a home, say twice a day or, worse, four times a day, would be prohibitive.

Other procedures that might require a nurse include routine catheter care, ostomy care, and tracheotomy care. Some younger disability activists maintain that, for them, a function like catheter care is as routine as any ADL function and that they should be permitted to teach and supervise a PAS worker in performing the necessary help. Along those lines, Bob Kafka of ADAPT, a relatively militant organization of disability activists, suggests that a distinction should be made between medical and nursing procedures and "health maintenance tasks."

> When we distinguish between "medical" and health maintenance tasks, it allows us to think differently about the delivery of long term services in the home and community. The focus would be on people with disabilities . . . needing health maintenance and support services rather than being seen as people who are sick or broken in need of "medical" services and professional fixing. . . . Health maintenance tasks include not only those tasks delegated by a health professional to an unlicensed personal attendant, but also a category of tasks that need no professional involvement. These are not activities of daily living in the traditional sense nor are they medical tasks. Intermittent catheterization, bowel programs and tube feeding are just a few examples. These are tasks that are a routine on-going part of the lives of many people with disabilities and their families. . . . Provision of these tasks are essential for the person to live in the home and community but do not necessarily need health professional involvement.[13]

A successful approach to in-home services requires that some midway position be developed that neither prohibits care attendants and in-home workers from doing any task that could be faintly construed as nursing nor allows untrained people to venture into nursing practice with absolutely no instruction or oversight. Some states have modified or clarified their nurse-practice acts in a way that enables nurses to teach people without nursing licenses how to do particular tasks for particular people. Often called "nurse delegation," this policy can open the way to a much wider range of services at home at a lower cost.[14]

Worker Rights
Another general set of concerns deals with the line workers and their rights as employees. Arguably, the person with a disability has the right to incur whatever risks are associated with going outside an agency to hire their own workers. At issue is the protection of salary and benefits for those workers. This matter, which has surfaced in policy consciousness in the period since 1990, is particularly sensitive when public programs and public money are paying for the services. Moreover, the Internal Revenue Service has issued criteria for defining self-employment that make it difficult to construe the independent personal care worker as self-employed according to the tax code. (To be independently employed, one ordinarily works on one's own timetable, receives little supervision, uses one's own equipment, applies a particular skill, and is paid by the job.) Ruling out self-employment means that the employers are either the consumers themselves or the

state program that pays the consumers. As an employer, the person with the disability is responsible for meeting a wide range of requirements for employees,
including payment of Social Security Benefits (regardless of the preference of the
employee) and observing workplace safety requirements. This can be an arduous
requirement for the person with a disability. For this reason, some public programs
have developed fiscal intermediaries to act as the employer's agent in cutting checks
and managing benefits and other employer functions. Some state programs, including two we profile below, have developed mechanisms for worker's compensation
for these employees. Some fiscal intermediaries also provide support and assistance
to the consumer regarding hiring practices, writing job descriptions, and supervising
workers.[15]

Consumer-Directed Care

Growth of the Movement

The term *consumer-directed care* has been in vogue since the late 1980s to signify
a general desire to put consumers in charge of their long-term care services. The
concept first emerged in communities of younger people with disabilities, perhaps
as an outgrowth of the welfare rights movements of the 1960s, but it is now being
actively pursued for older long-term care consumers. The first use of the term
cannot be pinpointed, nor can the term be precisely defined. Like many terms
attached to a social movement, it takes on a variety of meanings according to the
user. But the ideal of consumer-directed care has the power to revolutionize long-
term care. A review of how this term has been used and applied in the last decade
of the twentieth century illustrates how, although still controversial, the idea of
consumer direction has entered the mainstream of policy thought.

Consumer-directed care is sometimes contrasted to care delivered by home care
agencies, and it is sometimes further contrasted to care that is managed by an
external case manager who ascertains the need for services and purchases the care.
Others use the term to refer to consumer empowerment in general, which they view
as consistent with using an agency's services or a case manager. In 1993, the United
Seniors Health Cooperative published a consumer's guide on home care for older
people specifically, evoking the language of consumer rights and consumer empowerment to the broad range of home care programs available to consumers and
suggesting ways that older consumers could make the most of all forms of home
care, including that received from a home health agency, a homemaker/aide service,
a registry for nursing or personal care, and an independent worker. The preamble
stated: "if you need care at home you do not have to surrender control over your
life and let others tell you what you must do. You *do* have choices [emphasis in
original]."[16]

The proposed American Health Security Act of 1993 (the result of the Clinton
Health Care Task Force), used the term "consumer-directed services." The pro-

posed new benefit of "personal assistance services" for people of all ages was to be available in two forms: "agency-administered" and "consumer-directed." The proposed bill further stated: "Consumer-directed services are those provided by individuals who are hired, trained, and managed by the person receiving the services."[17] The intent of the Task Force was that *both* agency-administered and consumer-directed services be available and that consumers and their agents have the option of choosing the best solution for them. It does not appear that either form of personal assistance—consumer-directed or agency-administered—was meant to replace home health services that might be needed in connection with an acute health condition or with physical rehabilitation.

In 1994, the Administration on Aging provided funds to establish a 'National Institute for Consumer-Directed Home-and-Community-Based Services." The resulting institute, founded in 1995, was a partnership of the National Council on Aging, where the program was housed, and the World Institute on Disability (WID) in Berkeley, California. (WID itself was founded in 1983 by leaders of the Independent Living Movement and was meant to serve as a center for the study of public policy on disability and independent living.) The alliance of an advocacy organization for aging and an advocacy organization for disability in this enterprise testifies to the belief that services for older people needing long-term care could be made more responsive and effective by infusion of principles from the independent living movement created largely by young adults with physical disabilities such as, for example, spinal cord injuries.

The institute issued newsletters and position papers and, soon after its initiation, it changed its name "in response to the popular demand for brevity,"[18] to the "National Institute for Consumer-Directed Long-Term Services." With this change, two loaded words for some people with disabilities and their advocates (i.e., "home" and "care") disappeared from the title. Disability activists sometimes view the term "home" as restrictive (because needed services go far beyond the home) and the term "care" as patronizing or imprecise (because "care" implies an emotional bond, whereas "services" are more matter-of-fact and functional and arguably can be separated from the concept of "caring"). This view, however, is not unanimous. Some commentators believe that some element of a personal relationship is necessary to sustain both personal care worker and the consumer in the intimate tasks with which they are involved; in this view the challenge is "boundary maintenance," or the consumer's struggle to find a balance between viewing the worker as a family member or friend and viewing the worker as an employee.[19]

In 1996 the National Council on Aging, with funds from the Robert Wood Johnson Foundation, launched a research and demonstration initiative called Independent Choices: Enhancing Consumer Direction for People with Disabilities. Consumer direction was defined as "a philosophy and orientation to the delivery of supportive services whereby informed consumers assess their own needs, determine how and by whom these needs should be met, and monitor the quality of services received.'' It was stated to have four dimensions: *(1)* consumer control and direction of services as the primary decision maker, who assumes responsibility for controlling virtually all aspects of care or delegating responsibility to other individuals; *(2)* the availability of a service delivery system that offers the consumer meaningful choices and that can create new options outside the traditional service system; *(3)* the availability of appropriate information and support to inform the consumer about service options and the personal, legal, and financial issues associated with each; and *(4)* consumer participation in the policy-making process, including the design of the programs that serve them. Projects could apply to people of all ages with any defined service needs and in any care context. Specific suggestions were: providing consumers with options for cash benefits, vouchers, or debit accounts; developing consumer or provider cooperatives; developing fiscal or supportive intermediaries for consumer-directed services; and integration of consumer direction into managed care arrangements.[20]

In 1997, a wide range of projects were funded under the Independent Choices Initiative. These included projects attempting to bring consumer direction to the difficult area of care for people with Alzheimer's disease, a project to infuse consumer direction practices into traditional home health care, projects to bring a range of consumer direction into case-managed programs under Medicaid waivers (including cash and voucher arrangements), and research projects to articulate more precisely the nature of consumer preferences and the way consumer direction affects quality of care and quality of life.

In 1996, the National Institute on Consumer-Directed Long-term Care Services issued a fuller discussion of consumer direction. It reiterated the four dimensions: consumer control over decisions about their care, consumer participation in policymaking, availability of choices, and availability of information and support to enhance consumer direction. (The last two seem to be system requirements to support consumer direction.) The statement also enumerated five principles: *(1)* systems should be based on the presumption that consumers are the experts on their service needs; *(2)* different types of services warrant different levels of professional involvement (which recognizes that consumers must rely on professionals as the complexity of their service increases, though the consumers should still retain the right to participate in assessing need, evaluating options, and deciding on a course of action); *(3)* choice and control can be introduced into all service-delivery environments; *(4)* consumer-directed service systems not only support the dignity of people needing personal assistance, but can be less costly, when properly designed; and *(5)* consumer direction should be available to all, regardless of payer. The last principle asserted that people dependent on Supplemental Security Income (SSI) or who rely on public funding for their services should be able to direct services according to their preferences as much as people who pay privately for services. Inability to control the form of assistance received was characterized as ''dehumanizing.''[21]

Although consumer direction may seem to be poles apart from the Medicare home health program, some of its language and aspiration for people receiving publicly financed services have become part of deliberations at HCFA. In 1993 HCFA sponsored a conference on "beneficiary-directed" services. The then-administrator of HCFA, Bruce Vladeck stated: "The first and most difficult issue is that to build a client-centered, beneficiary-oriented long-term care system, the dollars should follow the clients. Funding should probably not be limited to a particular kind of provider or service, or to a particular bureaucratic category, such as 'skilled' level of care."[22] Illustrating this thinking, in late 1996 HCFA announced a small Consumer-Directed DME (Durable Medical Equipment) Demonstration under Medicare. This initiative responded to consumer complaints that physicians do not know how or what to authorize in the way of equipment that meets consumers' needs for comfort and convenience and that consumers incur unconscionable delays and out-of-pocket costs under the current mechanisms in order to receive equipment from certified DME vendors. The demonstrations, sponsored by Centers for Independent Living, would authorize consumers to purchase their own equipment within a budget while receiving advice and support to become more effective purchasers.[23]

The 1997 CASA bill, which proposed adding a qualified community attendant benefit for Medicaid clientele eligible for institutional care, calls for implementing Bruce Vladeck's injunction that the service should follow the beneficiary. The statute states that the attendant service should be available "under either an agency-provider model or other model" (the latter further defined to include vouchers, direct cash payment, or use of a fiscal agent in obtaining the services). The attendant service, furthermore, should be "selected, managed, and controlled by the individual."[24] Supporters of the CASA bill perceive these principles as pertinent to all Medicaid long-term care populations, including people with developmental disabilities and mental illnesses and elderly long-term care consumers.

This sketch of consumer direction is replete with resounding principles yet responds to common sense ideas of how many people would want to live if they had to live a disability. Moreover, it may make sense from a systems point of view. Flexible, user-friendly community-based services at relatively low cost could be the key to the future of long-term care outside facilities. In addition, consumer direction is thought to be the key to ensuring that the services fit into the consumer's desired lifestyle rather than forcing those who use services to adapt their lives to the service configurations. However, implementing consumer direction is easier said than done, especially making changes in policy so that the funding follows the consumer. Funds have already been invested in existing services, and vested interests surround them. Also it is difficult to begin a new model of benefits that follow the consumer while still paying for the old categorical model that funds specific service streams.

Finally, some people question whether older people really desire consumer direction, or at least they believe that more attention is needed to devising a model of consumer direction that is not unduly burdensome for older consumers, some of whom are sick as well as disabled. Commenting on this point, Elias Cohen suggests the existence of an "elderly mystique," something akin to the "feminine mystique," to which older people subscribe.[25] The elderly mystique is the belief that disability in old age spells the necessary end of mastery. Older people who become disabled, in this view, should no longer expect to "travel as they wish, eat what they want, engage in physically demanding activities, or exercise dominion over a work space or a group of people. They have no schedules they must keep." Noting that many younger people who face only a decade or less of life with increasing disability and deteriorating disease nonetheless exert personal and social advocacy on behalf of people with disabilities, Cohen concludes that the aging mystique rather than differences in remaining life expectancy accounts for observed differences between young and old in exercise of consumer control.

A lurking question with all consumer direction, furthermore, is how to handle the question of agency for people of any age who are incapable of directing their own care. A neat solution is to deem the consumer's agent, such as a guardian or conservator, to be designated to act in the consumer's interest. There is a growing literature, however, suggesting that guardians and conservators rarely act to promote the preferences or best interests of their wards, and some authorities even suggest that if at all possible, formal guardianships should not be sought.[26] This, of course, leaves in limbo who should be the responsible agent.

Agency Responses

Home health agencies and other home care agencies view the consumer direction movement with mixed reactions. Some home health agencies are actually developing programs that help support consumer direction. For example, an agency in Tucson, Arizona, has established a "Hire Private Help Program" whereby, for a flat fee, the agency recruits a suitable home care aide (doing the advertising, interviewing, reference checks, and criminal checks), provides brief initial training, gives the consumer a kit on the paperwork that must be handled, and provides support and backup. The consumer hires the aide directly and avoids the substantial overhead fee. If the consumer rejects the first three applicants sent, or if three hires fail to work out, an additional charge is affixed. Reporting on the basis of having made more than 300 such matches, the agency describes a win–win situation. The consumer quickly recoups the 1995 charges of $450 for finding a part-time worker, $750 for a full-time or live-in worker, and $1,050 for two workers because the agency would charge $130 a day for an assistant and $160 if that person were a nurse's aide, compared to about $80 and $95 in the private market.[27] Similarly, a Visiting Nurse Association in Dallas, Texas, reports its efforts to implement an Independent Provider Program funded under Medicaid for people with developmental disabilities, including doing the teaching and delegating necessary.[28] The authors express some scepticism that the program can work optimally because of low wages paid to the attendants during the training period and an inability to provide feedback to the attendants.

The National Association for Home Care has expressed official concern about states that have allowed independently contracted workers to provide a wide range of complex care procedures, including dressings, catheter care, suctioning, and nasogastric feedings. Recognizing the rights of individuals who are capable and desirous of "self-directing" their care but expressing concern that this model is being imposed on consumers, the Home Care Aide Association of America (HCAAA), a spinoff organization established in 1990 by the National Association for Home Care, has issued its own White Paper on the subject.[29] This organization's major concern is the rights of the workers, which includes rights to training, to be free of exploitation, to have a grievance procedure, to be working in compliance with state and federal safety laws. HCAAA affirms that "individuals who are capable of doing so and choose to do so should be permitted to self-direct care" but calls for quality standards to govern the process.

We have discussed the consumer direction movement with considerable detail because of its centrality to any system development for the next century. Professional paternalism, however well-intentioned, has become much less acceptable in home care and in long-term care in general.

Persuading Consumers to Use In-Home Services

Policy makers tend to fear that the same consumers who resist moving to a nursing home until the last possible moment will "come out of the woodwork" to use HCBS services at home if they become widespread public program benefits. Although it is pleasing to offer benefits that consumers actually like, the paramount need to control costs makes the idea of high demand frightening. But the surprising findings are that consumers often resist having help at home even when it is free. They frequently need to be persuaded to accept as much help as care coordinators recommend, or even to have any help at all. This mirrors the observation that people who need to buy most of their home care with their own funds because they do not qualify for subsidized programs are hesitant to spend the money.

It would be simplistic to interpret these reactions as evidence that help is unnecessary. Instead, it is important to determine the reasons for any rejection of proffered assistance. One likely reason is that consumers are reluctant to get in-home help because they perceive this as the beginning of a slippery slope that leads them to the nursing home. Once care providers, case managers, and government officials enter their lives, they may fear that their performance and their safety at home will be constantly judged. Another reason for dreading and resisting home help concerns the sanctity of the home and the desire for control within it. People do not welcome strangers in their homes. Some may have fears for the security of their possessions. They particularly do not appreciate caregivers who come in and take over, perhaps following a care plan devised by their agency supervisors or a case manager. Finally, those paying privately may be simply unable to purchase the kind of care they want at the times they want at a price they feel they can afford.

Although overt salesmanship for HCBS programs would be overdoing it, providers need to be sensitive to the objections and concerns that consumers may have, and program designers must try to develop programs in a form that consumers like. Some consumers need reassurance that taking help at home is not an automatic way station to a nursing home. They need to be given the opportunity to have a voice in selection, training, and job descriptions even when the worker comes from an agency. They need to be confident about who is being given a key to their home. They need to know whom to call if something goes wrong. If all these problems are solved, it is still unlikely that consumers will demand high levels of service. There seems to be a preference to get by with as little as possible, and to avoid unneeded dependency. Anyway, we recommend that the problem of oversubscription be faced when and if it happens. The first step is to develop programs that consumers like and that serve their needs well. Developing ways to control overuse is secondary.

Model State Systems

Some states have made substantial efforts to develop systems of service that increase the chances that someone needing long-term care will be able to receive it in the community and, to the extent possible, direct their own care. They have attempted to develop a wide array of options, to make the services user friendly, and to incorporate systemwide efforts to allocate resources and prevent overutilization. Some stellar examples are directed toward younger populations, such as programs for people with developmental disabilities in Alaska[30] and in New Hampshire.[31] In both those examples, low-income clients covered by Medicaid or the Medicaid waiver can draw upon a budget to organize care according to their own preferences. An agent, usually a family member, can assist when the client is unable to make judgments. These programs have demonstrated that people with substantial cognitive disabilities are capable of forging a program for themselves that pleases them, is not associated with untoward outcomes, and usually costs *less* money than the programs professionals would develop for them. Similarly, in Vermont a program has evolved for younger people with physical disabilities that relies heavily on a committee of helpers to develop the service allocation.[32] Although an assessment is performed that takes into account the actual minutes of help each functional task should require given the consumer's exact physical environment, nonetheless the peer assessors tend to be parsimonious in their allocation of attendant hours and their personal experience makes them credible gatekeepers.

For our more detailed examples, we draw upon states that have incorporated older people into statewide efforts to make in-home services more flexible and universally available. (It is somewhat easier to make those transformations with a younger clientele because so many fewer people will need the services).

Oregon's Waiver Program: Client-Employed Home Care

Late in 1981, Oregon received the first HCBS waiver and launched the series of programs that has made Oregon of great interest to many observers.[33] Due to the efforts of a well-organized senior lobby, legislation was enacted in October 1991 to create the Oregon Senior Services Division (later renamed the Oregon Senior and Disabled Services Division) to consolidate all aging and long-term care programs. Simultaneously, and also with support of the senior lobby, another bill called the "State Policy on Aging" was enacted. It made explicit that the following values would govern the delivery of services to seniors in Oregon: the right of free choice in planning and managing one's own care; access to a number of long-term care options; maximizing self-care and independent living; the right to live at home as long as possible; and the right to independence, privacy, and appreciation of individuality. Having these powerful concepts embodied in statute was extremely helpful in keeping the home care programs on course. Also invaluable was another principle included in the legislation that stated "it is appropriate that savings in nursing home . . . allocations . . . be reallocated to alternative services."

The funding vehicles to implement these brave new principles were the Medicaid program and the new Medicaid waiver program, supplemented by a gap-filling program for people age 60 and over funded by state money called Oregon Project Independence (OPI). The main difference between the waiver program and OPI is in income levels of the clientele; service needs and type of community services received are similar, but OPI clients typically have incomes too high to qualify for the Medicaid waiver, and they pay a sliding fee based on income for the services they receive.

The major mechanism for identifying clientele and allocating services were case-management units at the local level, which were empowered to allocate all publicly subsidized services including the nursing-home Medicaid program. Case management was usually housed in an Area Agency on Aging, which typically served a single county or sometimes multiple less populous counties. In some rural areas, where Area Agencies on Aging were not prepared to take on the functions of managing Medicaid, the Senior Services Division established local branches to do case management. All adults with physical disabilities were eligible for the program regardless of age, and the hope was that the case managers could unite the funding streams in a way that was seamless for the consumer.

The centerpiece of the waiver program is in-home services, and three-quarters of the in-home services are secured through the client-employed home care program. (The waiver also covers the service component, but not the rent, in three alternative housing settings—residential care, adult foster care, and assisted living. These kinds of services are discussed in the next chapter.) This program allows clients to hire, supervise, and fire their in-home workers. Addressing some of the concerns cited earlier about fairness to workers and burdens to consumers, the state pays the worker's compensation and FICA payments and cuts the checks on behalf of the client. The case-management units help the client identify a suitable in-home worker and perform criminal checks on all potential workers before they are hired. Clients may employ their relatives as in-home workers, though spouses cannot be hired unless they have been demonstrated to have left the workplace to give the care.

According to an analysis by Elizabeth Kutza, in 1995, 47% of Oregon's publicly subsidized long-term care population received in-home services (including from OPI), 25% received services in substitute homes (discussed in the next chapter), and 28% were in nursing homes. This represents a substantial reversal in the way Medicaid services are distributed in most states. At the time of her report SDSD purchased services as the agent for the consumer from 3,937 hourly housekeepers and 1,296 live-in attendants under the client-employed program and served another about 3,600 people under OPI. SDSD also contracted with twenty home care agencies, but agency-based home care was definitely perceived as supplemental or to be used when the client-employed program was inappropriate.

The Oregon program directly addresses the problem of developing cost-effective ways to receive help with routine nursing tasks. In accordance with the state Nurse Practice Act, nurse delegation is done by licensed nurses for each individual client as deemed appropriate by the nurse. The nursing task is delegated in writing to an individual nonlicensed provider who could be the client-employed home care worker.

Oregon evolved another unusual program that is known as *relative foster care*. In actuality, this is more like family-provided home-care than a congregate living situation. The designation *relative foster home* is used when a person needing services moves into the home of a relative (other than a spouse) who commits himself or herself to providing that care. In those instances, the home is especially licensed as a foster home and authorized to provide service to a particular consumer so that the relative may receive payment. In some ways it is the obverse of the client-employed home care program that permits payment to relatives who provide services to consumers who lives in different households from family caregivers.

A uniform comprehensive client assessment and a case-management capability are viewed as two necessary planks to hold the system together. Case management varies somewhat from region to region. In the more populous areas, case management may be specialized so that some highly skilled case managers with reduced caseloads devote their time to actively helping consumers move out of nursing homes and to working with clients considered at high risk—for example, people with Alzheimer's disease living in the community. The case management is meant to be enabling rather than intrusive, and ordinarily the caseloads are too large for anything other than biannual assessments and responses to client-initiated requests. But arguably the case-management program enables a highly flexible and varied set of programs with an emphasis on consumer control. Nurses who perform the delegation are typically hired as staff or consultants to the case management agencies.

As this book goes to press, Oregon is conducting an "Independent Choices" project wherein it is experimenting with a direct cash option. The case managers would provide advice and counseling to consumers who select this option but would no longer act as fiscal agent for purchase of services. Because the Oregon client-employed program offers substantial consumer control combined with consumer convenience, it will be of interest to see how many people still opt for the cash.

Wisconsin: Community Options Program

Unlike Oregon, Wisconsin does not have a fully integrated long-term care system where purchase of HCBS and nursing home services and licensure functions are embodied in the same agency. It does, however, have a long history of interagency cooperation. Starting out as a state with an extremely high proportion of seniors in nursing homes, it has evolved one of the most user-friendly home care systems in the country. Case managers are empowered to purchase anything (within their budget limits) that might make sense for the client and client preferences are emphasized.

Wisconsin's Community Options Program (COP) is operated at the county level in this seventy-two-county state. The Community Options Program started as a state-funded HCBS program and over the years added Medicaid waiver funding with the COP waiver for the elderly and physically disabled and an additional waiver for the developmentally disabled. As in Oregon, the goal is to make the funding seamless to the consumer, and case management is a major component of the program.

As in Oregon, the Wisconsin program is driven by a set of guiding principles, which are well known to all case managers and contracted providers. They are incorporated into the acronym RESPECT.

- *R*elationships. Relationships between participants, care managers, and providers are based on caring, respect, continuity over time, and a sense of partnership.
- *E*mpowerment to make choices. Individual choice is considered the foundation of ethical HCBS.
- *S*ervices to meet individual need. The emphasis here is on the notion that individuals want prompt and easy access to services tailored to meet their unique circumstances.
- *P*hysical and mental health. Services are intended to help people achieve their optimal level of health and functioning, including both physical and emotional health.

- *E*nhancement of participant reputation. Services maintain and enhance participants' sense of self-worth and community recognition for their value in every way possible.
- Community and family participation. Participants are supported to maintain and develop friendships and participate in their families and communities.
- Tools for independence. Consumers are supported to achieve maximum self-sufficiency.

The state COP program is designed to serve five target populations: the elderly, the developmentally disabled, the physically disabled, the chronically mentally ill, and chronic substance abusers. The elderly constituted 55% of the clientele in 1993. That year, however, the average expenditures per person per year were about $3,600 for the elderly consumers and $3,360 for physically disabled consumers in contrast to $6,700 for developmentally disabled consumers and $5,900 for chronically mentally ill consumers. The waiver programs spent substantially more per client. In 1993, there were 19,251 consumers served by all the programs: 9,118 clients were served by COP with total expenditures of $40.3 million; 7,625 were served by the COP waiver with expenditures of $52.1 million; and 2,508 were served under the developmentally disabled waiver with expenditures of $52.5 million. (Again, per-person expenditures on the developmental disability waiver outstripped those on the elderly waiver.)[34]

The hallmark of the Wisconsin program is flexibility in the way the COP and the waiver money is spent. Training for case managers highlights the stories of the innovative ways that plans have been pieced together. As in Oregon, case managers may authorize care from independent providers, though Wisconsin uses county-based fiscal agents rather than using the state as fiscal agent.

The Achilles heel of the program is its long waiting lists. The program leaders take the position that it is a mistake to keep dividing the available money among those who are eligible for services, likening that to doubling up clientele in nursing home beds. Consequently, in Milwaukee County, the largest region, the combined programs were serving almost 2,000 people in January 1995, but almost 1,500 more were waiting for assessment and more than 2,500 had been assessed, and deemed eligible for services, but were waiting for services to begin. This shortfall is a function of insufficient legislative appropriations. Nevertheless, the Wisconsin program is an almost inspirational example of how programs can be integrated at the local level and case managers can be motivated to act creatively and flexibly on behalf of consumers. The RESPECT slogan established an extremely broad purview. The Wisconsin programs take as their goal the full social and psychological well-being of the consumers. A quality assurance program built into the system endeavors to hold the program accountable for meeting each of the goals embodied in RESPECT.

Wisconsin program officials have been interested in better integrating their long-term care support programs with home health agencies in order to provide a more effective service to people with substantial health care needs, especially when they leave hospitals.

Washington State

The state of Washington offers a third example of statewide efforts to improve in-home options for elderly and physically disabled people.[35] The Aging and Adult Services Administration administers the programs through forty-six local field offices and fifteen Area Agencies on Aging, two of which are located on Reservations. As of late 1995, the field offices were staffed by 318 state employees, who manage the nursing-home program, perform case management, and do the initial eligibility for potential clients. The Area Agencies on Aging do the eligibility reauthorizations for clients receiving home care and also provide case management for that group.

Washington provides a variety of programs for people in their own homes. Some, such as home-delivered meals, are fairly standard nationwide. Others are truly targeted to those at high risk of entering nursing homes. As with Oregon and Wisconsin, the effort is to coordinate multiple funding streams on behalf of the consumer. The three major planks in the in-home services program are Chore Services, the COPES (Community Options Program for Elderly Services) waiver services, and the Medicaid personal care program.

Chore Services is a state-funded program that provides personal assistance to people with at least one need for personal care. The program predates Medicaid waivers, having been in existence since the 1960s. In 1995, it was budgeted to serve slightly more than 8,300 clients and spend $24.8 million. Those eligible for SSI and therefore Medicaid in Washington are not eligible for the program. The services are offered without charge, but those with higher incomes receive fewer services on the premise that they can pay for more of their services themselves.

In 1982, Washington received federal approval for a HCBS waiver, called the COPES. Eligibility was based on an income no more than 300% of the SSI standard ($1,460 in 1996) and nursing home certifiability. In addition to covering services in congregate care, adult family home care, and assisted living facilities (the kinds of programs discussed in the next chapter), the waiver covered case management and personal care. As in Oregon, the COPES program operates a client-employed in-home service and an agency-employed service. In 1996, the hourly rate for the client-employed program was $5.76 and the agency program was $10.08. The state pays both the employee and employer share of the FICA for the workers employed by the clients. COPES also has a live-in attendant program under the client-employed component of the waiver. In 1995 the program was budgeted at about $60.5 million predicated on an expected 5,440 clients, 3,838 of whom would receive in-home services.

Washington began a personal care program under its Medicaid plan in July 1989. It was designed to provide almost identical services to the COPES waiver, but to persons who were categorically eligible for Medicaid. Furthermore, these clients did not need to be nursing-home certifiable, though if they were, they would be entitled to greater payments. Under this program, there are three categories of in-home services: 24–hour in-home care given by independent providers, 86 to 116 hours of service a month, also give by independent providers, and less than 86 hours of services a month from agency providers.

The state has continuously worked to interdigitate the COPES waiver program and the Medicaid personal assistance program most effectively. In 1993 the COPES waiver was closed to new clients because the caseload was approaching the federal limits. Therefore, in 1994, Washington transferred all clients who were categorically eligible for Medicaid to the regular Medicaid personal care program. The COPES waiver program then reopened, but it only serves those with incomes between 100% and $300% of the poverty standard. With these changes, the Medicaid personal care program grew rapidly. In 1990, a year after it began, it served 4,550 clients and spent about $15.8 million. In 1995, the program was budgeted to serve 10,934 clients and spent $60.2 million. Obviously the Medicaid personal care mechanism allowed Washington to enormously increase the number of clients receiving long-term care services.

An important feature of the Washington program is a preadmission screening for all Medicaid applicants and those who will, if in a nursing home, spend down to Medicaid within 180 days. Program officials also have worked to develop a way to quickly qualify people for in-home Medicaid services. As we discussed in Chapter 4, nursing homes ordinarily receive reimbursement for a few weeks while medical eligibility is clarified, and, therefore, unless eligibility for HCBS services can be quickly determined, the bias toward using nursing homes increases. Also, since 1990, some of the local programs have developed vigorous efforts to become involved in the hospital discharge planning process to minimize the role use of nursing homes on discharge. Finally a great deal of attention has been given to developing quality assurance programs and training case managers to be the first line of defense in identifying and solving quality problems.

Case Management

All three state examples leaned heavily on locally based case management to give coherence to their system and especially to manage the in-home services programs. So too do many other states. Gradually a specification for the function of case management has emerged that includes at least these functions: screening and case-finding, comprehensive assessment (performed in the home), care planning, implementation of the plan (through purchase or authorization of services, referral and arrangements), monitoring, and reassessment at intervals. By now, several books have been written about case-management practice.[36]

Local case-management programs serve as well-publicized focal points for access to service. The case managers perform assessments that not only determine eligibility but also suggest the consumer's needs. They discuss with the consumer and family members how those needs might be met and in many programs actually purchase the services. In other programs they authorize the services, which are acquired from agencies also certified as vendors for the statewide program. At the programmatic level, case-management organizations bargain for favorable rates from care-providing agencies and establish and enforce quality standards. In many states, particularly where case managers actually make the purchases on behalf of the consumers, the case managers have substantial flexibility to arrange individually tailored programs.

In the approximately two decades since case management became a feature of HCBS programs, both under earlier demonstration projects and later operational HCBS waiver programs, substantial capacity has developed for effective case management. Also, many efforts have been made to refine and improve case-management programs and to discern, distill, and disseminate the essence of an effective case-management program. These efforts quickly identified one of the most difficult problems in implementing the ambiguous role of the case manager: reconciling the advocacy and counseling aspects of the role and the administrative and gatekeeping aspects.[37] Case mangers are, on the one hand, service providers, who directly assist the consumers. They are, on the other hand, an arm of program administration with responsibilities to use resources efficiently, to establish priorities, and to develop plans that are as inexpensive as feasible. Several issues concerning case management are worth highlighting.

Relationship to Care Providers
In general, the received wisdom about case management in HCBS services is that it should be separate from service delivery.[38] This means that organizations paid to give services under the waivers would be ineligible to provide case management. Case managers are thought to be less biased and more able to advocate for the consumer and the integrity of the state program if their organizations do not stand to benefit from the services ordered. For the most part waiver programs and statewide case-management programs in general have adhered to this principle, at least insisting on an arm's-length arrangement if some unit of a home care agency actually provides case management. There are notable exceptions. For example, the waiver and state-funded program in Florida selects a lead case-management agency in each county that is also usually a service provider. Similarly, the HCBS waiver program in New York is conducted through vendors that develop Nursing Home Without Walls programs. These vendors are often home care agencies and other providers; they undertake to provide case management and waiver services, contracting with other providers only as they deem necessary. But the more usual model lies in the other direction—that is, prohibiting those who do case management from also providing services.

Some home health agencies and state home care associations have expressed reservations or even had negative reactions to HCBS case management, and especially to the exclusion of direct-care providers from the case-management function. Complaints about case management independent from service provision include the following: The case management is redundant and therefore wasteful; it just duplicates the assessment, care-planning, and monitoring done by the home care agencies. The case management permits other professionals, often lesser trained, to interfere with the professional judgment of the agency-based professional. The clinicians at the provider agencies know the clients best and have the clinical skills to determine need, so they should do the case management.

The counterarguments in favor of separating case management from service include these: Care providers have an inherent conflict of interest that will lead to providing too much or inappropriate service. Providers are more interested in full caseloads and using all money allocated to the agency than in titrating services to meet changing client needs and moving people on and off the caseloads. Providers will be inadequate monitors of their own care. Providers have little experience or interest in managing care that crosses agency boundaries or continuing to manage care when the agency provides no service. Finally, the logic of providers being case managers disappears when what is being managed is a package of services that may involve multiple providers, including independently employed PAS workers who are not employed by any agency. For example, all three states that we profiled used some form of client-employed worker as an option. Indeed, one argument for the cost-effectiveness of the case-management function is that it has been instrumental in the development of creative, low-overhead care arrangements which are likely to be cheaper as well as more satisfying to the consumer.

Relationships between case managers and care providers are likely to be less acrimonious and may even be positive if the roles of all parties are carefully considered. In general, uncertified home care agencies that have arisen to provide a service under Medicaid and Medicaid waivers tend to report more appreciation of the case managers who send them business. For example, New York has a large number of licensed, uncertified home care agencies that act as vendors under Medicaid. South Carolina's waiver program, called Community Care Organizations, contracts with both home health agencies and personal care agencies, reporting a more amicable relationship with the latter. But Ohio and Pennsylvania have shown that the relationships can be positive, especially at the service level, if case managers modulate the intensity of their activity when the contracted agency is a home health agency with a nurse manager or an agency with a high complement of professional personnel and if the case managers are perceived as doing something useful for the agencies. Examples of useful activities are efforts to upgrade training for line personnel in the community, provision of technical assistance, and development of joint planning and partnership arrangements.

Search for Standards

Case management evolved as a function in practice settings. If HCBS case managers have professional degrees, they are usually social workers (with MSWs or, more likely, BSWs) or nurses. However, many are simply college-educated people with some human services experience who fell into the jobs. At issue now is the extent to which case management should be a credentialed enterprise with expectation of prior training and qualifications.[39] Case managers are also concerned about whether standards should be promulgated for caseload size and other features of the work environment. State programs also struggle with how to develop practical initial and ongoing training for case managers. With large state-wide programs, turnover is a constant. To obtain consistency in the program, current case managers need to be refreshed and new case managers socialized to the program philosophy and to a wide range of practical concepts and skills—how to use the assessment tools and make a care plan, how to cost out the care, how to work with families and vendors of service, and how to remain abreast of community resources.

A number of accreditation programs have been developed for case managers, and some long-term care analysts would prefer to establish credentials for the job title *case manager*, which would bind state programs and other employers of case managers. Others are concerned about any premature enunciation of standards and credentials, and the dangers of establishing yet another interest group in long-term care.

Intensity of Case Management

Some case-management programs have a lock-step process where each initial inquiry results in a full in-home assessment within a prescribed number of days, followed by a care plan that is monitored at prescribed intervals. Others allow more discretion to the case manager to determine how quickly to do the assessment and how frequently to monitor based on the circumstances of the case. Similarly, some programs would have the case managers remain rather distant from the consumers in terms of counseling and advising, leaving that to vendors. In other programs, case managers are meant to be salient figures to the consumer and would be perceived to be failures if the consumer were unaware of their existence and their roles.

The Ohio HCBS waiver program, which is known as PASSPORT, has evolved a triage system of case management based on perceived consumer needs. In this approach, some people who make inquiries receive information and perhaps a referral out with an open invitation to call again if they need further assistance. The notion here is that not every consumer needs full-blown case management. If not needed, case management is wasteful and possibly intrusive. In this program, various community agencies are all made well aware of the criteria for case management and waivered services. Therefore, these agencies can make referrals back to the HCBS program in an appropriate manner.

Individualization versus Protocols

An unresolved issue concerns the degree of standardization appropriate for case management. Some programs have strived to develop clear-cut criteria for various types and amounts of service based on information gleaned during the comprehensive assessment. If decision trees were honed to a fine science and if the assessment data were computerized, a machine could largely create the care plans. Such algorithms would, in theory, promote fairness in the use of services by minimizing individual decision-making.

But one of the complaints about the care plans developed by case managers is that they tend to be unimaginative, almost as though they were stamped out with a cookie cutter. Therefore, individualized efforts are particularly welcome to counteract that phenomenon. A useful midposition is to encourage creativity while developing some advisory protocols to help case managers deal with recurrent situations.

The Philadelphia Corporation for Aging, Pennsylvania's largest local case management agency, has provided particular leadership in this regard.[40] With grant funding, the agency developed protocols for common situations such as clients with memory problems living alone, clients who fall, clients suspected of being victims of abuse, clients with alcohol problems, clients who may have too many prescription medications, the depressed client, and so on. Each protocol describes how an assessment would identify the problem and suggests steps that should be considered based on resources in the community. A videotaped training module has been developed for each protocol. Although the system was developed to apply specifically to Pennsylvania, the demand for these protocols has been national. The advantages of the protocols are that they bring up-to-date information about medical conditions to the attention of case managers, who are usually social workers, and they obviate the need for each case manager to "reinvent the wheel" when they confront a particular problem. On the other hand, these protocols do not preclude creative care planning and individualized approaches.

Information Systems and Quality Assurance

HCBS case-management programs are becoming more sophisticated in using information at the individual and system level to improve their programs. To truly mine this potential, they need computerized assessments, and they would benefit from equipping their case managers with laptop computers. Several states, notably Alabama, Connecticut, and Indiana, moved into computerization early. The Indiana program in particular is impressive because of the variety and practicality of the reports that can be generated. The Indiana program, known as CHOICE (Community and Home Options to Care for the Elderly), is designed for long-term care consumers of all age and embraces acute care as well as long-term care services. The assessment information is perceived as the first step in a quality assurance system.[41] Therefore, the database also incorporates all the providers in the system and is able to display not only how well consumers are doing but also how well-paid caregivers are doing. During monitoring visits, case managers collect feedback on the providers, down to the particular care attendant, and can provide their vendors with information about complaints and problems.

Case managers have considerable potential to improve quality, as the Indiana example shows. Not all case-management programs are equally attuned to this dimension, however. The Ohio PASSPORT program has been dedicated to this topic, identifying and trying to overcome barriers to getting accurate information about consumer satisfaction. At one point, this organization, through a university consultant, tested out a "Nielsen-family" approach modeled after the well-known television ratings. Consumers who were designated as the Nielsen families and instructed to describe in minute detail what they liked and did not like about their experiences during a given period of time were able to overcome their reluctance to complain and to enter with enthusiasm into their responsibilities.[42]

Future of HCBS Case Management

In 1990 and again in 1995, Rosalie Kane promulgated ten commandments for case management that incorporated responses to many of the issues discussed above.[43] Still pertinent, they are:

1. Thou shalt not do case management unless the client needs it.
2. Thou shalt have only one case manager.
3. The case manager shall have authority over services.
4. The case manager shall do no direct services.
5. Case managers must calculate the costs of care. (The further explanation of this precept emphasized that they should calculate all costs of the plan including those borne by the consumer or other parties and become cost conscious.)
6. Remember the assessment: Do it wholly and as it is written. (This maxim responded to the well-documented tendency of case managers to be haphazard and perfunctory in their use of the assessment tool and to jump to conclusions about the consumer's needs and status.)
7. Care plans should flow from assessments. They should be individualized, yet contain standard responses to standard problems.
8. Thou shalt monitor, including when your client is in a hospital and discharged from a hospital to a nursing home. (Sometimes HCBS case managers have no system to learn quickly about the hospitalization of their client or relegate management during that period to hospital personnel. In fact, in the Washington State example illustrated, important decisions are made during this period and the effective case manager is on the scene.)
9. Thou shalt be flexible in service provision.
10. Honor thy client's preferences, so your days may be long as a case manager.

The fact that community-based case managers have the potential to follow these guidelines is a great strength of the HCBS case management function. A case-management program that cleaves to these general rules is likely to be a force toward redressing the balance of a state's long-term care system.

HCBS case managers are, however, becoming an endangered species in some areas. The threats to their continuation include providers who see them as superfluous and redundant, managed care organizations that are developing their internal care coordination capabilities (see Chapter 9), and some consumers who believe case management intrudes on their autonomy. Cash programs, to which we turn next, might be considered alternatives to case management. At the very least case management programs need to be conscious of their own costs, which vary widely in absolute terms and as a percentage of the costs of the services managed.[44] Important as case management is, it would be a travesty if more money were spent on management than on the services themselves.

Cash and Counseling

A true cash program is the ultimate in consumer control. In a cash program, the state government would assess long-term care needs at intervals and translate them into a cash payment for eligible long-term care consumers. The consumers would then be responsible for purchasing their own services. If they chose well and creatively, they might have resources left to put aside for a later time. If they chose poorly and ran out of money before the time period for which the cash allocation pertained, they would be out of luck.

Governments perceive the attractiveness of a cash option, especially if they can allocate lesser amounts of dollars than the average costs of services for those consumers who opt to have case-managed in-kind services. However, they also have qualms about cash programs in lieu of services for several reasons. First, cash is attractive. It is always the right size. Therefore, consumers who may be reluctant to use in-kind services are likely to collect any cash for which they are eligible. That being the case, the cost of the cash programs could swell because of the induced demand. Second, governments worry about the possibility that cash will be used inappropriately for purposes other than intended—for example, for liquor or movies. This would be especially worrying if the misuse of the cash became publicized and the government programs were involved in a scandal. The same concerns led most states to use food stamps rather than cash allocations for food, though Oregon cashed out its food stamp program in the city of Portland in the late 1970s with success (though on account of agricultural interests, renewal of the waiver was denied). Third, paternalistic officials may be concerned that the consumers would become prey to unscrupulous providers or abusive family members who take the cash but fail to provide adequate services. Finally, there are also concerns about whether governments could really walk away from the consumer who was left without resources. If such a hard-hearted stance proved emotionally or politically impossible, governments would end up paying twice.

Some states already have initiated small programs with cash benefits for certain targeted populations. Also, the Veterans Administration has long provided an "Aid and Attendant" benefit, which is supplied in the form of cash to certain eligible service-connected veterans with disabilities. The Aid and Attendant benefit seems almost always to be used to augment the income of the veteran's family and offset the costs of a family caregiver, usually the spouse. However, almost no systematic information is available about that cash benefit, or how it is used and how it is received.

Despite those concerns, considerable momentum developed in the 1990s for a test of a cash model for in-home services. Such models have been developed in Europe with considerable success (see Chapter 10), leading federal officials to wonder if they could be applied in the United States. A cash program would seem to allow maximally for consumers to hire their own workers in the pure PAS model and, if they chose, to hire family members. Furthermore, a well-designed program might guard against the possible abuses by providing substantial counseling assistance as needed to consumers who spend their own money to purchase their own services.

Therefore, a National Cash and Counseling Demonstration was initiated as a collaborative effort of the Robert Wood Johnson Foundation and the United States Department of Health and Human Services, through the Office of the Assistant Secretary for Planning and Evaluation (ASPE).[45] Four states—New York, New Jersey, Florida, and Arkansas—were awarded demonstration money to launch an initiative to cash out either Medicaid benefits or Medicaid waiver benefits, or both. The ASPE evaluation is rigorously designed as a randomized trial so that the cash and counseling projects can be compared to control groups of clients getting case-managed services as usual.

The United States context differs from the European in terms of cashing out benefits in one major way: The benefits cashed out in the United States are for low-income people on Medicaid or Medicaid waivers. Therefore, a number of complications arise. Clients move in and out of eligibility for Medicaid, and this eligibility is directly related to their incomes. Thus, a series of waivers were needed to ensure that these consumers would be able to preserve their eligibility for SSI, Medicaid, and food stamps despite the cash allocations. Furthermore, questions arose about whether consumers should be permitted to save any unexpended cash from month to month. State Medicaid programs are reluctant to allow their clients to accumulate money during a cost-cutting period where welfare reductions are at the top of the agenda. Then, too, Medicaid is specific about the kinds of expenditures covered, and some states felt that the client should be required to keep a record of those expenditures to prove that they are all related to care. Technically, under Medicaid, clients are prohibited from using the money to establish reciprocal relationships with family members (for example, buying a grandchild a bicycle in exchange for performance of shopping and errands, or paying the heating bill for a relative who in turn provides care). Many details of this nature needed to be worked out in each state. Initially, states developed plans that seemed to be cash with very long strings attached.

The "counseling" component of the demonstration could be a vehicle for providing consumers with useful assistance, especially at the outset of their efforts to purchase services, or it could be an intrusive function that exceeds the role of most case management. Still to be worked out on a state by state basis are the intervals and content of the counseling. Some states initially proposed frequent counseling, which included review of consumer budgets and the examination of their receipts. Initially, the counselors also seemed to be given the power to judge the success of the cash benefit and to terminate it if they thought the consumer was making poor use of the benefit. Obviously, cash surrounded with so many protections would not truly test the effectiveness of cash. The almost reflexive efforts of states to impose such constraints are inherent in the Medicaid programs.[46]

In 1997 most of the necessary waivers had been assembled to begin the demonstration, which will add a great deal of insight into the promise of cash benefits. Simultaneously, two other states, Ohio and Oregon, received Independent Choices grants to test cash payments. Thus, they too will be demonstrating adding a cash benefit to their waiver programs, though they will not be part of the main evaluation.

Family Programs

Some in-home programs are designed to help family members in their efforts to help the ultimate consumer of long-term care services. Programs with family caregivers as the intended clientele fall are often unclear about the purpose of their efforts.[47] Sometimes they seem to be designed to encourage family members to increase and sustain their efforts, sometimes they intend to improve the quality of the care family members provide, and sometimes they aim to ensure that no family caregiver is unduly burdened by the care they provide. Obviously, the goal selected is related to one's theory and understanding about family caregiving. For example, some people believe (against all evidence) that family members are deserting older people and need to be exhorted to pull their weight, and others believe that family members are burdened by their care-giving duties, suffering untoward social, psychological, financial, and even health effects.

The in-home services provided to family members fall into three main categories: *(1)* direct services to family caregivers, which include counseling and psychotherapy, training programs, and support groups; *(2)* respite programs, whereby their relatives receive small amounts of in-home care, day care, or institutional care to provide relief for the family member; and *(3)* direct payment of family caregivers.

The grab bag of direct services has not been well evaluated. There is evidence, however, that elderly family caregivers (spouses, adult children, and other relatives over age 65) have disproportionate health problems themselves and a high incidence of depression. Some programs are geared to ensure that family caregivers receive health checkups and treatment for physical and mental health problems. Support groups are often condition-specific—for example, for family caregivers of people with Alzheimer's disease or strokes. They seem to be regarded highly—

even as a lifeline—by those who use them, but many people either find attendance impractical given their caregiving responsibilities or prefer to get entirely away from their problems during their rare free time.

Training and education can be perceived as particularly helpful, but it must be the right content at the right time. There is little use to being offered a course in how to bathe a person who cannot transfer 3 years after one's spouse has suffered a stroke. When the consumer first incurs a disability or requires a new procedure, however, family members report that specific factual content about the condition and how to manage it is extremely helpful. In that regard, the physical therapists, occupational therapists, speech therapists, and nurses who visit from home health agencies often get rave reviews from family members because they offer instruction and reassurance at the right time.

Respite programs are an inexpensive public provision compared to provision of complete HCBS services for the eligible population. Their affordability, along with their consistency with "family values," helps account for their political popularity. It is relatively easy to persuade legislatures to fund efforts that provide limited help to families who are "taking care of their own." Some states, like Alaska, for example, have developed special respite programs targeted for caregivers of people with Alzheimer's disease. Many states include respite as a service under their HCBS waiver. Like other long-term care programs, respite programs often suffer from lack of goal clarity. For example, they may be evaluated in terms of whether the family caregiver who uses respite care has improvements in psychological well-being, whereas the respite program may be used to enable that family member to attend a funeral, have elective surgery, or merely run personal errands. Sometimes respite programs are rather poorly specified—for example, the respite may be available during weekdays, whereas the real desire of the family caregiver is to get away in the evening or on the weekend (e.g., to see grandchildren or go to church). One study of respite[48] showed that a great deal of counseling was needed merely to get family members to agree to accept respite, especially if they had experienced incompetent caregivers who upset their relative. The same study showed that consumers had a strong preference for in-home respite even when respite was needed for several days, whereas institutional respite is easier to arrange. Finally, for people not eligible for Medicaid or Medicaid waivers, most respite programs must be purchased privately or have heavy copayments. Family members cannot easily afford care that may equal or exceed $10 an hour. A common complaint of family caregivers is that they have difficulty finding inexpensive help to purchase for short periods of time. The few controlled evaluations suggest that respite services have an important value for those who use them but cannot claim major effects.

Direct payment to family caregivers can be accomplished through client-employed programs such as were described in our profile of Oregon, Wisconsin, and Washington. Some states that use agency models make arrangements for family caregivers to become employees of one of their agency providers. In some ways compensating family caregivers resembles a cash solution. It puts more money in the hands of the family unit. Opinions vary on whether family caregivers should be paid through public programs. Some commentators would answer affirmatively, noting that this is in part a woman's issue, that people who leave the labor force to care for relatives deserve compensation, and that relatives should have the same right to be compensated as strangers. Other commentators are concerned about altering the nature of voluntary exchanges within families and note that the quality and quantity of the service are difficult to monitor when the paid caregiver is a relative. They are also concerned about induced demand in a cash program for families, similar to the concerns about giving cash directly to consumers. And those who are particularly worried about elder abuse expect that cash to families will bring out the worst motivations. An extra complication arises when the family member who receives payment for care is also the guardian for a person who is adjudicated as incompetent and who needs long-term care. Some purists would consider this constitutes a severe conflict of interest, whereas others, ourselves included, would see no obstacle except on a case-by-case basis. The same case management that monitors all other providers could monitor the work of paid family caregivers.

We favor payment of family members under specific conditions. First, the family member should have left the workplace to give care. Second, they should be paid at the going rate for this care, not at their replacement costs in the labor force. And third, the ultimate consumer of the care, the person with the disability, must prefer to receive the care from the family member. With those protections, direct payment to family members seems a useful option.

Concluding Comment

This chapter has been free-ranging, dealing with a wide variety of programs and models for in-home services. If the chapter has seemed disjointed, so too are the services. Services available under Medicare are rarely coordinated with those available under Medicaid. Health-related in-home services, subsidized as they are by Medicare, are too expensive for private purchase. In-home services are often offered in a form that consumers do not value, and consequently refuse. Case management, a good idea, has sometimes been developed with competing case management systems. In fact, in the late 1980s, an entire national program called "The Living-At-Home-Project" was developed by the Commonwealth Foundation and a consortium of thirty-five other Foundations to address the gaps, duplications, and disconnections inherent in home care.[49] In that project grants were made to organizations in twenty large cities in order for them to make efforts to rationalize their home care capabilities in the geographic area. Most spent their funds on improving care coordination and interorganizational cooperation, developing information systems, and designing gap-filling programs, such as emergency assistance. The problems that the Living-At-Home Program tried to address are far from solved.

As this chapter has shown, consumer-directed models are coming into prominence with an emphasis on direct hiring of PAS workers. Yet, nobody believes that all in-home services to all consumers can be managed through PAS. Continued attention is, therefore, needed to infuse agency care with consumer direction principles. Also, the challenges of enticing, retaining, and nurturing the work force for in-home care should be high on the agenda for the next decade.

Consumers can and do benefit from a wide range of in-home services, and they are best organized according to some overall plan of care. At the same time, principles of consumer direction suggest that users of services themselves should be the ones who ultimately script those plans, though always within the constraints of funding availability and eligibility requirements.

Notes

1. In 1997, a bill called CASA (Medicaid Community Attendant Services Act) was introduced as H.R. 2020 by speaker Newt Gingrich. This would enable a new mandatory benefit under Medicaid for Qualified Community-Based Attendants, who, whether employed by an agency or directly by the consumer, would provide ADL or IADL assistance under the direction of the consumer. That bill used the term "attendant" more narrowly than the term personal assistant services (PAS) is sometimes used because PAS is sometimes broadened to include wide range of help for people with disabilities such as interpreter services, transportation, provision of equipment, and so on.
2. United Hospital Fund (1992). *Cluster Care: A New Approach to Home Care.* New York: United Hospital Fund.
3. Jette AM, Branch LG, Wentzel RA, Carney WF, Dennis DL, & Heist MM (1981). Home care service diversification: a pilot investigation. *The Gerontologist* 21:572–579.
4. Kane RA & Penrod JD. (Eds.) (1995). *Family Caregiving in an Aging Society: Policy Perspectives.* Thousand Oaks, CA: Sage.
5. See Vladeck BC & Miller NA (1994). The Medicare home health initiative. *Health Care Financing Review* 16:7–16; Mauser E & Miller NA (1994). A profile of home health users in 1992. *Health Care Financing Review* 16:17–34.
6. Ladd RC, Kane RL, Kane RA, & Nielsen WJ (1995). *State Long-Term Care Profiles.* Minneapolis, MN: National LTC Mentoring Program, Institute for Health Services Research, School of Public Health, University of Minnesota.
7. Goldberg HB & Schmitz RJ (1994). Contemplating home health PPS: patterns of Medicare service use. *Health Care Financing Review* 16:109–130.
8. Eisler P (1996). Buyer beware: the hidden risks of home health care. *USA Today*, November 11, pp. 11B–13B, November 12, 1A, 2A, 7A.
9. See Susik H (1995). *Hiring Home Caregivers: The Family Guide to In-Home Eldercare.* San Luis Obispo, CA: Impact; Werner AP & Firman JP (1993). *Home Care for Older People: A Consumer's Guide.* Washington, DC. United Seniors Health Cooperative; Alpha One (1994). *How to Manage Your Personal Care Attendants.* Portland, ME: Alpha One Center for Independent Living. A longer annotated list of such resource guides and where to order them is available through The World Institute on Disability, 510 16th Street, Suite 100, Oakland, CA 94612. Some of the resources are particular to how to hire an attendant in a particular state.

10. Litvak S, Heuman J, & Zukas H (1987). *Attending to America: Personal Assistance for Independent living.* Oakland, CA: World Institute on Disability.

11. Glickman LL, Brandt KJ, & Carol FG (1994). *Self-direction in Home Care for Older People: A Consumer's Perspective.* Boston, MA: Gerontology Institute, University of Massachusetts.

12. Sabatino CP & Litvak S (1995). *Liability Issues Affecting Consumer-Directed Personal Assistance Services: Report and Recommendations.* Oakland, CA: World Institute on Disability.

13. Kafka B (1997). When are medical tasks not medical tasks? InWagner DL, Nadash P, & Sabatino C. *Autonomy or Abandonment: Changing Perspectives on Delegation.* Washington, DC: National Institute on Consumer-Directed Long-Term Services, The National Council on Aging.

14. Kane RA, O'Connor CM, & Baker MO (1995). *Delegation of Nursing Activities: Implications for Patterns of Long-Term Care.* Washington, DC: American Association of Retired Persons.

15. Flanagan S (1994). *Consumer-Directed Attendant Services: How States Address Tax, Legal, and Quality Assurance Issues.* Cambridge, MA: SysteMetrics.

16. Werner & Firman (1993). See note 9.

17. Bureau of National Affairs (1993). Clinton Administration Description of President's Health Care Reform Plan, "American Health Security Act of 1993," Dated September 7, 1993, Obtained by the BNA September 10, 1993. Washington, DC: Bureau of National Affairs.

18. Institute changes name. *Consumer Choice* 1(3):5. (Newsletter of the National Institute on Consumer-Directed Long-Term Services). Washington, DC: National Council on Aging.

19. Eustis NN & Fischer LR (1991). Relationships between home care clients and their workers: Implications for quality care. *The Gerontologist* 31:447–456; Eustis NN, Kane RA, & Fischer LR (1993). Home care quality and the home care worker: beyond quality assurance as usual. *The Gerontologist* 33:64–73.

20. Robert Wood Johnson Foundation (1966). *Independent Choices: Enhancing Consumer Direction for People with Disabilities.* Princeton, NJ: Robert Wood Johnson Foundation.

21. National Institute on Consumer-Directed Long-term Services (1996). *Principles of Consumer-Directed Home and Community-Based Services.* Washington, DC: National Council on Aging.

22. Vladeck B (1995). Long-term care: the view from the Health Care Financing Administration. In JM Wiener, SB Clauser, & DL Kannell (Eds.), *Persons With Disabilities.* Washington, DC: The Brookings Institution.

23. HCFA announced consumer-directed DME demonstration (1996). *Consumer Choice* 1(3):2. (Newsletter of the National Institute on Consumer-Directed Long-Term Services). Washington, DC: National Council on Aging.

24. See note 1.

25. Cohen ES (1988). The elderly mystique: Constraints on the autonomy of the elderly with disabilities. *The Gerontologist* 28 (Suppl):24–31.

26. Kapp MB & Detzel JA (1992). *Alternatives to Guardianship for the Elderly: Legal Liability Disincentives and Impediments.* Dayton, OH: Wright State University School of Medicine.

27. Clinco JB (1995). *The agency's role in hiring private help. Caring Magazine* 14:76–77.

28. Suther M, Rogers J, & Wassenich L (1995). The CLASS program: self-directed care. *Caring Magazine* 14:72–75.

29. Home Care Aide Association of America (1995). White paper: guiding principles governing the delivery of long-term care. *Caring Magazine* 14:70–71.

30. Ladd RC (1996). *Long-Term Care in Alaska: Recommendations for Reform.* (Report Submitted to the Alaska Department on Aging, November 1995). Austin, TX: Ladd.

31. Nerney T. & Shumway D (1996). *Beyond Managed Care: Self Determination For People With Disabilities.* Concord, NH: Institute on Disability, University of New Hampshire.

32. Reinardy J, Kane RA, & Mollica RL (1994). *CAILS Assessment Project: Background Data.* (Report prepared for the Vermont Department on Aging and Disabilities). Minneapolis, MN: National LTC Resource Center, Institute for Health Services Research, School of Public Health.

33. Oregon was chosen along with Wisconsin and Washington for a GAO study of model programs; see United States General Accounting Office (1994). *Medicaid Long-Term Care. Successful State Efforts to Expand Home Services While Limiting Costs.* (GAO/HEHS-94-167, August 1994). Washington, DC: Government Printing Office. It was also chosen along with Washington and Colorado for an AARP study of three states with cost-effective community programs. See Alecxih LMB, Lutzky L, Corea J, & Coleman B (1996). *Estimated Cost Savings from the Use of Home and Community-Based Alternatives to Nursing Facility Care in Three States.* Washington, DC: American Association of Retired Persons. For descriptions of Oregon's programs see Kutza EA (1995). *Long Term Care in Oregon.* (Paper prepared for the 1995 White House Conference on Aging and distributed by the National Association of State Units on Aging). Portland, OR: Portland State University Institute on Aging; and Ladd RC (1996). *Oregon's LTC System: A Case Study by the National LTC Mentoring Program.* Minneapolis, MN: University of Minnesota Institute for Health Services Research.

34. These figures were supplied to Richard Ladd by the Wisconsin Bureau of Long-Term Care Support during a 1995 site visit to that state as part of the fact finding efforts of the National Long-Term Care Mentoring Program housed at the Institute for Health Services Research at the University of Minnesota School of Public Health and incorporated in an unpublished document available from that program.

35. Richard Ladd visited Washington in late 1995 as part of the fact-finding efforts of the National Long-Term Care Mentoring Program, housed at the Institute for Health Services Research in the University of Minnesota School of Public Health. The figures cited in this section are drawn from an unpublished report available through that office.

36. Applebaum R & Austin C (1990). *Long-Term Care Case Management: Design and Evaluation.* New York: Springer; Quinn J (1993). *Successful Case Management in Long-Term Care.* New York: Springer.

37. For discussion of the ethical issues that arise because of the tensions between advocacy and gatekeeping, see Kane RA & Caplan AL (Eds.) (1993). *Ethical Conflict in the Management of Home Care: The Case Manager's Dilemma.* New York: Springer; Kane RA, Penrod JD, & Kivnick HQ (1994). Case managers discuss ethics. Dilemmas of an emerging occupation in the United States. *Journal of Case Management* 3(1):3–12; Kane RA (1992). Management in long-term care: it can be ethical and efficacious. *Journal of Case Management* 1(3):76–81; Dubler NN (1992). Individual advocacy as a governing principle. *Journal of Case Management* 1(3):82–86; Browdie R (1992). Ethical issues in case management from a political and systems perspective. *Journal of Case Management* 1(3):87–89; Clemens EL & Hayes HE (1997). Assessing and balancing elder risk, safety, and autonomy: decision-making practices of health care professionals. *Home Health Care Services Quarterly* 16(3):3–20.

38. This discussion is drawn largely from a research project sponsored by the United States Office of Technology Assessment. See Kane RA & Frytak J (1994). *Models for Case*

Management in Long-Term Care: Interactions of Case Managers and Home Care Providers. Minneapolis, MN: National LTC Resource Center, University of Minnesota School of Public Health.

39. For results of a project to develop standards for case management sponsored by the Robert Wood Johnson Foundation, see Geron SM (1994). *Guidelines for Case Management Practice Across the Long-Term Care Continuum.* Bristol, CT; Connecticut Community Care.

40. Amerman E, Graub P, & Schneider BW (1992). *Clinical Protocol Series for Case Managers.* Philadelphia, PA: Philadelphia Corporation for Aging.

41. Kinney ED, Freeman JA, & Loveland Cook CA (1994). Quality improvement in community-based, long-term care: theory and reality. *American Journal of Law and Medicine* 20 (1&2):59–77.

42. Applebaum RA, & McGinnis R (1992). What price quality? Assuring the quality of case-managed in-home care. *Journal of Case Management* 1 (2):9–13.

43. Kane RA (1995). Capacity-building for case-managed LTC systems: Getting specific about advocacy and gatekeeping. In RA Kane, MO Baker, & L Starr (Eds.), *Issues in Capacity-Building for Case-Managed LTC Systems; The Nitty-Gritty For States.* Minneapolis, MN: National LTC Resource Center, University of Minnesota School of Public Health.

44. Kane RA, Penrod JD, Davidson G, & Moscovice I (1991). What cost case management in long-term care? *Social Service Review* 65 (2):281–303.

45. Mahoney KJ & Simon-Rusinowitz L (1997). Cash and counseling demonstration and evaluation: start-up activites. *Journal of Case Management* 6(1):25–31.

46. Cameron K, Lagoyda R, & Nadash P (1996). *Cash and Counseling Technical Analysis: The Counseling Component.* Washington, DC: national Institute for Consumer-Directed Long-Term Services, National Council on Aging.

47. For a full discussion of these issues see Kane RA & Penrod JD (Eds.) (1995). *Family Caregiving for an Aging Society: Policy Perspectives.* Thousand Oaks, CA: Sage.

48. Lawton MP, Brody EM, & Sapperstein A (1991). *Respite Service for Alzheimer's Caregivers.* New York: Springer.

49. Bogdonoff MD, Hughes SL, Weissert WG, & Paulsen E ((1991). *The Living-At-Home Program: Innovations in Service Access and Case Management.* New York: Springer.

6.

Combining Housing and Services

As the cliché has it, everyone needs a place called home. Home health programs, home care programs, personal-assistant services, day care, home modifications, and a host of other offerings in the armamentarium of long-term care are predicated on the long-term care consumer having a place to live. Moreover, almost since the advent of Medicare and Medicaid in 1965, long-term care analysts have set as a goal that long-term care clients continue to live in their own homes. Movement to a nursing home or other institution has been perceived as a last resort when a care plan cannot be arranged at home for anything resembling a reasonable cost.

What does living in one's own home actually mean? Surely, it cannot exclusively mean remaining in the home where one has spent most of one's lifetime, perhaps rearing children there. Many older people change their residences when their children are grown or when they retire from the labor force. Perhaps the cost of maintaining a largely empty house has become prohibitive. Perhaps the relocation is designed to support a new lifestyle—simplified and smaller space, or multiple spaces (even using a summer home or manufactured housing as part of the plan). Adult-only retirement communities such as Sun City and Leisure World have had some appeal, as have trailer-court communities in sun-belt areas.

When people need additional services or perceive themselves as in frail health, residential relocation may be stimulated all the more. For example, people move from farms and villages to more settled areas to be closer to health services, and many people move closer to adult children, siblings, and other relatives. Also, people with disabilities seek living environments that are easier to maintain, that are adapted to physical limitations (for instance, without stairs), and where the need for ongoing maintenance of the home and grounds is less.

Although many services can be provided in a person's home, the cost of home care includes paying for the travel time of those providing the care. People living some distance from the origin of the services, especially for care that must be given frequently and in small aliquots, may be forced to consider some type of relocation to render that care more affordable. Congregate living offers a means to reduce the unit cost of home care while providing reasonable amounts of privacy and independence.

People often must move their residences specifically because they need long-term care. Might it be possible for them to move into housing situations where they can readily receive services and still maintain the sense of living in their own homes? This depends on what we encompass in the meaning of words like "home" and "home-like." As America becomes urbanized, growing numbers of people call an apartment, condominium, or town house "home." Traditional single-family dwellings are less common. Proximity to neighbors, sharing of facilities (such as, for example, a laundry, a pool or recreation center, a lobby, a party-room, a garden, or a barbecue), and sharing of services (such as garbage collection, utilities, and maintenance) do not transform that home into an institution. Nor does rental as opposed to ownership transform homes into institutions. This chapter considers the challenge of creating places for long-term care where people with substantial disabilities can live and receive services and still feel "at home."

Conceptual Background

For many years, long-term care programs have been sharply bifurcated into HCBS and nursing home programs. The thrust of public policy has been to develop the former services to ward off use of the nursing home and to do so in such a way that the public costs can be controlled. But, as we have already pointed out, a nursing home can be an efficient location in which to receive care because of the economies of scale involved. Assuming that some long-term care clients will need to move away from their current home, an ideal long-term care system would present a range of options for new living quarters where services could be received and daily life would still go on in a normal manner. (Despite the fact that people live in them, nursing homes were never even envisaged as housing since they evolved on a hospital prototype.) A "home care model" might be plausible in congregate living situations, whether that care is delivered by program staff, outside home care agencies, or some combination. Consider that home care providers face a need to balance travel time with care time and that some of its inefficiencies and resultant high price relate to the cost of travel time. If enough people reside in the same congregate community and use the same home care providers, home care could become much more efficient.

What is expected of such residential care settings and how might they be judged? The best known residential care setting is the nursing home, sometimes called a health care facility or a long-term care facility. Nursing homes are defined through the evolving federal rules that hammered out the requirements for facilities that would be reimbursed under Medicare and Medicaid. It is now easier to recite the requirements that nursing homes must meet than to conjure up a positive statement about the nature and purpose of a nursing home. In contrast, other residential settings, including small group homes (sometimes called adult foster homes) and board-and-care settings (sometimes known as assisted living), are regulated at the state level with all the variation that we mentioned in earlier chapters.

Some advocates see this unsettled situation, characterized by a proliferation of sometimes ill-defined care settings and a lack of overriding federal regulation, as dangerous to the health and financial well-being of the consumers. In contrast, we tend to view the emergence of new care settings as a promising phenomenon that may promote better ways of combining housing and care. To further explore this promising prospect, we need to ask what we, as a society, expect of those settings that provide services along with housing. Should the living spaces resemble a hospital (where the housing is secondary, almost incidental to the needed services) or should it resemble an apartment, where concerns about housing are primary? Need housing and services be provided as a fixed pair? Might not the quality of housing be allowed to expand with a person's income regardless of the services provided? Should those who operate the housing component and the hotel-like functions also be responsible for the care services, or should responsibilities be divided? And where does individual consumer choice figure into the paradigm?

Keren Brown Wilson introduced a useful way of thinking about the requirements of a setting for housing and services, which takes into account both the housing and the care dimensions.[1] As shown in Figure 6.1, she envisages the essential nature of an assisted living setting as a three-legged stool, each with two prongs. One leg is a homelike residential environment, which, in turn, encompasses home-like public space and home-like private space. A second leg is a capacity for service, which entails a capacity for meeting routine or regular needs of the consumer and meeting more specialized needs that might arise. Furthermore, routine needs can sometimes be met through scheduled services—for example, for baths or administration of medications—and sometimes must be met on an unscheduled, ''as-needed'' basis (e.g., toileting assistance or general supervision for safety.) The final leg is maximum control and choice for the consumer, which, in turn, includes choice and control over the use of the private space (what is kept there, how it is arranged, what is done there and when, and who enters) and control and choice over the care plan (the timing of services, the nature of services, refusing unwanted services, and deciding when to remain or leave the setting).

We will return to Wilson's rubric (home-like residential environment, service capacity, and philosophy that promotes consumer choice and control) as we consider, first, the nursing home and how it might be improved and, second, the range of new residential services that have emerged, largely courtesy of the private market. The perennial challenge is to retain *both* the service capacity and the home-like environment, which seem to work against each other, especially as service providers aspire to greater efficiency and quality control. Finally, the philosophy

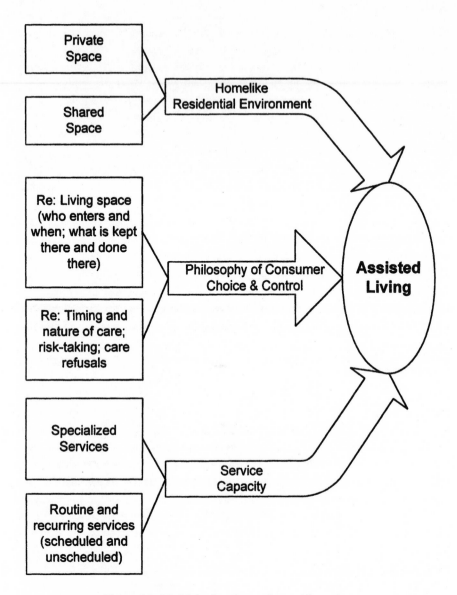

Figure 6.1. Model for housing settings with services.

of respect for consumer choice and control, always a challenge in long-term care even when consumers are in their separated homes, is harder to maintain when the consumers seem to be captive residents or tenants in a community that is staffed to provide them with care.

Some trends already blur the sharp distinctions between home care and so-called institutional care. Some care "institutions" are much becoming more home-like, offering private apartments where residents can enjoy privacy and a modicum of control. Some home-care providers give service to residents of assisted living settings; such services either complement the services provided by in-house staff, or even act as the main mechanism for care. Some state Medicaid programs pay for the services in alternative residential settings under their HCBS waiver programs, leaving the charges for room and board to be covered from the income and resources of the consumer. (This splitting is sometimes referred to as unbundling or separating the charges for housing from the charges for services.) If such unbundling were applied to nursing home settings as well, and if no regulatory constraints were imposed against high levels of care in alternative residential settings, current nursing home residents might well choose more home-like housing arrangements. Even without the unbundling, some nursing homes have already responded to the market pressures created by competition for privately paying long-term care consumers (who currently have more choices) by offering private rooms with private baths.

One of our goals is to transform the situation that currently requires so many people to live in nursing homes as we know them. Therefore, we see the blurring of boundaries between home care and "institutional care" as a positive development.[2] We also welcome any transformations of nursing homes from within. Nevertheless, we recognize that the policy strategy of unbundling charges for housing and for services and encouraging blurred boundaries between home care and institutional care has a potential pitfall: It is possible that some of the new residential settings have or will have all the problems currently associated with nursing homes. This risk renders it even more imperative to articulate what is meant by home-like environments, service capacity, and a philosophy that respects consumer choice, control, and dignity.

Nursing Homes

We turn first to the nursing home, where about 1.6 million Americans live, to consider what life in a nursing home is like, how it might be improved, and for whom it might still be "appropriate." With that as a backdrop, we can then examine other residentially based forms of long-term care and the challenges associated with developing and maintaining a home-like quality in places where people congregate for long-term care.

Even when they deliver impeccable quality of care, typical nursing homes cannot be construed as homelike settings. The shared sleeping space, cramped quarters, hospital-like physical arrangements, and institutional rules that govern daily life make a mockery of the cherished concept of home. The dread of nursing homes among prospective clientele is palpable. As part of a national study, researchers at participating sites polled more than 3,000 seriously ill hospitalized elderly patients to find out how willing they would be to live in a nursing home. Over a quarter of the respondents (26%) indicated they would be very unwilling to live in a nursing home and a startling 30% indicated that they would rather die than live in a nursing home; only 7% stated they would be very willing to live permanently in a nursing home.[3] Yet many long-term care clients who dread and avoid nursing homes cannot afford to organize the care they need in their current homes because the quality of their current living is poor and because the cost of the home care they need is prohibitive. They have to go somewhere else.

Two very different kinds of problems have been documented in nursing homes. First and most important, these institutions tend to be the antithesis of a home; they are built, staffed, and regulated as health care settings, and expectations for the behavior of residents are similar to expectations of hospital patients. Second and paradoxically, health care in these health care settings to which people have relocated because of health-related functional impairments tends to be inadequate. In short, nursing homes usually fail to respond to the basic needs of people to obtain a reasonable quality of life.

Nursing Homes as Living Environments

The litany of problems with nursing homes as places to live is familiar. Anthropologists and sociologists have documented the conditions well.[4] Past and present nursing home residents and staff members have also borne witness to the conditions in autobiographical or fictional treatments.[5] The evocative titles of these books— for example, *Uneasy Endings, Limbo, Ends of Time, A Home Is Not a Home*—tell the stories of sharing rooms with successions of not necessarily compatible strangers, crowded conditions, rigid routines, patronizing attitudes, healthful but unappetizing meals presented unattractively; programs that are designed for a lowest common denominator of functioning and often seem more suited for children; forced mingling of cognitively intact people with cognitively impaired people; and relentless protection that transfers into lack of privacy even in a bathtub. Activities tend to be compressed into weekday, daytime hours; morning starts ridiculously early, dinner is at an unfashionable four-thirty or five o'clock. Boredom and a sense of the unnatural prevail. Trips outside are construed as events. The stuff of ordinary life—music, conversation, newspaper reading, pets, gardening—is transformed, even in enlightened facilities, into therapies—music therapy, reminiscence therapy, current events discussions, pet therapy—and they are scheduled events with assigned participants. Homogenized religious activities, often stripped of their symbolism, are brought to the residents, sometimes on the wrong day of the week. Residents become detached from their pasts, and their current actions and reactions are charted as "behaviors." When guests come from the outside, residents are rarely empowered to offer them a comfortable chair, let alone a cup of tea and refreshments.

This picture is stark, but not unrealistic. Thus, Sheldon Tobin describes the maintenance of a sense of personal identity as one of the major challenges for nursing home residents.[6] An interview study with cognitively intact nursing home residents in forty-five nursing homes in five states found that the respondents gave high priority to their wish to control access to the outside world, such as use of the telephone and trips away from the home, and that they also tended to unsatisfied with the extent of control they could exercise over the timing and conduct of ordinary events, such as getting up, going to bed, eating, and bathing. Many also wanted to summon and interact directly with their physicians rather than through the intermediary and interpretive role of nursing staff. Moreover, staff with direct responsibility for care shared the view that control and choice over these somewhat mundane matters were important to residents but held pessimistic views about the likelihood of offering more choice to residents.[7]

The primary responsibility of nursing staff is to provide residents with care according to the care plan and keep residents protected. With working days full of routines and tasks (dubbed "bed and body work" by sociologist Jaber Gubrium[8]) to be performed under the general supervision of nurses, staff have little discretion or opportunity to innovate or individualize. Personnel is the major cost in nursing homes, yet line staff are hard pressed to respond to requests for what is perceived as extra nursing attention, such as, for example, unscheduled trips to the toilet or help getting in and out of bed upon request—let alone to respond to more socially oriented requests.

Efforts have been made to create communities in nursing homes and to emphasize resident governance and social solidarity,[9] but with only mixed success. In the last analysis, nursing homes are at best accidental and artificial communities. Consumers are rarely there through positive choice and must co-exist in close proximity to others who share similar needs for care rather than similar interests.

Nursing Homes as Care Settings
The dominant staff of long-term care institutions are nurse's aides, who are supervised by nurses. Medical direction, required by law, is often perfunctory. Preventive, diagnostic, or medical treatment in nursing homes tends to be inadequate. Somehow our society has not yet learned how to deliver primary health care effectively to people with chronic health problems who live in residential settings. Health authorities sometimes forget that the landscape of chronic illness is punctuated with acute illness, including both new problems and exacerbations of old problems. Nursing home residents bring all the classic challenges of geriatric medicine that are discussed in more detail in Chapter 8. They require, for example, appropriate and parsimonious use of medications; management of incontinence and the underlying problems that cause it; detection of acute illnesses such as infections

and heart disease when they present in atypical ways; vigilant guarding against iatrogenic problems that result from the therapies themselves; consciousness that foot care, hearing, vision, and dental care may improve functional abilities; and detection of untreated depression.

Ironically although nursing homes are health care settings, residents currently receive relatively little medical or health-related care. Interaction with physicians, sometimes to the distress of the residents, is formalized and mediated through the nursing home staff. Few nursing-home residents have found a way to consult with physicians as they might have done as an outpatient. Moreover, the amount of attention from nursing staff is also likely to be minimal. Based on data from multiple states, Alan Friedlob pointed out that nursing-home residents receive on average only 70 minutes of care a day from all nursing personnel, and only 5 minutes from a registered nurse.[10] This hardly sets the stage for active attention to health conditions.

Although residential institutions for long-term care should be built upon a social model, permitting ordinary lives of the residents to continue, therapeutic lethargy is hardly appropriate. Vigorous attention to health needs and health improvements should be possible without sacrificing social conditions. At present, too many institutional settings for the elderly fail on both the social and health care dimensions.

Toward a New Classification

Perhaps the greatest pitfall of the nursing home is that it is forced to be all things to all people. Heterogeneity of residents is a given. Residents differ from each other in health status, prognosis, expected length of stay, and cognitive abilities. Some are there for rehabilitation, some to die, and some have taken up permanent residency for an expected lengthy stay. They also differ in age (a 75-year-old has as much of a generation gap with a 95-year-old as a 35-year-old with a 55-year-old), culture, religion, education, interests, and preferences. And, unlike apartment complexes or even hotels, these disparate individuals are thrust together in shared sleeping and living spaces.

Health care policy makers have made a science out of classifying patients according to illness levels and care needs. These acuity indexes or, as the jargon goes, case-mix adjustors, are used to establish appropriate staffing levels and payment rates.[11] Although perhaps useful for hospital care (which nobody pretends is home), classification of nursing home residents tends to group people by characteristics that have little to do with whether they would enjoy living as neighbors, let alone roommates. We reject out of hand the idea of classifying nursing home residents at all if it follows that they will be routinely moved around the facility as their conditions change. However if groupings are to be made, we consider it useful to do so in a way that helps predict the desirable qualities of a residential care environment for the particular subgroup of clients and the kind as well as amount of care and staff support they might need. For that purpose, we would separate clientele now in nursing homes by their differing capacity for personal autonomy, their prognosis, and the likely duration of their need for care.

Table 6.1 presents a crude classification of people who might need care in group residential settings but have no need for the intensity of hospitals. The table over-simplifies complexities in the real world where people do not fit neatly into categories; it is designed to stimulate discussion about optimal kinds of residentially based programs rather than to present precise, measurable categories.[12]

At the far end of the spectrum are those relatively few nursing home residents who, for all practical purposes, have no interaction with their environments. They are comatose, in vegetative states, or experience Alzheimer's disease so advanced that they are virtually moribund. Beyond providing decent physical care out of respect for that individual's personhood and the sensibilities of family, little else can be done. Their quality of life cannot be improved. A hospital-like ward where efficiencies can be maximized may well be a suitable environment for such people. Designing residential environments to maximize convenience and efficiency of staff and minimize cost seems appropriate here. One cannot distinguish this group by likely duration of the need for care or by length of stay. Some people live only a short time in this "twilight zone," whereas others live for many years in comatose or moribund states even when respirators are disconnected.

Other nursing home residents are ill and need acute care and monitoring during a period of convalescence. They may also need help with personal care and housing for a period of time. They can receive care in their own homes, if two conditions are met: The monitoring and medically oriented care they need is intermittent and, therefore, can be mustered in individual homes, and the patient has sufficient resources or family help to assist with functional needs during this period of time. Often, however, circumstances require the consumer to move for the convalescent period. If the time is sufficiently limited and the consumer understands the nursing home stay as temporary, he or she may be willing to tolerate hospital-like conditions. However, the accounts of some older people who experience short stays in nursing homes during convalescence reveal that the experience can be perceived as traumatic as well as unpleasant. For example, a respondent in one of our studies recounted having had eleven different roommates during a 6-week nursing home stay, five of whom died in his presence. Other respondents recounted being frightened by other residents with dementia or humiliated by being lined up and undressed in the corridor for showers. Reasonably planned convalescent care should be able to avoid much of this hardship.

Still other nursing home residents need a course of rehabilitation, for a hip fracture, a stroke, or a spinal cord injury, as well as varying degrees of help with daily living until maximum functional abilities are attained. If an expensive rehabilitation team, specialized equipment, and a complex daily schedule is required, or if the individual lacks home support for routine care needed during this period, then the person may need to relocate to receive the care efficiently. The optimal

Table 6.1. Consumer Characteristics Related to Care Needs and Environmental Requirements

Consumer characteristic	Care needs	Predicted duration	Autonomy capacity	Environmental requirements
Terminal illness	Pain control; management of symptoms; possible high tech	Short	Moderate; fluctuating	Psychosocial support & physical comfort; takes weakness, low energy, & debility into account
Convalescence—e.g., postcoronary; post-surgery	Monitoring; personal care & daily living help while recuperating	Short	High	Maintenance of lifestyle; consumer may be willing to trade off normal lifestyles for health care monitoring and recovery
Comatose; vegetative	High to moderate; possible high tech	Uncertain	None	Inexpensive; convenient for staff; patient does not interact with environment at all and has no requirements
Rehabilitation potential—new condition—e.g., strokes, fractures, spinal cord injuries	Varies by condition; data not good on necessary inputs for results; personal care & daily living help	Usually short	High	Therapeutic environment to create physical challenge and morale; consumer may be willing to trade off normal life style for rehabilitation results
Chronic condition—cognitively alert	Personal care and daily living help; primary care monitoring; acute care and rehabilitation as new conditions warrant	Long	High	Permitting autonomy, dignity, privacy, and normal lifestyles; no enforced mingling with cognitively impaired
Chronic condition—cognitively impaired	Personal care and daily living help; oversight and supervision; acute care and rehabilitation as new conditions warrant; intermittent	Long	Moderate or low	Tailored to dementia; maximize function and orientation, minimize environmental demand, and offer protection

environment, whether in a private home or an institutional setting, needs to be therapeutically designed for the particular kind of rehabilitation being undertaken. Even though the consumer may be willing to trade off some aspects of lifestyle for the hope of recovered physical abilities, the amenities of the living environment and the opportunity for normal social interaction surely should make a difference. Morale is, after all, associated with rehabilitation success.

Substantial numbers of nursing home residents needing heavy levels of care are terminally ill but, for one reason or another, cannot receive care in their own homes. Until their last days and weeks, however, their physical and social environment for living out their lives is important. The environment needs to be geared toward privacy, comfort, normal lifestyles, and psychological support. They also are likely to need skilled management of pain and discomfort and may or may not need high-tech interventions. They may need an environment conducive for family members to gather and be with them and each other during the months, weeks, days, and hours before their deaths.

The last two rows of Table 6.1 depict the large numbers of residents (perhaps half of all those admitted to nursing homes) who are likely to need help with personal care and daily living for long periods of time or indefinitely. These are people with chronic illnesses and disabilities who have completed a recuperative period or course of rehabilitation and still have need for care, as well as those for whom no rehabilitation is feasible. It is useful to divide this group into people who are cognitively intact and those who are not. The environment is important for both, but the details if an optimal environment may differ.

People who have physical disabilities but retain the ability to direct their lives need a living environment that permits them to live meaningfully, exercise choice, and maintain social ties and familiar lifestyles as much as possible. The physical environment should use features and technology in architectural design and furnishing to help people compensate for impairments in mobility, communication, strength, dexterity, or sensory abilities.[13] The living environment should also permit people the privacy, control, and flexibility that anyone would desire in their own home or apartment. We earlier pointed out the modest amounts of attention that nursing home residents receive on average from the care staff, including nurses, licensed practical nurses (LPNs), and nursing assistants. Of course, these small amounts of nursing-staff total time—amounting to about an hour and a half a day— are distributed across the entire day and night and are hard to replicate at home for a reasonable cost. Yet, these small amounts of care and oversight can surely be arranged in such a way that the quality of life be less compromised than in a typical United States nursing home.

Older people with cognitive limitations also seem to thrive in normal living environments that permit them to exercise whatever capabilities they have for self-direction, but they also seem to benefit by safe living settings that have cues for orientation and are not unduly complex. Those who have moderate or greater dementia will need and want reminding, suggestions for how to spend their day, and intermittent attention initiated by staff; they are unlikely to be able to make many decisions. The physical environment may need to be adapted for safe wandering and features that promote way-finding.

Whether cognitively or physically impaired only, a large range of people in nursing homes appear to benefit by a normal, "unmedicalized" environment. Many such individuals seem to thrive in small family homes or adult foster homes[14] as well as in assisted living settings where they have their own apartment, but where the staff supervision and structure are increased to provide cues for daily activities and oversight for safety.[15] Even in nursing homes, in part because of the need to create a less disturbing environment for people without dementia,[16] the trend is decidedly toward special care units for people with Alzheimer's disease where environments are simplified and no undue demands or strictures are placed on the resident.

Improving Nursing Homes

Although many people now cared for in nursing homes could be more happily served in other residential settings, the search for alternatives is no reason to neglect positive changes within nursing homes themselves. Such changes can address the living situation, the care situation, or both. Often nursing home providers have become convinced that pervasive regulations, limited budgets, and fixed physical configurations preclude doing anything at all to improve the lives of nursing home residents.

Even within the constraints of shared rooms, heavy disability levels, and relentless pressures of care routines, both life and care in nursing homes can be improved. Supporting this contention are three decades of both isolated and systematic efforts to make changes that can improve the lives of nursing-home residents. Perhaps because of the paucity of stimulation and individual attention in nursing homes, most small-scale studies of interventions tend to show measurable benefit for the residents, regardless of what the intervention is or its intended effect.[17] Reform efforts have been directed toward both lifestyle issues and care issues. Many of the former have entailed increasing the control and choice for nursing home residents or developing ways that nursing-home residents can have greater access to the world outside the nursing home. That can be accomplished both by bringing outsiders in, or, more satisfactorily if the resident's condition permits, by arranging for the resident to leave the facility to pursue their own interests. Too often residents leave nursing homes only for health-related activities.

To improve care and health status, structural changes have been put in place to improve primary care for nursing home residents. Some rely on nurse practitioners, who are either employed by the nursing home or by the primary care provider or health care plan. Affiliations between nursing homes and schools of nursing also are helpful in creating a positive clinical atmosphere.[18] Continence training programs have had positive results; some of these not only attempt to modify the behavior of residents, but also the behavior of staff who need to keep to a toileting schedule.[19] In another example, a Canadian nursing home performed a randomized trial of physical therapy for a stable nursing-home population (as opposed to those undergoing formal rehabilitation), finding positive functional outcomes even for people previously presumed to be unable to benefit from therapy.[20] Generally speaking, any efforts that increase attention to the health status of nursing home residents tend to be useful, and this includes teaching nursing home staff how to make systematic observations and what to do with the information.

In the 1970s, Robert Kane demonstrated the utility of this approach in a group of nursing homes in Utah.[21] In some homes, the research team took on primary care for the Medicaid residents, using a nurse practitioner as the lead, backed up by physicians, pharmacists, and social workers. An important hallmark of the approach was the initiating of a recording system and a set of benchmarks of progress that could be used by staff with low literacy levels. In turn, nursing assistants were taught to distinguish between information that needed to be brought to the immediate attention of a nursing supervisor and information that could be communicated through more routine channels. The entire program of health care proved in the demonstration nursing homes proved cost-effective compared to the regular care received by Medicaid residents in other Utah nursing homes.

Some efforts to improve health care in nursing homes involve modification of the financial arrangements for medical care and even hospital care for nursing home residents to create better incentives to provide timely and high-quality care for resident populations. Some such programs are discussed in Chapter 8, which deals with the relationship between LTC and acute care. Highlighted below are some efforts that do not necessarily involve capitation or altering basic financial arrangements for nursing homes.

Alzheimer's special care units. At least 50% of nursing home residents are estimated to suffer from Alzheimer's disease or some form of cognitive impairment. Critics point out that nursing homes have not been geared to meet the needs of that large group. Often people with dementia experience the nursing home as a complex living situation with bureaucratic arrangements, and institutional-style physical spaces that could exacerbate confusion. Typically, programming and environments in nursing homes are not designed for Alzheimer's disease. Moreover, people with dementia who become labeled as having "behavior problems" may experience further restriction of their activities.

Many nursing homes have responded by developing special care units (SCUs) for people with Alzheimer's disease. Such SCUs began appearing even in the 1970s, but the widespread proliferation of the programs took place in the 1990s. An SCU is at minimum a geographically separated part of the facility that is dedicated to serving people with Alzheimer's disease. Some of its special programming is made possible because of its targeted population, but SCUs at their best are "special" with regard to the training and skills of their staff; the purposeful design and use of the physical space, the furnishings, and other appointments in the environment; and their special programs tailored to people with dementia. SCU programs are often characterized by a great deal of one-on-one attention of staff, but frequent, short, structured activities are also typical. The physical environment may be simplified and cut down to size by having most meals and activities right on the unit. SCUs may use music and exercise programs to good purpose, capitalizing on long-range memory that permits pleasure in old songs, a seemingly innate enjoyment of music, and the restless energy that many people with dementia exhibit. Some SCUs feature safe indoor and outdoor wandering paths; the very features that would be obstacles for people with physical impairments in wheelchairs or walkers can present interesting environments for people with dementia.

Finally, SCUs often are organized so as to engage family members in the care and life of the program. Some SCUs attempt to create a biography of the resident so that staff will have a sense not only of who the resident is but who the resident was prior to being diagnosed with dementia; one program combines family involvement with the creation of the biography, which family then present to staff. This biography task helps family members bring closure to their decision to use the nursing home and is seen as having good effects for both residents and their caring relatives. (Developing techniques to remind nursing home staff that residents are people with lives and interests is a technique that should be widely applied. Although these biographical devices were developed especially for demented residents, they can be usefully employed in various forms for all.)

Nursing homes seldom serve all their residents with dementia in their SCUs. Selection criteria for SCUs vary, as do the philosophies of the particular unit. Some SCUs concentrate on ambulatory people with dementia, especially those whose behavior is difficult in the nursing home as a whole, and move people to another part of the nursing home if they become wheelchair-bound or reach a terminal stage. Other SCUs undertake to care for the person until they die or leave the nursing home. Some SCUs have structured themselves to minimize stimulation, whereas others seek to create a stimulating environment.

The jury is still out on the effectiveness of SCUs. Because of their variation in nature, philosophy, and target group served, the expected outcomes would be particular to the SCUs' goals and activities. In general, however, it would seem sensible to identify some easily observed indicators of well-being that have face validity. In an SCU, one would expect that observable distress should be minimized and observable pleasure maximized. Perhaps, one should also expect that people with dementia would sleep well (without benefit of sleeping pills), that use of psychoactive drugs would be rare, and physical restraints would be almost nonexistent. Also not clear is whether SCU care needs to be more expensive than other nursing home care. Although originally marketed vigorously with a higher price tag than usual care, some analysts argue that the care should not necessarily be more expensive even though the money may be distributed differently.

Some people also argue that the SCU assists people without dementia by removing from the immediate environment people whose behavior might be disturbing to them or whose diminished competence interferes with social activities. This benefit also seems logical and likely, but because SCUs almost never treat all or even most nursing home residents with dementia, their full effect would not be felt as long as cognitively intact people are still living in close proximity to people with dementia on the regular units. On the negative side, some advocates for people with dementia fear that their loved ones will become isolated and neglected on SCUs. They see the ultimate ideal as infusion of the best principles of dementia care throughout the facility, a strategy that is feasible for many of the elements, but not for the physical environment, and which may have a negative effect on the quality of life of people in nursing homes who do not have dementia.[22]

The Eden alternative. Unlike SCUs, which depend in part on bricks and mortar, the Eden Alternative is a philosophy that can be applied in existing facilities without altering the buildings. Its founder, William H. Thomas, is a physician who became medical director of a traditional nursing home in upstate New York by dint of becoming a practitioner in a small community. Appalled by the isolation and loneliness of the residents and the stultifying atmosphere driven by routines, he gradually evolved his "Eden Alternative" as an approach to promote human flourishing in nursing homes.[23] By now well publicized in the popular press, the Eden Alternative has been associated with making deep-seated changes in the nursing-home climate and the expectations of all who are involved—residents and staff. Animals, birds, and plants are omnipresent in facilities that have adopted the Eden Alternative, and mechanisms to bring children into the facilities are encouraged. Although journalists tend to pick up particularly on the idea of a nursing home as a habitat for companion animals (typically hundreds of birds and substantial numbers of cats in a 100-bed facility), the philosophy of the Eden Alternative goes much deeper. The idea is to create an atmosphere where spontaneity is possible; where loneliness, helplessness, and boredom are combated directly; and rigid hours for routines and activities are minimized. Nurse's aides and housekeepers are involved in the care, and efforts are made to empower frontline care attendants so they in turn are free to individualize decisions for the clients. In a 1997 *Washington Post* article,[24] Judy Thomas, a partner in the Eden Alternative efforts, offers the following prescription: "End the rigid hours residents must keep for meals, baths, and bedtime; let them sleep in some mornings if they choose. Throw out the time clock and let workers schedule themselves."

The Eden Alternative has so far been associated with a reduction in depression and medication use and higher retention rates and less absenteeism among staff (helpful testimony in a cost-effectiveness age). The main effects are harder to quantify, however: sounds of laughter, a sense of energy and purpose, a sense of family. Missouri and North Carolina have both taken steps to "Edenize" their facilities, with North Carolina "dangling grants of up to $25,000 to encourage facilities to adopt Eden techniques." Several large nursing home corporations are also planning pilot projects using Eden Alternative principles.

Improving quality of life. The pendulum has swung somewhat away from consideration of quality of care in nursing homes to considerations of quality of life for nursing home residents. Accordingly, nursing homes are increasingly expected to enable dignity, privacy, a sense of identity, continuity, social involvement, and meaningful social relationships for their residents. The Eden Alternative is just one approach to transforming nursing into more habitable developing places.

Most efforts related to quality of life try to restore control and choice to residents and help them realize their own goals. In one facility, for example, residents interviewed prospective nursing assistants as part of the hiring process. Some efforts build on residents' particular skills or wisdom, for example, having them serve as history or language teachers to school age children or even college students. One facility that bills itself as a "regenerative community" has a daily meeting in the dining room after breakfast where anyone may raise issues of concern or interest.

All such efforts to break with customary role and expectations for passivity among residents are welcome. However, the key to success is to avoid giving way to complacency after small successes. It has been pointed out that true reform in the quality of nursing home life requires nothing short of culture change.[25] Such change is slow and painstaking. Similarly, as Chapter 7 suggests, it is dangerous to allow simplistic markers to stand in for concepts like dignity, meaningful relationships and the other attributes of a good quality of life. It makes a mockery of these goals to consider them met by a few easily measured facility practices and policies. In truth, only the residents can attest to their own quality of lives, and facilities where staff routinely ask residents about their quality of life (or, in more usual language, about the extent to which their lives are good) and how their lives could be improved have already taken an important step towards the goal of improving quality of life.

Adult Foster Homes

An adult foster home is a small group residential setting, housing just a few residents. (It also goes by other names, such as small group homes, family care homes, domiciliary care homes, and, in one state, homes plus.) The usual range is three to six residents, and the settings resemble private residences in most respects. States typically license adult foster homes and promulgate rules about the requirements of the environment and the personnel, and shape the setting by their admission and retention rules that enunciate the kinds of residents the facility is permitted to serve and those it must not serve. States that pay for adult foster care through Medicaid or other reimbursement programs have another way of shaping the service: The amount they choose to pay dictates the levels of disability that can be served.[26]

Adult foster care homes closely resemble private homes in the community. In the most typical model, the owner of the home or someone hired by the owner lives there and directly provides the cooking, housekeeping, and care services the resident needs. Meals are served family style, and family members come and go in the setting as partners to the care. Adult foster care homes are a cottage industry of sorts. Typically, foster homes cannot make a profit unless they have a lean staff—perhaps limited to family members of the foster care provider and a few hired helpers for peak hours. Such foster homes obviously cannot use an elaborate division of labor; they depend on a flexible ability to handle whatever needs to be done. Ordinarily, they will be unable to care for Medicaid or low-income clientele with heavy levels of disability unless state regulation permits nursing functions to be done by foster care personnel without nursing licenses or unless (for Medicaid) reimbursement is high enough to permit contracting with nurses. (The latter is unlikely since few states would undertake the higher risks they believe are associated with foster care without the lure of lower public costs.)

A variant of adult foster care is the "corporate" or "chain" model, where one firm owns several adult foster care homes and staffs them with live-in providers. The corporate office may provide some common services—shopping that relies on bulk purchases, nurse consultation, transportation, and so on. The advantage of the corporate model is its ability to bring more services to the foster home clientele and perhaps provide backup and support services. The disadvantage is the potential erosion of the home-like atmosphere. A further variant of corporate foster care used shift staff rather than a live-in manager; some states would prohibit this model in their licensure, however. Some states attempt to provide support and quality control for adult foster care programs by licensing oversight agencies, which, in turn, have responsibility to recruit foster care providers, train and supervise personnel, and even match them with clients. This strategy, for example, was adopted in the initial rules established by the State of New Jersey, but it is under reconsideration as this book goes to press.

Adult foster care homes have proven particularly suited for people with dementia, who may benefit by the small scale and the familiarity of the home-like setting. They may also be adaptable to rural areas that might have difficulty supporting a larger program. Relatively few evaluations of adult foster care have been performed, and the service modality has only recently emerged as a setting for middle-class people. An early program run by Queens Hospital in Hawaii proved beneficial to people leaving the acute care hospital, but the program reported some difficulty in persuading family members that "some other woman" could care for their relative where they themselves were not able to do so. Another issue that arose in Hawaii was cultural. Most of the clientele for the foster homes were of Japanese or Anglo ancestry and many of the foster care providers were originally from the Phillipines. In the intimacy of the family group, these disparities sometimes led to unsatisfactory arrangements.[27] Foster care homes are in plentiful supply also in upstate New York and one evaluation reported a highly satisfied clientele.[28] Other evaluations of adult foster care are under way in Washington and in Michigan.

The state of Oregon made adult foster care one of the first planks in its efforts to identify viable alternative to nursing homes. Oregon defines an adult foster home as a care setting in a residentially zoned area that may be licensed to care for one to five people, where meals are taken family style, and where a resident manager lives in the setting. From the beginning of its HCBS waiver in 1981, Oregon covered services in adult foster care under the Medicaid program. The stimulation of a public payment source accelerated the growth of foster homes, and the option, which is about two-thirds the price of nursing homes, proved popular in the private market. Since the program stabilized in the late 1980s, about two-thirds of the residents have been paying privately for foster care, and a 1989 evaluation showed that those privately paying clients were even more disabled on average than the Medicaid clients, all of whom had to be deemed nursing home certifiable to qualify for the service.[29]

By that time, foster care had become a mainstream, middle-class option in Oregon, available in elaborate upscale homes and in modest surroundings. In this cross-sectional study where researchers collected original data to look at both privately paying and Medicaid residents, the functional outcomes were comparable for the two settings and social and psychological outcomes seemed to favor foster care.[30] Further longitudinal studies were done using data collected by case managers for the Medicaid population only. Here functional abilities tended to be stable in both foster care and nursing homes, but among those who experienced a change in physical functioning, improvements were more likely in nursing homes and declines more likely in foster care.[31] Although the authors still concluded that adult foster care was a viable choice for long-term care consumers, the results introduced a cautionary suggestion that health care and rehabilitation efforts should not be neglected in adult foster care, which is very much a "social model" of care.

Assisted Living

Assisted living is a relatively new umbrella term for any residential setting that goes beyond the family home qualities of adult foster care, that provides real personal care, and that is not licensed as a nursing home. Like adult foster care, assisted living is defined through state licensure policies. Some states view assisted living as a step on a continuum for people not disabled enough to need nursing homes, whereas others view assisted living as a viable choice for people with the same disability levels as nursing home residents. States also vary as to the requirements and prohibitions they build into the physical environments. To add complications, a few states use the term assisted living to refer to a model of service regardless of where the consumer lives. Thus programs designed to promote "aging in place" could bring assisted living services into any private home or apartment or group residential setting where the consumer lives, including single-rooms-only residential hotel and public housing. (Minnesota instituted this approach.) In this book, we consider assisted living more narrowly to refer to congregate living settings with services attached.[32]

Oregon is a bellwether state for assisted living, having made an early effort to articulate its elements. There, any entity licensed as an assisted living facility (ALF) must offer a single-occupancy apartment (which may be a small studio apartment) with a full bathroom inside the apartment, a refrigerator and a stove or microwave, individual temperature controls, a locking door, and voice-to-voice communications. In contrast to these prescriptive rules for the environment, rules for services are much less specific. The facility must offer three meals a day and provide or arrange the array of personal care and nursing services that permit people to stay in the setting almost indefinitely, and at least one staff member must be awake and on duty at all times. The philosophy of promoting dignity, choice, privacy, independence, and normal lifestyles is built right into the regulations.

Oregon's rules for Assisted Living were published in 1990 when the state had only three licensed ALFs. Since then this service sector rapidly expanded to more than 90 licensed ALFs in 1998. Most are staff models, meaning that most care services are supplied by personnel employed by the ALF, supplemented by services from home care agencies and hospices from time to time. Oregon-style ALFs are controversial. Some critics believe that the privacy provided and the unprotected access to showers, microwaves, and refrigerators are unsafe for people with nursing-home levels of impairment. Some believe that the amenities are unnecessary and frivolous. For example, if most residents don't cook real meals, skeptics ask why they need kitchenettes. Yet another criticism is that the privacy is isolating and that roommates would be preferable. We touched on our own opinions about these issues already in Chapter 3. Indeed, the privacy and the autonomy-enhancing features of assisted living in Oregon mean that the model has many of the same advantages as being in one's own apartment dwelling.

Assisted living usually has two component prices, one for the real estate rental and meals, and one for the care services. For privately paying individuals, most ALFs list a variety of rental rates for room and board based on the size and location of the unit. These rates are typically based on single occupancy with an additional charge if another person lives in the unit. That add-on charge for the second person covers the extra housekeeping services and the meals; it is ordinarily much less than for the first person in the unit. Facilities vary as to the amount of services that are incorporated in the basic rate for room and board; most include some general oversight, an activities program, and weekly housekeeping and laundry. Many include transportation to doctors and scheduled transportation to shopping areas; some include the services of a health clinic, and a few include a minimum amount of personal care. After the basic rental package, the prices for services escalate according to the needs of the individuals and the amount of service they choose to purchase. (For example, some people may need extensive laundry assistance because of incontinence but decide that a family member will do that laundry rather than incorporate it into the bill.) Typically, ALFs establish three or four levels of service over and above their base rate. Alternatively, some programs charge according to a point system where each point on the assessment of the resident translates into a sum of money. The average private-pay rates for ALF residents in Oregon are less than 80% of the average private-pay rates for nursing-home residents.

Oregon's Medicaid program pays for services in ALFs if the resident is eligible for nursing-home care under Medicaid. Residents pay a fixed minimum for the rent portion from their social security income, in some instances receiving a small SSI supplement from the state if their own income fails to cover the rate. Medicaid rates for ALFs are established at five levels. As of January 1, 1998, these ranged from currently established at five levels ranging from $999.70 to $2,063.70, with $420.70 of that construed as the price for room and board, ordinarily paid for by residents from their retirement incomes. ALF operators point out that the combined rent and service income that they can receive from Medicaid residents is substantially lower than their charges to private pay residents. In some markets and some firms, therefore, ALF operators limit the proportion of people on Medicaid whom they accept. Nevertheless, some ALFs have 50% or more of their residents on Medicaid, and statewide about a third of the residents are supported by Medicaid.[33]

Some states, such as Washington, New Jersey, Texas, and Arizona, have followed the Oregon pattern and reserved the term assisted living for programs that assure privacy and some similar amenities. But many states, including those that reimburse or plan to reimburse assisted living under Medicaid, license shared accommodations as well as single-occupancy accommodations as assisted living. Also, the fully contained apartment is far from a universal standard. Some board-and-care homes comprised of small single or shared sleeping rooms with bathrooms down the hall also can be licensed as assisted living in some states. Recalling the three-legged stool presented earlier in this chapter in Figure 6.1, we argue that the residential living environment and the philosophy of care cannot be achieved in some of the settings licensed as assisted living in some states. Note, too, that some states have discouraged staff models of assisted living (partly by instituting rules that require many services to be performed or supervised by a nurse). Thus, in some states, the norm is that most personal care and nursing services is brought in by arrangement with home care agencies. This contractual model as opposed to a staff model is not in itself a problem in achieving the three elements of a good residential setting with services. However, it may be more expensive to mount the service capability when outside home care providers are utilized for routine personal care and medication management and few services are provided by the staff of the assisted living facility.

Blending Housing and Services

The assisted living programs described in the previous section are an example of blending housing and services in new ways to create a full range of services in a homelike residential environment. The blending involves both "bundling" and "unbundling." Some services are typically bundled into the housing. Indeed, if each person living in an ALF organized his or her own services separately, all the efficiencies would disappear. On the other hand, for payment purposes providers can and do distinguish between their room and board and "hotel" services and their care services. Thus, governmental programs and private insurers can choose to treat the two sets of payments separately, a disaggregation that is not feasible currently for nursing homes.

If such new blends of housing and services are to become widespread, viable options for many people now in traditional nursing homes, some potential problems must be resolved. Otherwise there is a danger that the societal promise of assisted living will be broken. For instance, assisted living could largely be developed as an option for the wealthy, and, within that framework, prices are likely to be all that the market can bear. Alternatively, assisted living could be developed as an option for people with few service needs. Or, in yet another scenario, assisted living could be developed by bringing services into board-and-care homes without the emphasis on privacy, dignity, and normal living situations that make the concept attractive. To avoid these various problems, sustained policy attention is needed.

Health Services Within a Low-Price Social Model

Oregon has achieved its lower price for assisted living services compared to nursing homes in large part through eliminating rules and permitting flexible approaches to staffing. In particular, the delegation of nursing services, described in Chapter 5 apropos of home care, also applies to staff in assisted living settings, adult foster care settings, and virtually any setting other than a hospital or nursing home. If a registered nurse teaches a caregiver to do any care task and vouches for that delegate's ability to do it properly, the delegate may then perform the function without close supervision by the nurse. It is up to the nurse to decide whether the task can be safely delegated to that individual and to establish what kind of oversight might be needed. If the nurse performs the delegation properly, she is not liable for any malfeasance on the part of the person who had been delegated to do the task. Nursing trade associations and policy makers are giving serious thought to the extent to which nursing practices should be modified to permit more delegation of nursing tasks in HCBS. Against it from nurses' perspectives are the usual guild considerations that no professional wants to work their way out of a job, concerns about legal liabilities, genuine concerns about the safety of the consumers, and fear that the policy would be used inappropriately and coercively to cut costs. On the other hand, some nurses note that delegating authority can be empowering for nurses, enabling them to use their full range of skills, and "keeping them in the loop" where arrangements have previously simply bypassed them. Both the hopes and the anxieties that surround this issue were reflected in the title of a 1996 conference on the subject, called "Autonomy or Abandonment: Changing Perspectives on Delegation."[34]

Policy makers and the general public are not comfortable relaxing standards for the credentials of those who minister to vulnerable people needing long-term care, especially frail older people. There is still a strong belief that credentials themselves are the best way to guarantee quality of input and good results. Experimenting with another model of group residential care for the same people who might be in nursing homes without the minimal protections nursing homes offer strikes some advocates as foolhardy. The credentials of those doing nursing tasks are not the only issue at stake. ALFs may have only one person on duty at night for a group of twenty or so residents. Clearly, this single person cannot accomplish two-person transfers or deal simultaneously with two emergencies. Oregon-style ALFs often achieve their efficiencies by using generic, cross-trained workers, expecting almost anyone to be able to step into any job (a personal care attendant can run laundry loads at night, a cook can assist in transferring a resident) and staffing up and down for peak times of day. The environments are organized to facilitate easy movement for people with disabilities and easy communication (e.g., through voice-to-voice communications between staff and resident's apartments and state-of-the-art call systems).

What is really at stake in resolving this issue and many others is determining what kind of a place a group residential setting for people with long-term care needs should be. Is it like a private apartment in a building where many of the other renters also have long-term care needs? Is it like a full-service hotel, which has expanded its "room service" to include personal care and nursing services? Or is it like a hospital or nursing home? If it is like the first two, it is not expected that all problems that might arise can be anticipated and solved in advance. More help will need to be brought in when a large number of people have a lot of care needs at night. With an emergency, staff and or residents will summon paramedics by calling 911 just as people do in their own homes. Assisted living settings will have some advantages of easier access to nursing and other health personnel and standardized procedures and competence in handling some recurrent emergencies, but all risks will not be minimized by having a large staff of credentialed health workers around the clock. But if the model is a hospital or a current nursing home, then the loss of autonomy for the residents is expected to be compensated for by guaranteed protection.

Privacy and Amenities: Their Value and Price

Our vision of the residential care setting of the future offers private occupancy in at-least studio-size apartments with familiar features of home contained therein: a refrigerator and cooking setup, and a full bathroom. Is this realistic as a policy goal? First, it goes against the puritan grain to make subsidized accommodations for low-income people too comfortable. Taxpayers and the legislators representing them question whether they should subsidize even small self-contained apartments in lieu of the multiple-bed rooms they have subsidized in nursing homes since 1965. Kitchenettes are said to be wasteful if the residents have their meals prepared for them by the program. Second, some providers believe that long-term care consumers should not be isolated behind closed doors. Rooms in nursing homes are never locked, and rarely closed. Even though the convention is to knock before entering, the fact that they are largely shared gives them a somewhat public quality. Staff and visitors come in and out more readily than when the unit is known to belong to one person or one couple. This quasi-public nature of the space is seen as an advantage by those who truly worry about the safety of residents who cannot be easily and quickly supervised. Similarly, full bathrooms and kitchenettes may be seen as opportunities for injuries from scalding water, slippery shower floors, or stovetops. Because we have become so accustomed to the privations of the nursing-home room, we have also come to see this form as a prudent way to provide care. Oddly, it is almost as though the shared, minimalist space is considered natural and the small, private, self-contained apartment an aberration that has to prove itself.

The case for privacy needs to be made on two levels: value and price. Its intrinsic worth to the consumer needs to be established. Then, there follows discussion about what such privacy would cost, and who would bear those costs.

The case for the intrinsic value of privacy is easily made. Heath professionals and long-term care providers sometimes speak positively about the friendship and companionship that can occur among roommates in nursing homes and the way roommates sometimes help each other out. But there is absolutely no empirical evidence to suggest that these positive reactions to shared rooms tend to occur or that companionship and helpfulness are promoted by forced shared rooms. On the contrary, all available evidence converges to state the opposite.[35] People not yet in a facility dread the shared space above most things, and people already in facilities say they would much prefer to have private rooms and baths, and would be willing to accept much less in the way of planned programs and activities in exchange. People with Alzheimer's disease are often unable to speak for themselves on this issue, but many of their advocates believe that they too would, on the whole, flourish better if not forced to share living space. Certainly people who are cognitively intact dread the thought of a roommate with Alzheimer's disease, though, in fairness, they are opposed to any roommate who was previously unknown to them. Nursing home residents do not react to forced proximity to others by forming intimate or close relationships. On the whole, intimacy and friendship flourish when privacy is available. Older people forced to share rooms in nursing homes and board-and-care homes put up with it. They assume it is inevitable. They do not "adapt" or come to like it. Many tell poignant stories about the indignities and problems about their experiences with shared rooms and baths.

The sticking point, therefore, is price. The price charged to private and public payers is in part a matter of what the market will allow, but clearly there is some minimum sum required to produce the care at all. Is this minimum sum much greater for private space than for shared space? Industry groups attest that private rooms and baths are prohibitively costly. What they probably mean, however, is that it might be prohibitively costly for them to convert existing stock into the new form. It is useful, however, to separate the costs of new developments from those of retooling existing programs.

According to one analysis, modeled by considering a 39-unit building under more or less expensive construction and more or less favorable lending arrangements,[36] the difference between building for 78 residents in 39 units versus 39 residents in 39 units would range from $6.30 a day to $3.20 a day per tenant. This slightly higher construction cost and, therefore, higher debt service was projected to be offset by sharply lower operational costs in the single-occupancy apartments.

Among the reasons for greater costliness in operating shared facilities were higher maintenance (since frequent roommate switches cause more wear and tear and more need for moving assistance; higher housekeeping costs (because higher needs or preferences from one resident lead to spending more resources on both); higher costs in maintaining common-use areas and more demand for entertainment; increased needs for highly paid staff to deal with conflict resolution and behavior management; higher demand for tray service in rooms since the time a roommate is in the dining room is the only time the other roommate can be assured of being alone; and greater dependence on residence-provided snacks.

By far the greatest extra cost of shared space, however, relates to the costs of vacancies and the difficulties in roommate matching. If a unit is vacant for a week more because of the difficulty in finding a new occupant, a whole year's savings on the development and construction costs are more than wiped out. Individualized services such as personal care and nursing, of course, are charged according to the individual's need, and it is presumed that the staff will be sufficient to perform the services for which residents are billed. These services should cost the same whether the person receiving them lives alone in their unit or with someone else.

Based on these kinds of analyses, it seems unnecessary to cleave to shared space as a norm. Nor does it seem necessary for those providers who do offer private units to conceptualize this as a deluxe feature worthy of vastly inflated prices and unaffordable for people living on SSI alone. In any transition, political concerns would be voiced by those providers who already had invested in double stock. For example, if nursing homes were required to switch to small private apartments or even private rooms and baths, the cost of refurbishing and new plumbing would be out of reach for most. Similarly, if a state developed an assisted living benefit that could only be used in apartment-style facilities, many existing board-and-care homes could not convert their premises to take advantage of the new subsidy. Nonetheless, the policy changes need to begin somewhere. Over the last 30 years, while arguments about hardships to existing nursing homes prohibited new rules on the subjects, many new facilities were built, mostly relying on shared occupancy.

First the political will needs to be summoned to create a standard of privacy, and then the details of how the policies will be phased in will follow. Some states may wish to provide incentives for firms that retool, while others will feel no obligation to protect part of any particular industry. States that subsidize long-term care in various residential settings will need to resign themselves to paying a price predicated on single occupancy. On the other hand, states will need to steel themselves to come up with what they view as a fair price rather than to allow facilities to set the price based on their self-reported costs.

The question remains as to whether some people simply cannot benefit from privacy, either in a nursing home or assisted living, nor from any of the other environmental amenities proposed. One might argue that extremely debilitated people, those who are comatose or virtually moribund, need not have an apartment and that their living arrangements and furnishings should be organized to facilitate the convenience and comfort of staff who tend them. There would still be a concern for the human dignity of the people receiving care, however, and for the dignity and feelings of family members who came to visit them. Even hospitals, where the stay is temporary, seem to be moving toward privacy. There seems to be an enormous advantage in switching the presumption to one that says that all residential care facilities, even nursing homes, will be eventually based on a norm of private accommodations. People who want to share would be the exception, though sharing would not be prohibited, and such people would achieve some economic advantages through sharing.

How to Regulate

As new models for residential care are developed, a key challenge will be determining how and what to regulate. It is tempting to build on the models already in place, most notably the nursing home. That kind of thinking begins with all the nursing home regulations as a given. The questions that follow are: Do we need all these regulations? If not, why not, if the populations served have similar disabilities? What regulations and expenditures can be dispensed with? More useful, however, would be a broad, fresh dialogue that examines how to construct protections for vulnerable long-term care consumers wherever they are.

Regulatory policy poses a serious dilemma. One the one hand, the desire to create a different type of institution argues for regulatory reform that would allow for more flexibility and would encourage more attention to quality of life issues. However, many of those looking at the emerging ALFs fear that these institutions may become the reinvented nursing homes and that we may have to relive the history of catastrophe and regulatory response that marked the last two decades. Some of the harshest critics of proposals for more regulatory flexibility are the consumer advocates who are not prepared to yield any of the ground they have worked so hard to win. While they can acknowledge the potential benefits of a regulatory environment that attends to individual resident preferences, they fear that concessions will lead to exploitation.

Nursing homes argue from another perspective. They call for level playing fields. The danger of leveling the playing field, however, is creating another generation of nursing homes.

Regulators need to hold someone accountable. Who would be accountable for care in newly configured residential settings? How would the responsibilities be allocated to the living setting itself, to any home care providers who work in the setting, to any medical personnel with patients in the setting, and to any community-based case managers who oversee the care of Medicaid clients in the setting? These difficult questions cry out for resolution.

Separating Payment

Throughout the chapter we have alluded to the separation of payment for the hotel functions and the care functions. Though such separation is occurring already in various jurisdictions, the basis for the separation is sometimes arbitrary. It is almost as though the housing payment, at least for the public sector, is constructed by looking at the lowest subsidized incomes in the community and determining what should be a fair proportion for rent and what is a decent minimum income for the person to have remaining for personal expenditures. We will see in Chapter 10 that various other countries that have universal benefits for nursing home care but maintain heavy consumer cost-sharing have done something similar. They establish a price that seems to make sense for the room and board portion that is within the means of the poorest pensioners and the rest of the daily rate is considered service.

To some extent the determination of what portion of a nursing home's costs are attributable to room and board and what proportion to service can become an arbitrary accounting exercise. Some states have attempted to micromanage nursing home budgets, allocating specific proportions of the homes' costs to specific activities. Once a base price for room and board is established (either based on estimated real costs or linked to minimum ability to pay), the market can be allowed to grow to permit persons with different amounts of wealth to purchase differing levels of accommodation amenities, as presently occurs in the general housing market.

From a consumer perspective, the advantage of separation of services and room and board is that they have much more flexibility and power in the marketplace. They can presumably take their room-and-board money and move elsewhere, and their service dollars can be expended wherever they live.

An unresolved dilemma remains: Who keeps the difference in potential costs under different models of care? For example, if it is cheaper to treat someone in an assisted living setting (even with additional services brought in) than in a nursing home, can the ALF contract for the nursing home rate? Can the client pocket the difference? Or does the state attempt to base its payments on some estimate of costs? In the case of private payment, the situation is simple. People retain what they do not spend. In the case of publicly supported care, the problem is more complex. Take the most extreme case: Suppose that a patient and her family decided to forgo care that was deemed appropriate. Can they keep the cost of that care? Under a proposal for cashing out benefits they could (assuming, of course, that the cash-out were not deeply discounted), but in all other instances they could not. It seems unlikely that our system will accept any approach other than a cost-based approach unless we move to some form of capitated long-term care (where the same problems will be faced but at a lower level within the capitated organization) or unless we permit active cashing out of benefits (with the concomitant problem of what to do if the money is spent unwisely).

Concluding Comment

The landscape is now dotted with improved residential care settings where long-term care is available. It remains a great challenge to combine an adequate service capability (including both routine and specialized services) with a homelike environment and a philosophy of client control and choice. The "subversive" effort to create an organization that is 180 degrees different from today's nursing home will be incomplete until this problem is solved. At present, some assisted living programs boast pleasant apartment-style amenities, but people cannot remain once their needs increase beyond a minimal level, whereas other assisted living programs that do offer substantial care do so in double-bedded rooms that constitute no improvement on a nursing home. Furthermore, new residential care needs to be provided within the means of people with modest incomes and governmental subsidies for poor people. A new and positive paradigm for care in residential settings has been advanced over the last decade. It would be a sad result if the dominant assisted living models ended up offering none of the improvements in homelike residential settings and philosophy yet offered a distinctly poorer level of service than does the typical nursing home.

Notes

1. Wilson KB (1996) *Assisted Living: Reconceptualized Regulation to Meet Consumers' Needs and Preferences.* Washington, DC: American Association of Retired Persons.
2. For a discussion of the potential advantages of blurred boundaries between home care and institutional care, see Kane RA (1995). Expanding the home care concept: blurring distinctions among home care, institutional care, and other long-term care services. *The Milbank Quarterly* 73(2):161–186.
3. Mattimore TJ, Wenger NS, Cesbiens NA, Teno JM, Hamel MB, Liu H, Califf R, Connors AF, Lynn J, & Oye RK (1997) Surrogate and physician understanding of patients' preferences for living permanently in a nursing home. *Journal of the American Geriatrics Society* 45 (7):818–824.
4. The rich repository of ethnographic studies by anthropologists and sociologists dealing with nursing home care and life tends to treat both the struggles of the people living in nursing homes and the struggles of people working in them. See, for example, Diamond T (1992). *Making Gray Gold: Narratives of Nursing Home Care.* Chicago: University of Chicago Press; Foner N (1994). *The Caregiving Dilemma: Work in an American Nursing Home.* Berkeley, CA: University of California Press; Gubrium JF (1993). *Speaking of Life: Horizons of Meanings for Nursing Home Residents.* Hawthorne, NY: Aldine de Gruyter; Gubrium JB (1975). *Living and Dying at Murray Manor.* New York: St. Martin's; Savishinsky JS (1991). *Ends of Time: Life and Work in a Nursing Home.* New York: Bergen & Garvey; Shield RR (1988). *Uneasy Endings.* Ithica, NY: Cornell University Press; Schmidt MG (1990). *Negotiating a Good Old Age; Challenges of Residential Living in Late Life.* San Francisco: Jossey Bass.
5. Laird C (1979). *Limbo: A Memoir About Life in a Nursing Home by a Survivor.* Novato, CA: Chandler & Sharp; Newton E (1979). *This Bed My Center.* Melbourne, Australia: McPhee Gribble; Sarton M(1973). *As We Are Now.* New York: Norton; Tulloch GJ (1975). *A Home Is not a Home: Life Within a Nursing Home.* New York: Seabury Press.
6. Tobin SS (1991). *Personhood in Advanced Old Age: Implications for Practice.* New York: Springer.
7. Kane RA, Caplan AL, Urv-Wong EK, Freeman IC, Aroskar MA, & Finch M (1997).

Everyday matters in the lives of nursing home residents: wish for and perception of choice and control. *Journal of the American Medical Association* 45:1086–1093.

8. Gubrium (1975). See note 4.

9. Barkan B (1995). The regenerative community: the Live Oak Living Center and the quest for autonomy, self-esteem, and connection in elder care. In LM Gamroth, J Semradek, & EM Tornquist (Eds.), *Enhancing Autonomy in Long-Term Care: Concepts and Strategies* (pp. 169–192). New York: Springer; Kari N, Hayle P, & Michels P (1995). The politics of autonomy: lessons from the Lazarus Project. In LM Gamroth, J Semradek, & EM Tornquist (Eds.), *Enhancing Autonomy in Long-Term Care: Concepts and Strategies.* (pp. 155–168). New York: Springer.

10. Friedlob A (1993). The use of physical restraints in nursing homes and the allocation of nursing resources. Unpublished doctoral dissertation, Health Services Research, University of Minnesota.

11. Fries BE (1990). Comparing case-mix systems for nursing home payment. *Health Care Financing Review* 11:103–120.

12. This classification was first presented in Kane RA (1996). The future of group residential care. In Organization for Economic Co-operation and Development (OECD), *Caring for Frail Elderly People: Policies in Evolution.* (Social Policy Studies No. 19). Paris: OECD.

13. Regnier V (1996). *Critical Issues in Assisted Living.* Los Angeles: National Resource and Policy Center on Housing and Long-Term Care, University of Southern California Andrus Center on Gerontology.

14. Kane RA, Illston LH, Kane RL, Nyman JA, & Finch MD (1991). Adult foster care for the elderly in Oregon: a mainstream alternative to nursing homes. *American Journal of Public Health* 81:1113–1120.

15. Kane RA & Wilson KB (1993). *Assisted Living in The United States: A New Paradigm for Care for the Frail Elderly?* Washington, DC: American Association of Retired Persons; Regnier V, Hamilton J, & Yatabe S (1995). *Assisted Living for the Aged and Frail: Innovations in Design, Management, and Financing.* New York: Columbia University Press.

16. U.S. Congress Office of Technology Assessment (1992). *Special Care Units for People With Alzheimer's and Other Dementias: Consumer Education, Research, Regulatory, and Reimbursement Issues.* (OTA-H-543, August, 1992). Washington, DC: Government Printing Office.

17. See Kane RL & Kane RA (1987). *Long-Term Care: Principles, Programs, and Policies.* New York: Springer, Chapter 8 for a review studies that illuminate correlates of well-being for nursing home residents. Some such studies were designed to improve residents' sense of control over their environment. Even small interventions seem to lead to positive results.

18. The "teaching nursing home" is an example of fruitful collaboration between facilities and schools of nursing. See Schneider EL, Wendland CJ, Zimmer AW, List N, & Ory, MG (Eds.) (1985) *The Teaching Nursing Home: A New Approach to Geriatric Research, Education, and Clinical Care.* New York: Raven Press; Aiken L, Mezey MD, Lynbaugh J, & Buck C (1985). Teaching nursing homes: prospects for improving long-term care. *Journal of the American Geriatrics Association* 33:223–229.

19. Schnelle JF, Newman D, White M, Abbey J, Wallston KA, Fogarty T, & Ory MG. (1993). Maintaining continence in nursing home residents through the application of industrial quality control.*The Gerontologist* 33:114–122.

20. Brzybylski B, See D, & Watkins M (1993). *A Study of the Outcomes of Enhanced Physical Therapy and Occupational Therapy Hours Offers to Long-Term Care Residents in a Nursing Home.* (Report to the Alberta Long-Term Care Branch). Leduc, Alberta: Salem Manor Nursing Home.

21. Kane RL, Jorgensen LA, Teteberg B & Kuwahara J (1976). Is good nursing home care feasible? *Journal of the American Medical Association* 235:516–519.

22. The Alzheimer's Association has released several documents suggesting the ideal features of an SCU, notably in Alzheimer's Association (1992). *Guidelines for Dignity; Goals of Specialized Alzheimer's/Dementia Care in Residential Settings.* Chicago: Alzheimer's Association. In September 1991, the National Institute on Aging began a ten-project initiative on SCUs for Alzheimer's disease. Under that initiative, several evaluations of the effects of Alzheimer's SCUs were funded. See Ory MG (1994). Dementia special care: the development of a national research initiative. *Alzheimer's Disease and Associated Disorders* (Suppl):389–394 for an overview of the study. Also the entire Supplement is devoted to articles about aspects of that Initiative.

23. Thomas WH (1994). *The Eden Alternative: Nature, Hope, & Nursing Homes.* Sherburne, NY: Eden Alternative Foundation.

24. Levine S (1997). Creating an Eden for seniors: nursing home movement stresses quality of life. *Washington Post*, November 21, A1, A 35–36.

25. Many of the accounts of culture change in nursing homes in the United States were gathered by Carter C. Williams, a social work consultant and the guiding spirit for an organization known as the "Pioneers in Nursing Home Culture Change. See various chapters in Gamroth, Semradek, & Tornquist (1995), Note 9, for examples of specific efforts. Also see Fagan RM, Williams CC, & Burger SG (1997). *Meeting of Pioneers in Nursing Home Culture Change, March 14–16, 1997.* Rochester, NY: Lifespan of Greater Rochester.

26. For a full description of the range of adult foster care homes around the country, see Falconer D, Jensen A, Lipson L, Stauffer M, & Fox-Gage W (1996). *Adult Foster Care for the Elderly: A Review of State Regulatory and Funding Strategies,* Volumes 1 and 2. Washington, DC: American Association of Retired Persons.

27. Braun K & Rose C (1986). The Hawaii geriatric foster care experiment; impact evaluation and cost analysis. *The Gerontologist* 26:516–523.

28. Sherman SR & Newman ES (1988). *Foster Families for Adults; A Community Alternative in Long-Term Care.* New York: Columbia University Press.

29. Kane et al., (1991). See note 14.

30. Kane et al., (1991). See note 14.

31. Stark A, Kane RL, Kane RA, & Finch MD (1995). Effect on physical functioning of care in adult foster homes and nursing homes. *The Gerontologist* 35(5):648–655, 1995.

32. Malachi RL & Snow I (1996). *State Assisted Living Policy: 1996.* National Academy for State Health Policy. Portland, ME. U.S. Department of Health and Human Services.

33. The data provided here come from an in-progress evaluation of Assisted Living in Oregon, funded by the Robert Wood Johnson Foundation and directed by Rosalie Kane.

34. An invitational working conference, "Autonomy or Abandonment: Changing Perspectives on Delegation" was held on October 24– 25, 1996, and sponsored by the American Association of Retired Persons, the American Bar Association's Commission on Legal Problems of the Elderly, the American Nurses Association, the National Association for Home Care, the National Council on Aging, the National League for Nursing, the National Council of State Boards of Nursing, the Veteran's Administration, and the World Institute on Disability. The long list of sponsors reflects the interest in the topic. Panelists from Oregon, Washington, Texas, and New York presented different state approaches to achieving desired flexibility in nursing programs for long-term care, and spokespeople for various disability groups presented strong views in favor of increased delegation. Wagner DL, Nadish P, & Sabatino C (1997) *Autonomy or Abandonment: Changing Perspectives on Delegation.* Washington, DC: National Institute on Consumer-Directed Long-term Services; National Council on Aging.

35. See Kane RA, Baker MO, Salmon J, & Veazie W. (1998). *Consumer Perspectives on*

Private Versus Shared Accommodations in Assisted Living Settings. Washington, DC: American Association of Retired Persons. This report summarized information available in the published literature and presented the results of focus groups conducted by the authors. Among the published literature most relevant to the subject, see: Hawes C, Green A, Wood M, & Woodsong C (1997). *Family Members' Views; What is Quality in Assisted Living Facilities Providing Care to People with Dementia.* Chicago: Alzheimer's Association; Jenkens R (1997). *Assisted Living and Private Rooms: What People Say They Want.* Washington, DC: American Association for Retired Persons; Lawton MP & Bader J (1970). Wish for privacy by young and old. *Journal of Gerontology* 25 (1):48–54; Pastalan LA (1970). Privacy as an expression of human territoriality. In LA Pastalan & DE Carlson (Eds.). *Spatial Behavior of Older People.* Ann Arbor, MI: University of Michigan Institute on Aging; Shoeman FD (Ed.) (1984). *Philosophical Dimensions of Privacy: An Anthology.* Cambridge, MA: Cambridge University Press; Tetelbaum M (1996). *Evaluation of the LTC Survey Process.* Boston, MA: Abt; and Teresi JA, Holmes D, & Monaco C (1993). An evaluation of the effects of co-mingling cognitively and non-cognitively impaired individuals in long-term care facilities. *The Gerontologist* 33 (3):350–358.

36. Wilson KB (1997). What cost privacy for developers and operators? Paper presented at the Annual Scientifics held on Meeting of the Gerontological Society of America, Philadelphia, PA, November 17, 1997.

7.

Quality and Accountability

The United States has made more sustained efforts to set standards for acceptable quality of long-term care services, and to hold programs accountable for meeting those standards, than other countries. Despite all these efforts, good quality has eluded definition, let alone universal achievement. In part, the conceptual problem is rooted in the highly personal and subjective reactions that people have to their care and their life circumstances. The long-term care consumers' view of quality combines a personal and internal response to the events and conditions they experience with a basic expectation that the technical quality meets some standard. Few long-term care consumers have stopped to ponder the trade-offs they might be willing to make if they had to choose between technical quality of care and quality of life. They presume they can obtain both. Despite much of the current rhetoric about the need to choose between these concepts, there is no reason to assume that the consumers are wrong in their basic belief that they can and should have both.

A long-term care consumer's satisfaction is a subjective experience that can be judged and attested to by nobody other than the person most concerned. The implications of this are that opinions need to be solicited from those who can express themselves, and every effort must be made to heed and interpret the nonverbal communications of those who cannot express themselves. Those who provide care and those who plan and finance it must, in all good conscience, adopt consumer satisfaction as a paramount goal. Yet, consumer satisfaction is an insufficient test of quality for several reasons.

Beyond satisfying the consumer, care must meet technical quality requirements, some of which the consumers may be incapable of judging. This care must achieve a quality standard even when the consumers are incapable of communicating satisfaction or dissatisfaction at all or of forming any opinion. Care must also meet objective standards even if a self-effacing consumer is willing to settle for whatever is offered. Some objective definitions of quality are needed to set the societal compass and, thereby, develop, improve, and judge programs. Long-term care is, indeed, an intensely private matter, but, paradoxically, it is also a matter of public policy. Public policy demands efforts to arrive at some sort of consensus about when quality has and has not been achieved.

Medical versus Social Approaches

Defining and assuring quality in long-term care is rendered more difficult because the care is a hybrid of health care programs and social programs. In an albeit oversimplified way, Table 7.1 presents the contrasting ways that health programs and social welfare programs are regarded, and hints at the implications for quality assurance.

Goals

Before one can define adequate or excellent long-term care, one must be clear about just what long-term care is supposed to achieve. Previous chapters have described the difficulties in reaching societal consensus on this very point. As a hybrid between a social program and a health program, long-term care is subject to varying and competing emphases by well-intended authorities who give priority to one or another goal. As the table suggests, health programs typically emphasize achievable therapeutic goals related to physical or mental health, whereas social programs take a broader view, extending to social and even spiritual well-being (often collapsed into the idea that the program is judged by the "quality of life" of its clientele). Health care authorities themselves argue over the emphasis to give to competing health goals such as prolonging life versus controlling pain. Considering long-term care as a social program introduces other goals, such as maintaining social and psychological well-being. However, psychological and social well-being cannot be the only goals. Long-term care is also a health-related program with legitimate important objectives related to the consumer's functional abilities and health status.

Another important distinction is based on whether long-term care services are themselves expected to result in measurable "clinical" improvements or whether they are meant to provide services that address unmet need caused by functional impairment and, through that vehicle, help the individual achieve other life goals, whatever they mean. In this chapter and in Table 7.1, we refer to the latter approach as *compensatory* and the former as *therapeutic*, a distinction previously introduced in Chapter 5.

The compensatory approach emphasizes that an individual should be able to live as full a life as possible despite functional dependencies. Its success can be measured by the extent to which personal care and technology have compensated for

Table 7.1. Quality in Health Programs and Social Programs

Feature	Health	Social	Hybrid
Goals	Health, safety (emphasis on physical and mental health). Care is meant to achieve therapeutic goals	Quality of life (can include social and spiritual well-being). Care is meant to compensate for impairment so consumers can achieve life goals	Multiple and conflicting goals. Therapeutic and compensatory approaches both crucial
Role of expertise	Professions identify health problems and solutions. Strive for objective appraisals of quality	Consumers determine their own well-being. Subjective appraisals most important	Both consumers and professionals have quality assurance roles; both subjective and objective information is important
Role of consumer choice	Consumers may consent to or refuse care but boundaries of necessary and appropriate care are set by professional guidelines	Consumers as citizens are free to make all choices within legal limits. Constraints on consumer choice relate to legal and functional competence and rights of others	Confusion about extent to which consumer choice is the major goal, especially when public money is being expended on care
Time horizon	Relatively short term. Discrete activities and concept of episodes of care	Relatively long-range. Many "cases" never close	Short-term and long-term approaches both needed. Readjustments of short-term activities within long-term framework
Public roles	Some public responsibility to ensure access to and quality of care	Residual public responsibility only. Low-income workers unlikely to be able to afford minimally adequate quality	Minimum standards for training of health workers likely to be relatively high and standards for housing quality & privacy likely to be relatively low
Paradigm	Discomfort associated with treatment is worth it in expectation of beneficial result	Care is seen as the end in itself, or care is seen as a means for consumers to achieve personal goals	Retain focus on current situation but without forsaking expectation of benefit from good care
Expectations	Results of treatment should lead to a status at least as good as before the illness	Good treatment should delay decline in relevant outcomes	Maintain expectation of positive effects of treatment (at least slowing rate of decline) but not enough to deemphasize current situation

the impairments. This philosophy is directly related to placing a high value on achieving a high quality of life. Long-term care is seen as more than just a treatment, but rather as a means to allow a person to experience as full a life as possible, maximizing those things that are most important to that person. The therapeutic approach holds that measurable improvements in physical, cognitive, affective, or social functioning can sometimes result from long-term care. Although it is unrealistic to expect that all people with long-term care needs will improve in functioning, good care should delay the rate and extent of functional decline. An emphasis on potential improvement counteracts the therapeutic nihilism often prevalent among long-term care providers and emphasizes the "science" of long-term care practice. Such a goal orientation offers a more attractive rationale for supporting efforts to improve (and to invest in better) long-term care. Thus, the therapeutic approach is more likely to be associated with technical measures of quality, often classified as quality of care.

These two aspects of care—the therapeutic and the compensatory—are often mistakenly portrayed as polar opposites. In fact, both approaches are needed. Neglecting efforts to improve functioning and well-being is unconscionable, especially when (as is often the case for long-term care) relatively inexpensive interventions can result in great differences for the clientele. Depression can often be treated, sensory impairment and mobility problems can be alleviated, incontinence can be reduced. Simply compensating for such disabilities without trying to improve the client's status is indefensible. On the other hand, long-term care has purposes beyond the therapeutic, and it retains those purposes even when therapeutic goals are impossible. Located on that awkward boundary between a health program and a social program, long-term care providers must guard against viewing the client's entire life as simply a therapeutic plan.

Similarly, the distinction between the terms *quality of care* and *quality of life* is dysfunctional. The two concepts have more in common than many people realize. An operational definition of quality of life usually includes attention to physical functioning, pain and discomfort, as well as psychological well-being, social relationships, social activity, and satisfaction. These are the same elements that are used as building blocks for examining quality of care in terms of outcomes. Proponents of quality of life may go on to suggest that these elements are necessary but not sufficient. Quality of life includes a larger perspective that can permit someone with quite limited abilities to enjoy, nonetheless, a positive outlook and a genuine belief that his or her life has value and meaning. Some commentators refer to this as a spiritual dimension.

Professional versus Lay Judgments
Specialized expertise plays a greater role in health programs than in social programs, both for setting standards and assuring the standards are met. In contrast, consumers themselves are the best, and some would say only, arbiters of their quality of life. Long-term care must be judged by both objective standards (some

of which are technical) and also by subjective standards. The latter are crucial because long-term care shapes the lives of the people who are served. Only the persons receiving the care and help can judge how it enhances or interferes with their happiness, productivity, and social lives. For relatively nontechnical services, such as cooking and cleaning, the consumers are best able to evaluate whether they are done well and according to specifications that they or others may have developed. The consumers are also best able to judge whether the manner and timing of giving personal care is dignified or demeaning, comfortable or painful, convenient or inconvenient. However, consumers alone cannot be expected to determine whether new health problems are identified in a timely way and whether new or old problems are treated appropriately. For example, a client may be unaware of the steps to avoid infection, the way medications interact, or a host of other matters.

Time Horizon

Long-term care is a continuing, and sometimes a lifelong process, rather than a product or a discrete event. It is also a pervasive phenomenon, having an impact on many areas of life. Thus, quality inevitably has many dimensions and the rankings of their relative importance can change. Different aspects of quality may take precedence, even in the mind of the consumer, at different times. Because of the long time horizon, those who ponder quality often look beyond the current moment to possible future negative consequences. In the name of quality, long-term care consumers are commonly asked to forgo present comfort or contentment in order to forestall accidents or dangers that could create potential subsequent exacerbations of disability. The emphasis on the long time horizon tends to result in highly protective efforts to shape the client's present life in the name of safety and health. For example, this emphasis could lead to professionals insisting on a therapeutic diet in home-delivered or institutional meals, regardless of whether the client likes the food. Clients with gait problems could be discouraged from undertaking any activities that would put them at risk for a broken hip or from going anywhere unaccompanied. A 95-year-old could be urged to forgo the current pleasures of her familiar setting for a pressured longer life expectancy in an environment where emergencies could be better handled.

If a long-term care program takes a stance that gives priority to client independence and choice, issues arise about how to consider and count the extra falls and broken hips that will probably occur. Will these be perceived as demerits for the program by the clients themselves, their family members, or external judges? Long-term care clients tend to have difficulty prioritizing being safe and protected versus their desire to be free to pursue activities as they please. One study showed that although about one third of a large group of clients chose one or the other of these values, fully a third of the group wanted *both* freedom and protection and could not get beyond their ambivalence to make a choice.[1] If clients are thus conflicted, it is small wonder that providers opt for what they perceive as the safety route. Sometimes those perceptions are, themselves, based on mistaken data. For example, during the 1970s and 1980s, nursing home staff believed and communicated to clients and families that physical restraints designed to prohibit residents from moving (in less euphemistic language, tying up the elderly) promoted safety. Leaving aside the negative psychological consequences of restraints, recent data show that physical restraints cause as much physical harm as they prevent and that accidents of people in restraints are often more serious than those of people not restrained.[2]

Public Provision and Standards

Long-term care is heavily regulated for several reasons. A substantial portion of this care uses public finds to pay private, often proprietary, providers. Public expenditures to private vendors usually require regulations. When the beneficiaries are viewed as vulnerable, public concerns are magnified. When the history of the service is marked by scandal, public trust is low.

As a social program, long-term care is subject to the profound ambivalence in American society about the level of excellence that should be guaranteed for social services. The American taxpayer is particularly loath to spend public money for low-income people on anything judged as an amenity or frill. Ambivalence is present even about the threshold for access to health services for low-income people. Once access to health services is achieved, however, most agree that technical standards need to be met for health procedures and the training of health personnel. For example, an x-ray or a surgical procedure is expected to meet quality standards regardless of the income of the patient or the patient's payment source. If a procedure requires a licensed nurse for a high-income person, a licensed nurse is required for a low-income person.

On the social side of long-term care, however, many of the gradations of attention and environment that comprise some people's views of quality can be interpreted by others as imposing too high a standard for public expenditures on housing, food, and personal niceties. Mandating single rooms with full bathrooms inside the consumer's own living apartment may be considered a pampering of the poor and a deterrent to personal saving to buy a better quality of amenity. Members of Congress and of state legislatures have been known to publicly deride long-term care programs that would offer "maid service" to every American with a disability.

Despite concerns about frivolity, two factors press for a reasonably high standard for the quality of long-term care as a social program. First, the users of long-term care are not a relatively small, readily stigmatized group. They are, by and large, everyone who survives into their 80s and 90s, all our grandparents and great-grandparents, our future selves. In many instances, long-term care users are people who fall into the historically popular category of "deserving poor." They played by life's rules but their life expectancy and functional problems eventually exceeded their ability to pay for meeting their basic needs. Policy makers tend, therefore, to be less pejorative and judgmental about social welfare programs for older people with disabilities than for their younger counterparts (though a fear lurks that wealthy older persons may take advantage of programs designed for those who fall below the income and asset "safety nets"). Second, one can successfully redefine some of the so-called amenities in long-term care as aids to independence and self-sufficiency. For example, privacy and access to a bathroom, a refrigerator, and a stove could be viewed as necessary to exercise independent living skills. Pursuing this line of argument can become somewhat dangerous, however, since, if carried to an extreme, it would relegate all aspects of social life to the therapeutic category.

One last caveat about emphasizing quality of life. The enthusiasm for recognizing quality of care can be a two-edged sword. The term *quality of life* means different things to different people. For some, especially those to whom it is a new concept, it is equated with the onset of disability. Economists and epidemiologists, for example, have introduced the concept of quality-adjusted life years (QALYs) as an intermediate stage between health and death.[3] In effect, disability is treated as an outcome in the same way as death, and years until the point of disability are considered quality survival.[4] This technique is flawed in two important ways: *(1)* Disability is often incorrectly treated as an irreversible phenomenon. *(2)* More important in the present context, virtually all of the population receiving long-term care would be effectively written off under this approach because they are already disabled. Although disability indisputably has a strong bearing on a person's life, it is shortsighted to declare that a person is bereft of quality of life because of a disability. Indeed, such thinking ignores the important effects that long-term care can have on just this aspect of life.

Inevitably, long-term care is a blend of health-oriented and socially oriented efforts. In approaching quality assurance, one must grapple with this duality and satisfy the requirements of each. With that caveat in mind, we now consider the steps in a quality assurance program and how they might best be regarded for a long-term care program.

Steps of Quality Assurance

Quality assurance requires three seemingly simple but extraordinarily difficult steps: defining adequate or excellent quality of care or services in the first place; assessing care and services to determine whether those quality standards are being met; and correcting problems when quality shortfalls are noted.[5] In the 1990s, more emphasis has been placed on a process of continuous quality improvement (CQI) or, alternatively, total quality management (TQM). Both CQI and TQM have taken on an almost cult-like aspect among enthusiasts for the approach, but they do reflect an important effort to make quality improvement meaningful. When done properly CQI is a rigorous process.

What then is CQI, and how does it differ from quality assurance as usual? Although standard-setting, assessment of care, and correction of problems (the three steps just reviewed) are pertinent to CQI, these processes in CQI are designed to continuously upgrade care as opposed to making sure that care meets a minimum standard. Borrowed from a western understanding of Japanese business principles, the organization dedicated to CQI is infused with commitment to quality from the top management down and from the bottom up in terms of seeking input and creativity from actual work groups at the lowest levels of the organization. The strength of this approach lies in never being satisfied with having reached the end of the quest for better quality. The twin dangers lie in never achieving an acceptable level of quality despite improving or, worse, in accepting "improvement" in lieu of real meaningful change.

Defining Quality

Ultimately quality must be defined in terms of operational standards that can be measured. This is much harder to do for attributes of a service like long-term care, compared, say, to attributes of a manufactured product. Quality indicators or criteria are commonly expressed in one of three ways: as structure, as process, or as outcomes.

Structure. Structural criteria refer to general attributes of a program that need to be in place for it to be said to be of adequate or high quality. Most of the time the importance of these elements is based on professional beliefs about what attributes are necessary to produce quality. Such elements may include the training and experience of staff, the ratios of staff to clientele, the physical plant and equipment, the record-keeping system, and various organizational structures (e.g., quality assurance committees, ethics committees, utilization committees, emergency evacuation procedures, infection control procedures, and so on). These elements can be evaluated for the program as a whole. In long-term care, quality assurance first was applied to nursing homes, and detailed criteria were enunciated for such elements as the minimum sizes of the spaces, the heights of the railings, the temperature of the water, the role definitions for various personnel, and countless other elements.

Process. As the term suggests, process criteria examine what is done for the consumers and how well it is done. The standards for such activity are usually expressed in terms of words like "necessary" and "appropriate." The underlying premise of process criteria is that following them will result in better outcomes. However, this premise, like that for structural criteria, relies more on professional belief than on empirical findings. Criteria can be written about the need to perform certain activities in response to specified conditions or they can be express in terms of how well various specific procedures are carried out. Process errors can include both errors of commission (i.e., unnecessary care) and those of omission (i.e., necessary services that were not received). Some process criteria are rather general, and some are minutely particular, relating to the steps in care for a particular diagnostic condition or the way to administer a particular drug or carry out a procedure. Process criteria are sometimes elaborated into orderly protocols for how to assess and treat a particular condition (sometimes called *guidelines* or *care pathways*). Care can then be audited as to whether the logic of the protocol was followed. For example, Did the assessment examine specific issues? In the presence of certain assessment data, did the care provider follow up in a specific way?

Process criteria are popular because they are usually based on professional beliefs about what is the right thing to do. Caregivers find comfort in knowing they did the correct thing, even if it led to a less than desired result. The more complicated the situation, the more difficult it is to know what is the right thing to do, or that it will make a difference. Thus, writing guidelines for treatment is much easier in clear-cut situations, but most chronic care cases must deal with multiple problems simultaneously. In these instances, it is harder to define specific rules of proper procedure.

Judging the process of care can likewise rely on specific explicit criteria (e.g., was an evaluation done when a bad event occurred), but when the situation is complicated it is hard to get a real feeling for the quality of the care provided from a simple list of explicit criteria. No single answer is necessarily correct or sufficient to capture the nuances of care. One may have to rely on the judgment of experienced clinicians to determine the overall quality (and appropriateness) of what was done.

Process measures are especially useful in situations when one does not want to have to wait for a bad event to occur to identify a problem area. For example, procedures for good infection control in long-term care facilities should be monitored in the absence of evidence that a facility-borne infection has spread. Another valuable use for process measures is to address areas where certain ways of giving care are intrinsic to the concept of good care—for example, treating clients with respect and dignity and, acting kindly, honestly and reliably. In another context, we have called these attributes of care "enabling criteria."[6] They are aspects of care which are dictated by common sense and decency, and that should be taken for granted. Consumers tend to enumerate those qualities when asked what they view as important in a helper or caregiver. Their lists include: someone who comes on time; someone trustworthy, who does not steal; someone kind, polite, and gentle; someone compatible with them who seems to care about them; someone who performs tasks competently or as the consumer likes them. These attributes are hard to measure through process indicators, though an observer of a care situation can sometimes note their presence or absence.

Outcomes. The shift to an outcomes focus is already underway in other parts of health care. Effectiveness and outcomes management have become contemporary watchwords. It is at least as feasible to implement an outcomes-based system in long-term care. Indeed, long-term care has several advantages for this approach. Not only is the relationship between current practices and outcomes less well established than in acute medicine, because things unfold more slowly in long-term care, there is an opportunity to intervene proactively when unsatisfactory outcomes are detected. Because quality of care and quality of life are so closely intertwined in long-term care, an accountability system that incorporates both is preferable to separate approaches.

The appeal of outcome criteria is that they seem to emphasize what is most important—results. The reason why outcome criteria are not embraced more enthusiastically is that the good or bad results may not be associated with the services provided. Herein then lies the Catch-22. Providers of care do not want to be judged by outcomes that they consider to be outside of their control, but they are content to be judged by process measures that may have little to do with improving outcomes. Because outcomes are based on the probabilities that a given client will do better as a result of the care received, when outcomes are used to describe quality, they must be expressed for groups of consumers; using group averages describes the overall effects but takes into account those cases where the outcomes may have been unavoidable. One can do a very good job without being successful every time. Thus, actual outcomes for the group must be viewed against expected outcomes. Using expected outcomes incorporates the concept of adjusting for differences in the makeup of the client populations served. Some clients will have poorer prognoses than others; some will be more resistant to treatment or less likely to improve because of other circumstances. For example, the death rate in a cancer hospital should be higher than in a general hospital. Depression rates—even suicide rates— should be greater in a group of people with histories of mental health problems and treatment than in the general public. Likewise, outcomes are usually limited by the client's ability in that area before receiving the treatment. Remember the old joke about the patient who asks the doctor if he will be able to play the piano after the operation. (It depends on whether he could play it before.) In the jargon of long-term care, taking into account characteristics of the population being served is called *case-mix adjustment.*

An outcomes approach requires an epidemiological perspective.[7] Outcomes are meaningful for groups rather than individuals; they reflect averages. Because outcomes are based on probabilities, they are best interpreted when the actual outcome is compared to an expected value. The latter should be derived from statistical analyses based on actual experience with large numbers of cases, but some outcomes practitioners are content to at least begin the process by establishing norms based on clinical experience.

Basically, the outcomes of care are the result of several factors, illustrated in the following conceptual equation:

$$\text{Outcomes} = f \text{ (baseline status, patient demographics, patient clinical factors,}$$
$$\text{environment, treatment)}$$

The goal of outcomes assessment is to isolate the effects of treatment by accounting for the contributions of the other factors. Any determination of outcomes must take cognizance of the level at which the patient began. Especially in long-term care, it is unlikely that the client will do better than to recover his or her status prior to the inciting event. Two types of client characteristics play an important role in determining outcomes. Demographic variables include the obvious attributes of sex and age, as well as more subtle roles of education and economic status; the category also includes various measures of social support and the availability of informal care. Clinical characteristics reflect concerns about diagnoses, cognitive and functional ability, and severity of illness. In some cases, the level of specificity may include defined physiologic parameters, such as blood glucose levels or blood pressure, or the presence of pressure ulcers. Environment describes both the physical and social environment. It may reflect access to care as well as living situation. Treatment usually means formal care, in which case the extent and type of informal care become part of the environment. Treatment can be described in many ways. It should include at least measures of amount and type.

Outcomes can be expressed through a variety of measures. Although there is active debate about which measures are most appropriate for which types of clients, this argument may miss the real target. More error is likely introduced by poor use of existing measurement and weak analysis than through the specific choice of measures. Too often the measures used are not used well. The specific questions are not asked systematically. Instead, staff may decide unilaterally that questions are too stressful for the client and attempt to intuit the client's likely response had they actually been asked, or the questions may be indirectly posed.

There is general agreement on the domains that should be encompassed in assessing the outcomes of long-term care, although the relative weights to be placed on these various domains are open to more debate. The domains include:

- Physiological function (e.g., blood pressure, pressure sores)
- Pain and discomfort
- Physical function (ADLs and IADLs)
- Cognition (some would argue that this domain is more often a modifier than an outcome; but many clinicians would argue that while little can usually be done to improve it, treatment, such as overmedication, and care environments can make it worse)
- Affect (i.e., emotional state)
- Social participation (in activities that are meaningful to the client)
- Social interaction (a relationship with at least one person with whom the client feels intimate; some would expand this to include relationships with pets)
- Satisfaction (with both the care received and the setting in which it is delivered)

Methods are available to measure each of these domains by obtaining information directly from clients.[8] Techniques are likewise available to develop predictions of expected outcomes as a basis for comparison.[9] In some cases, clients may not be able to provide this information. Proxy informants can be used for some domains but are meaningless for others. For example, proxies cannot really measure satisfaction for a person with dementia. In the latter instances, these domains should receive a zero weighting in developing a summative score. Efforts to ascertain the value weights to be placed on the various domains suggest that most of the relevant constituencies in society generally agree about the relative importance of these different types of outcomes, and even agree that these weights will differ with the clients' underlying condition.[10] Nonetheless, it is often preferable to employ a specific set of value weights designed to fit the situation at hand, rather than using some predetermined set. It is even possible to incorporate individual client preferences, as long as they are determined in advance of the outcome assessment.

Choosing criteria. Each type of criterion has a rightful place in the long-term care quality assurance toolkit. Structural criteria, we argue, are sometimes overdone. Many of the innovations that we described in Chapter 5 and Chapter 6 require relaxing certain orthodoxies about the kind of personnel needed to perform various tasks. They may even require relaxing environmental codes originally seen as protecting consumer safety. On the other hand, structural criteria can be used in the service of genuinely promoting a better quality of life. In the last chapter, recall that we argued for requirements mandating single-occupancy accommodations in long-term care settings.

Although we tend to favor outcome criteria, we emphasize that outcomes should not be construed narrowly as health, functional, and safety outcomes. The principles of outcomes assessment can be readily applied to a variety of measures, including those that address quality of life. As always, the measure of success is not necessarily improvement; the delaying decline can be a significant achievement. Furthermore, health and safety outcomes must be achieved with some attention to process since long-term care shapes everyday life for the clientele. An accident-free group of consumers is a good outcome, but not if it is won at the expense of virtual imprisonment.

Setting a standard. For each quality indicator, some standard of acceptable performance is needed. Those thresholds can be set very high, even to the point of zero tolerance of deviation. For example, in a long-term care program of adequate quality, there should be absolutely no instances of staff abusing clientele or stealing their possessions. Some people would also say there should be zero instances of new bedsores appearing in nursing-home residents, or zero instances of administration of the wrong medication. On the other hand, some falls are to be expected in an elderly but mobile population. Some rate of depressive mood is to be expected in any population and, therefore, in a group of long-term care consumers. Part of making operational definitions is setting the standard for acceptable performance. Sometimes this issue is finessed by using statistical standards—that is, comparing a particular program's performance to the performance of all other programs and determining whether it falls above or below the statistical average on indicators of interest.

Assessing Quality

Armed with criteria and standards, we can examine care to see if the standards are met. Numerous detailed questions can be asked about how long-term care should be assessed. First, what is the source of information? Should one rely on a passive system of taking complaints initiated by consumer and their families, or is a more active system needed? If the latter, who actually gathers the information—registered nurses, social workers, lay inspectors? How is such information gathered? From the records maintained by the program staff? From interviews with program staff? From interviews with consumers and their family members? From direct observation of care and care settings? (Some would argue that a lot can be learned about quality, at least in a residential program, by walking in and using one's senses—how does it smell, how does the food taste, is the temperature comfortable, how do the residents look, are they dressed, what about the noise level, does staff treat residents politely, are call buttons answered?)

Then, too, how often should care be observed or consumers polled? What kind of sampling framework should be developed to inspect care? How can feedback be gathered about the most invisible care—care that occurs at night, the quality of social interactions between caregivers and long-term care consumers in the latters' homes? How can feedback be gathered about the quality of care received by people who cannot speak for themselves because of dementia or some other disability? How, even, can outcomes be assessed for people with substantial cognitive impairment? And how can the quality assurance system avoid being bogged down by the sheer weight of data collection and analysis? Although we hold quality dear, we certainly do not advocate spending more money on quality assurance than on care itself.

Long-term care, especially long-term care provided in the home, relies on paraprofessional workers and tends not to have an elaborate standard for a written record. Gathering information from the record may therefore understate the quality of care given. Moreover, if a system is developed so that quality of care will be gathered from written records without other verification, the danger is that the records will receive much better care than the people. On the other hand, we are enthusiastic about the ability of well-used information to improve care and would encourage the use of computer technologies to create records that trigger providers to perform necessary care.

We recommend a mixed approach to quality assessment that includes audits of routine records, surveys of cognitively intact consumers, and direct observations of care and care settings. We recommend that some responsive complaint mechanism be in place but that proactive efforts also be undertaken to examine quality. Also, when consumers are asked about quality, the questions need to be posed in a way such that they understand and in a context where they are comfortable being candid. This is easier said than done because so many older long-term care consumers prefer not to complain, or are not sure what standard they have a right to expect, or fear reprisals in response to complaints, or are grateful for any services they do receive. Some consumers feel so dependent on the continued presence or continued goodwill of their caregivers that they would hardly dare complain.

Correcting Problems

When quality problems are found, what then? Correcting problems that are uncovered is the true test of a quality assurance system. Failing to take steps to fix problems is comparable to making a diagnosis but never implementing a plan of care. Difficult as it is to set standards, assessment will always reveal some problems with whatever standards are used. And, difficult as it is to conduct the perfect assessment of care, any assessment tool will reveal some problems. What recourse is then available?

Corrective actions may involve both carrots and sticks. At the positive end of the spectrum, training programs, consultation, provision of role models, rewards for good performance, prizes and publicity for best programs—these are all benign and positive strategies for achieving improvement. Negative sanctions include firing an employee (if the sanction is applied by a provider) and fines, decertification, removal of accreditation, or removal of a license if the sanction is imposed by a regulator or accrediting body. Legal remedies through criminal or civil courts are also possible though taking such actions is cumbersome and expensive both for public bodies and private citizens.

Historically, authorities have been reluctant to penalize a facility by closing it down or depriving it of financial resources because the already disadvantaged consumers may suffer most from such actions. On the other hand, pouring resources into a weak institution in an effort to improve its quality creates a host of perverse incentives. Some critics suggest that the market can best correct poor quality because consumers will vote with their feet. This is only possible, however, if consumers have somewhere to run to. If the supply of long-term care programs is kept down through regulation of entry into the market, then market forces cannot exert much influence over quality.

The corrective action component of quality assurance in long-term care seems to be the weakest of the three steps. In part, concerns about fairness and due process for providers tend to trump concerns for consumers' well-being. Also, public authorities have few resources to vigorously undertake improvements of programs or vigorously prosecute offenders. The latter have every incentive to threaten litigation. The greater the potential penalty, the more likely the resort to litigious strategies. Also, especially for long-term care consumers living at home, the accountability for action is sometimes unclear. It is not always clear who should be responsible to ensure quality when several providers are involved in care. For that matter, the focus of responsibility for the poor outcomes in the individual case may also be unclear. Long-term care is often a continuous process with many players. Affixing responsibility can be a fruitless quest, but in the end someone or some organization must take responsibility for the results of the care provided.

Approaches to Quality Assurance

Thinking about quality another way, one can identify a number of broad approaches to improving the quality of long-term care and establishing accountability for results. These include: consumer approaches, regulatory approaches, provider-initiated approaches, educational efforts, and systemic approaches. These five approaches are not mutually exclusive. They can and should coexist and be mutually reenforcing.

Consumer Approaches

Well-informed, politically empowered consumers with vehicles through which to complain are an important part of assuring quality. Certainly, unwary consumers have used their purchasing power badly, whether they have been buying insurance policies, hiring in-home personnel, or choosing a nursing home. Efforts to educate consumers directly, and to inform them of their rights, to inform them of reasonable costs for services all are elements of a strategy to promote quality. Consumer complaint lines either established by provider organizations or by outside agencies can also enhance consumer power. Although each state is mandated to have such complaint lines, they seem to be only lightly used.

Perhaps the best known mechanism to enhance the consumer voice in long-term care is the National Long-term Care Ombudsman Program.[11] Every state is required to establish a long-term care ombudsman office with legal responsibility for taking complaints and mediating problems on behalf of residents in board and care facilities and nursing homes, who are the group perceived as most vulnerable. Some ombudsman programs also function in the home care arena. Ombudsmen are expected to be consumer advocates, to treat consumer complaints confidentially, and to take as their causes the causes of the consumers themselves. Ombudsman programs are unevenly funded from state to state and locality to locality and are chronically underfunded. Nonetheless, some ombudsman programs have played a very important part in improving quality for long-term care consumers, often moving ''from case to cause'' with efforts to deal with systemic problems through legal or legislative action. To be maximally effective, ombudsmen need to be sheltered from conflict of interest (their paychecks should not depend on the same government agencies that pay for the care they oversee), they need access to legal counsel, and they must have some reasonable level of funding. Occasionally, also, ombudsmen have been a force for reflexive conservatism, especially when regulatory protections seem to be undermined.

Regulatory Approaches

Regulatory approaches are the most familiar, and we have in many ways been discussing them throughout this book, especially at the end of Chapter 4, where we point out the variation in state regulations. Federal and state governments establish the conditions under which programs are allowed to operate and are paid through public subsidy. States may license professions and health occupations and they may license health and social service agencies. They also inspect agencies to make sure the conditions of licensure and payment are being met. They establish the criteria for their waiver programs, including the quality standards agencies must meet to participate in the program. Regulation is, of course, a blunt instrument. It is better at eliminating egregiously bad performance than upgrading all performance.

Criminal checks for employees is a form of quality regulation that came into prominence in the 1990s. Fanned by concerns about the caliber of people going into the homes of vulnerable long-term care consumers, especially under client-directed, nonagency types of programs, some states have required that all personnel who are reimbursed as individual providers receive such criminal checks. Some states have gone further to mandate criminal checks for all personnel employed by licensed home care and residential care agencies. With this strategy comes a set of specific concerns. Who should bear the costs of the criminal checks? How can they be organized to avoid delays in starting services? How can information be gathered adequately across various state and federal jurisdictions? Most perplexing, what is to be done with the information, once gathered. What kinds of brushes with the law should preclude an individual from working in long-term care, for how long, and who should make those decisions? What civil rights interests need to be taken into account when criminal records are sought?

It is often suggested that regulations constrain the very consumers that they seek to protect, rendering certain services unavailable at a price they can afford or restricting consumer options in other ways. But regulations can also be directed toward empowering consumers. For example, certain forms of disclosure and informed consent can be mandated through regulations. So, too, can consumer governance structures and complaint mechanisms. Regulations can also mandate that providers establish quality assurance mechanisms, while leaving the details up to them.

Provider-Initiated Approaches

Regulatory approaches and even, to a large extent, ombudsman-type approaches are largely reactive. Although they may attempt to prevent problems, they mostly deal with problems that have already occurred. And regulators may not necessarily even learn about problems until well after correction is feasible. In contrast, providers of care could develop their own mechanisms to avoid problems, to detect problems early, and to correct quality problems as they arise, aided by their own information systems and perhaps by their own trade organizations. Certainly, leaders among long-term care providers, be they nursing homes, assisted living settings, home care organizations, or case-management organizations, all advocate this kind of approach. Partly their preference is derived from the proverbial aversion any business has to regulation, and partly out of genuine and reasonable conviction that the best improvements come from the creative efforts of providers themselves.

Regulations, they point out, also tend to stifle positive innovation. The CQI and TQM approaches mentioned at the beginning of the chapter are a provider-initiated approach to quality.

There are indeed a wide variety of strategies that providers can and do use to improve their own quality. In a study of home care agencies, for example, we identified the following kinds of efforts: audits of records systems, surveys of current and former consumers, efforts to recruit and retain high-quality personnel, orientation and staff development efforts, mechanisms to collect and redress consumer complaints, monetary incentives for performance of personnel, explicit ways to observe and supervise personnel on the job and implement performance standards, and monitoring of their own outcomes through information systems.[12] Some of these approaches were more conducive to large firms.

In the aftermath of the 1987 reforms for nursing home quality assurance, a standardized approach to resident assessment was developed and mandated to be used quarterly as a vehicle for record-keeping and care-planning, known as the Minimum data Set (MDS).[13] Although imposed from outside, some facilities are now experimenting with proactive ways to computerize and use the information from the MDS as an active way of monitoring and improving quality.[14] At issue is the extent to which a provider-driven approach such as is being proposed should replace outside regulation of nursing homes. Also at issue is whether the MDS should be moved to other residential care settings, even small foster homes and board-and-care homes, with the resultant financial costs and costs in terms of formalizing a more socially oriented system.

Educational Approaches

Some educational approaches are long-range indeed, geared to the continuing education or even the basic education of health professionals, such as nurses, physicians, and social workers. Some shorter-range educational approaches are tied to regulatory efforts—for example, when a state mandates that nurses' aides or home care attendants have a specified number of hours of training from training institutions that also meet specified standards. If requirements for certain educational levels or training experiences are adopted in regulations, these are examples of structure criteria, as discussed earlier. We are skeptical of these credentialing approaches. They may achieve a certain standard by weeding out those who will not even withstand 60, 90, or 100 hours of training, or whatever is mandated. But typically, the training requirements are too skimpy to have much meaning, especially if they are not reinforced by good working conditions, well-structured jobs, and ongoing supervision, feedback, and training.

Systemic Approaches

Case management. Quality can also be improved through system changes. Along those lines, some propose that case managers from outside the long-term care system can promote quality and minimize poor quality through the way they perform their regular functions. They could do this through judicious use of their purchasing power at the level of the individual client and the case management system and through the way they monitor the well-being of the individual clients and use their information systems at the community level. Some skeptics question whether case managers can really have this function if they also have responsibility for conserving public dollars through parsimonious care-planning. Other more optimistic commentators think that an external case management system could obviate much of the need for regulation of providers. We do think case managers are a potential force for quality assurance in long-term care, with some caveats. First, case managers would need to consciously adopt this quality assurance role, something research tells us they rarely do at present.[15] Second, they would themselves need to meet a quality standard for how they perform their jobs. Unfortunately, this latter problem seems to be approached at present through self-credentialing of the case-management industry and through rather arbitrary standards for caseload size and other structure criteria that are not clearly linked to outcomes.

Contractual approaches. Another rather radical way of looking at long-term care quality is as a matter of contract between providers and consumers. In this model, the consumer or the consumer's agent enters into a contract with a care provider who specified what services the provider will undertake to give, under what conditions, and for what price. Also specified are the circumstances, if any, whereby that provider would cease to give care. Contracts could be quite individualized or they might be standard—like standard rental agreements. Some providers favor this approach as a way to eliminate unwanted regulations. But some consumers also see advantages in a contractual model whereby they could specify the terms of their agreements and have redress if the contracts are breached.

Paying for quality. The discussion of quality and the ways to assure it can culminate in a plan to use quality as the basis for paying for care. Essentially, one can argue that the payments for most services are currently based on some combination of process and structure. At least to the extent that certain types of personnel and certain levels of effort are expected. In the case of nursing home care, until recently federal regulations required that the payment of such care be adequate to cover its costs. Many states calculated the costs based on a formula that determined how many minutes of care from what kinds of personnel were needed to meet the service needs of clients with various attributes. In effect, the payment system was determined by staffing guidelines that were, in turn, based on observations of how much time, on average, was devoted to different types of clients. No one ever stopped to ask if that pattern of care was associated with good outcomes or if there was evidence suggesting that more or less (or a different mix of) care might lead to better results.

Indeed, this sort of case-mix reimbursement can create a number of perverse incentives for poor outcomes. First, it relies entirely on the current state of care, which no one has established as being correct. For example, if it should take more time than the averages reflect to work with a client to motivate that person to do more for herself, or if it takes more time to supervise a client with dementia to do a task rather than just doing the task for the person, the assigned value of the care may be grossly underestimated. Indeed, in case-mix reimbursement systems dementia care is often the least expensive, not because it requires the least amount of time but because it has received the least amount of time. Second, if carried to its logical extremes, case-mix reimbursement creates exactly the wrong incentives. Making clients more independent lowers their reimbursement rates. Care providers will do better financially by making their clients more dependent.

At a minimum, payment principles should not oppose quality goals. The next logical step to bringing payment into line with quality would be to base payment on quality. More specifically, one might well consider paying more for better outcomes. Because payment should also recognize case mix (some types of clients do require more care than others), some combination of approaches is needed. Probably the most reasonable compromise is to base the payment on clients' initial status and to use some form of bonuses or penalties tied to achieving expected outcomes. The size and extent of the bonus/penalty payments could vary with the degree to which the expected outcomes were met or exceeded, or one could employ less precise categorical measures. (For example, providers get the payment of the goal is met and are penalized if the achievement falls below a fixed percentage of the target.)

Designing monetary incentives for outcomes and building them into state reimbursement policy is difficult. In the 1980s, the state of Illinois made an effort to encourage positive outcomes through their payment of nursing homes in a Quality Incentive Program (QUIP). Nursing homes could voluntarily decide to compete for add-on payments related to achievement of any or all of six "outcome" standards. Unfortunately, most of the "outcomes" measured really were process or structural measures; for example, a pleasant environment was measured by the surveyors, and presence of a goldfish aquarium tended to ensure earning the incentive payments on that outcome. The chief real outcome criterion was resident satisfaction. Unfortunately, the measured satisfaction was so invariably high in all the facilities striving for the incentive payments that failure on this criterion was almost impossible. The evaluation of this QUIP program pointed to these problems.[16]

Safety versus Freedom

An overriding issue in quality assurance for long-term care is how to balance pursuit of safety versus respect for individual freedoms, and what to do with the bad results. Almost invariably public officials state that their objective is to maximize the choice and control of the long-term care consumer. But almost invariably the rules that begin at the highest level in the state and that percolate down to every care provider emphasize safety. As we indicated as we discussed the persistent beliefs in long-term care, nobody wants an injury or care scandal on his or her watch.

In a variant of contracting, Keren Brown Wilson proposes "managed risk contracting" as an ongoing way for providers and consumers to communicate about risks that seem inherent in various care plans so that consumers or their agents can make informed decisions about the risks that they want to incur.[17] This concept is attractive in many ways, though largely untried. Case examples of managed risk contracts have largely been derived from programs in Oregon, especially assisted living programs. Even there providers and advocates are divided about the merits of the concept as a vehicle for respecting consumer autonomy and as a vehicle for protecting providers from liability.

At its best, a managed risk contract is used when providers identify behavior or preferences of the consumer that they believe are injurious to health or safety. The managed risk agreement provides a structured vehicle for providers to raise their concerns, describe the risks they think the consumer is incurring, and discuss alternatives to minimize the risks. Ultimately, the consumers make their choices and all parties sign on to the agreement. If managed risk contracting were ever to become widespread, other details would need to be clarified. For example, does the consumer have the right to waive all risks, or would some kind of tolerance on the provider's part be tantamount to negligence? Is it coercion if a particular program does not have sufficient staff to provide adequate care and consumers are forced to choose between leaving or accepting the risk. Who should inform consumers about risks? What about people with impaired decision-making capabilities? Should their agents be able to enter into a managed risk agreement for them, and if so on what basis should such agents make their judgments?

Reaching a Societal Consensus

The difficulty arises when the discussion moves from theoretical descriptions of ideal conditions to more practical problems of administering programs. What are the minimal standards that society will accept as adequate care and how much more will it pay for better results? Although we pride ourselves on living in a democracy, it is not a state of full equality. A well-established principle is that society will permit people to pursue individual goals with few restrictions and to pay as much as they wish for services that provide them with whatever satisfaction they seek, but obligations of publicly provided services are more constrained. (Even the Declaration of Independence guarantees only pursuit of happiness, not happiness itself.)

Long-term care has a different history from other health care in terms of quality regulations. Whereas groups like hospitals, physicians, nurses, and social workers established professional societies which undertook to create a set of performance standards, professionalization came late to long-term care. As a result standards for quality were imposed from without. Regulations arose from a combination of factors: a perceived need for standards to oversee public programs, a series of scandals, and the absence of any internal structure to dictate policies around quality or assume responsibility for assuring it.

As in so many other areas, much of the work on quality issues in long-term care has been shaped by reactions to nursing homes. Long-term care has been shaped by regulations. Regulations have been shaped in turn by professional norms and a strong sense that long-term care recipients need to be protected. Indeed, the early history of nursing homes immediately after the implementation of Medicaid was rife with various types of exploitation and scandal.[18] Perhaps due to the continuing regulatory efforts, however, modern long-term care is quite different from its progenitors. It is more professionally populated. These professionals have, in turn, contributed to the contemporary problem of creating a large array of regulations that dictate professional norms for a variety of services and situations.

Because regulations often arise in response to problems, especially well-publicized problems, they are usually written to avoid future catastrophes. As a result, quality of care is more likely to be defined as the absence of bad events than the presence of good ones. The first line of defense in establishing a regulatory program is to assure that bad things do not occur. Advocating for good aspects may be seen as desirable but unaffordable.

Most regulatory efforts are thus designed to identify the "bad apples." This emphasis has a number of unfortunate consequences: *(1)* It subjects the majority of care providers (who are doing a good or at least adequate job) to unnecessary scrutiny; *(2)* it directs attention to a limited set of measures; *(3)* it creates a false sense of quality that suggests that staying out of trouble is equivalent to doing a good job; and *(4)* it creates, or supports, a negative image of the field by not identifying positive goals.

Regulations can address any of the three principal ways of measuring quality: structure, process, and outcomes. Although some aspects, like fire safety, do address the actual physical structure, most structural elements refer to organizational issues such as staffing (numbers and level of training) and administration (committees, record keeping). The basis for validating structural and process requirements should be whether they lead to better outcomes. Outcomes can be expressed as the results of care or the states one seeks to achieve by giving care.

Most regulatory efforts have been directed at structure and process. These two components are most comfortable to administer. They offer a set of activities that can be prescribed. In effect, they limit the provider's responsibility. Good care is defined as doing the right things. Indeed, one can do the right things and still obtain poor results just on the basis of chance or because the client was uncooperative.

Although this regulatory effort is designed to assure a sufficient level of safe care, it suffers from two major disadvantages: *(1)* The majority of the regulations are based not on empirical evidence of what activities are associated with better outcomes but on professional judgments, which quickly approach dogma. *(2)* Strict statements about what should be done for whom become rapidly restrictive at a time when long-term care dearly needs innovation and creativity. Especially because so little has been proven about how to deliver the best care (and there is every likelihood that more than one way is available to achieve this end), it is premature to ossify the process.

In a situation where public funds are used to support private (especially proprietary) care of frail persons, regulation is inevitable. The issue is not whether to regulate but how. Methods should be devised to provide accountability in the context of maximum freedom to innovate. When there is little concordance between the process of care and its outcomes, most reasonable observers would suggest that it makes more sense to focus on the outcomes. Ironically, human nature tends to do just the opposite. Faced with uncertainty, we often tend to become more dogmatic.

The problems of regulation have been exacerbated by the growth and diversity of long-term care programs. As new forms of care have emerged, they present both an opportunity to escape from the heavy regulatory burden that has been layered on the nursing homes and a challenge to assure the adequacy of the quality they provide.

These new forms of care pose a paradox. To the extent that they represent alternatives to nursing home care, the nursing homes have called for a level playing field. Nursing homes find it understandably hard to compete if they must meet higher (or more limiting) standards than the new forms of care. On the other hand, if the new forms of long-term care are forced to follow the demands of nursing-home regulations, they will inevitably come to resemble nursing homes and thereby lose whatever advantages they offer as more innovative, flexible, and client-focused care. One solution would be to revise the rules for long-term care altogether to create a new playing field. If the emphasis is shifted from defining the process and structure of care to focusing on the outcomes, programmatic flexibility can be achieved without forfeiting accountability.

Once one has the ability to compare actual and expected rates of various outcomes, the nature of the discussion shifts. Attention is directed away from a model that tends to emphasize the elimination of untoward events to one that features the achievement of positive outcomes, expressed as both quality of care and quality of life. Caregivers, who often see only the gradual decline of the people they serve, may now be helped to see just what difference their care actually makes by comparing the client's course with what would otherwise have been expected to occur.

Summary

Everyone is in favor of quality but no one seems quite able to define it, let alone measure it. The difficulties in assessing quality cannot become an obstacle to using it as a central element in developing new policies for long-term care. In effect, two forces shape care delivery: payment and regulation. These two major influences cannot send out discrepant messages. Especially in light of the press to find new and better ways to deliver long-term care, great care must be taken not to champion extant orthodoxies. This strategy implies placing more emphasis on elements of outcomes than on structure and process. Indeed, this approach facilitates innovation while providing accountability. Emphasizing outcomes also forces society to address important questions about what is valued in long-term care. Such an outcomes system will not come into place until more systematic information about long-term care is routinely collected and analyzed.

A balance of emphasis must be found between relying on professional and consumer perspectives. The focus on the consumer includes both consumer-directed and consumer-centered perspectives. Outcomes may be the best place to seek that balance, because there is more opportunity for consensus, or at least more to be gained from dialogue about the differences in these perspectives. Central to both consumer perspectives are dignity, autonomy, continuity of preferred lifestyle, right to take risks, and consumer satisfaction. Outcome measures must include these concepts.

Quality definitions and quality assurance strategies should presuppose a cognitively intact client capable of using information to make decisions. Many persons with cognitive impairments have family members or others who could act as their surrogates in planning care.

Emphasizing outcomes over structure and process does not mean abandoning the latter concepts altogether. Where good evidence supports the linkages between what is done and its effects, process measures can be used effectively, although some leeway must remain to seek alternative means of achieving the same ends. In some areas, the process is the central element. Much of long-term care is based on principles of respect and compassion. These qualities are best measured directly rather than by trying to catch their reflections in outcomes.

Some structural elements seem obvious. In our view, privacy, including single-occupancy living quarters, and autonomy-enhancing features in residential long-term care environments are not luxuries, but rather basic quality expectations.

Service components of quality must include access to appropriate and technically competent care as needed, ability of care providers to identify and respond to a change in clients' physical condition, and ability to bring services to clients as their care needs change or increase. Consumers should not be required to move repeatedly among programs and care settings to have their needs met. A competent and caring labor force is crucial, but it cannot be generated by mandated training alone. Screening and selection, supervision, and job restructuring are needed.

Detection of quality problems requires a mixture of active efforts to seek information about quality of care and reactive responses to complaints. These detection strategies should be both internal and external to the activities of care providers. Care coordinators (or case managers) who are independent of care providers can play an important role. However, to do so, these case managers must consciously monitor the quality of care and must themselves perform in a high-quality way.

Correction of problems should be emphasized over mere detection. A graduated system of education, consultation, mediation, and sanction should be used to achieve prompt correction of serious problems and to remove incorrigible providers from the market. Ideally, payment incentives can reenforce quality goals.

Although it may be difficult to combine quality and payment regulations into a unified approach, at least our system should try to avoid internally inconsistent strategies. We may not be able to pay directly for better outcomes, but we should be able to use information about outcomes to inform consumer decisions. At a minimum, we should not champion payment systems that create rewards for achieving poorer outcomes.

Notes

1. Degenholtz H, Kane RA, & Kivnick HQ (1997). Care-related preferences and values of elderly community-based long-term care consumers: can case managers learn what's important to clients? *The Gerontologist*, 37:767–776.
2. Kane RL, Williams CC, Williams TF, & Kane RA (1993). Restraining restraints: changes in a standard of care. *Annual Review of Public Health* 14:545–587.
3. Katz K, Branch LG, Branson H, Papsidero JA, & Greer DS (1983). Active life expectancy. *The New England Journal of Medicine* 309:1281–1224.
4. Rogers A, Rogers RG, & Branch LG (1989). A multistage analysis of active life expectancy. *Public Health Reports* 104:222–226.
5. Kane RA & Kane RL (1988). Long-term care: variations on a quality assurance theme. *Inquiry* 25:132–146.
6. Kane RA, Kane RL, llston LH, & Eustis NN (1994). Perspectives on home care quality. *Health Care Financing Review* 16:69–90.
7. Kane RA (Ed.) (1997). *Understanding Health Care Outcomes Research.* Gaithersburg, MD:Aspen.
8. Kane RL, Bell R, Riegler S, Wilson A, & Kane RA (1983). Assessing the outcomes of nursing-home patients. *Journal of Gerontology* 38:385–393.
9. Kane RL, Bell R, Riegler S, Wilson A, & Keeler E (1983). Predicting the outcomes of nursing-home patients. *The Gerontologist* 23(2):200–206; Garrard J, Kane RL, Radosevich DM, Skay CL, Arnold S, Kepferle L, McDermott S, & Buchanan JL (1990). Impact of geriatric nurse practitioners on nursing-home residents' functional status, satisfaction, and discharge outcomes. *Medical Care* 28(3):271–283.
10. Kane RL, Bell R, & Riegler S (1986). Value preferences for nursing-home outcomes. *The Gerontologist* 26:303–308.
11. Harris-Wehling J, Feasley JC, & Estes CL (1995). *Real People Real Problems: An Evaluation of the Long-Term Care Ombudsman Programs of the Older Americans Act.* Washington, DC: Institute of Medicine.
12. Kane RA, Frytak J, & Eustis NN (1997). Agency approaches to common quality problems in home care: a scenario study. *Home Health Care Services Quarterly* 16:21–40.
13. Morris JN, Haws C, Fries BE, Phillips CD, Mor V, Katz S, Murphy M, Drugovich ML, & Friedlob AS (1990). Designing the national resident assessment instrument for nursing homes. *The Gerontologist* 30:293–307.

14. Zimmerman DR, Karon SL, Arling G, Clark BR, Collins T, Ross R, & Sainfort F (1995). Development and testing of nursing home quality indicators. *Health Care Financing Review* 16 (4):107–127.
15. Kane RA & Degenholtz HB (1997). Case management as a force for quality assurance and quality improvement in home care. *Journal of Aging and Social Policy* 9 (4):5–28.
16. Geron SM (1991). Regulating the behavior of nursing homes through positive incentives. Ananalysis of Illinois' Quality Incentive Program (QUIP). *The Gerontologist* 31 (3):292–301.
17. For one of the only published descriptions of this philosophy, see Kapp MB & Wilson KB (1995). Assisted living and negotiated risk: reconciling protection and autonomy. *Journal of Ethics, Law, and Aging* 1:5–14.
18. See Mendelson MA (1974). *Tender Loving Greed: How the Incredibly Lucrative Nursing Home "Industry" Is Exploiting America's Old People and Defrauding Us All*. New York, NY: Random House; Moss FE & Halamandaris VJ (1977). *Too Old, Too Sick, Too Bad: Nursing Homes in America*. Aspen Systems Corp.

8.

Acute Care for Long-Term Care Consumers

By acute care, we mean hospital care and the full range of physician and medically related preventive, treatment, rehabilitation, and palliative services delivered inpatient, outpatient, in-home, and in long-term care residential settings. For some seniors, medical care may be coordinated by a primary care provider (PCP), usually internists or general practitioners, often backed up and made efficient by nurse practitioners and other nonphysician personnel such as pharmacists. Also part of acute care are the services of all physician specialists who practice with older people in hospitals and community—for example, cardiologists, urologists, orthopedic surgeons, and oncologists. Mental health services for people with definable mental illnesses also fall under the acute care category.

Although the term *acute care* is useful as a contrast to long-term care it may be somewhat misleading. Society as a whole (and especially those receiving long-term care) is more likely to suffer from chronic conditions than acute ones. Over two-thirds of national health expenditures are spent on care for chronic conditions.[1] For those with two or more chronic illnesses and conditions the annual costs of medical and hospital care were sixfold higher than for those with acute conditions only. Thus, in this chapter we are focusing on acute care for people receiving long-term care with the recognition that most, though not all, this acute care will be dealing with the ramifications of chronic conditions as either primary or contributing aspects of the problem.

Geriatric medicine is a subspecialty of internal medicine and of family practice. Although geriatrics is often viewed as a primary care specialty and some patients receive their primary medical care from a geriatrician, for the most part, geriatricians practice as consultants. Geriatricians provide brief clinical assessments and interventions on referral, do programmatic consultation, and train medical students and others in the principles of working with the elderly. The numbers of geriatricians are still far too scanty for any other role.[2]

The relationship between acute and long-term care is intimate. Virtually all people have episodes when they need medical care. People receiving long-term care, with their greater likelihood of having more and more severe chronic illnesses and conditions, are more likely to need medical attention than the average older person; but health care should not be the overriding aspect of their lives any more than it is for the rest of us. Yet, as we keep emphasizing, a health-driven system of care, the nursing home, has been the dominant model of long-term care for many decades. The most bitter irony in this situation is that, despite this "medical model" of life, nursing home residents have received some of the worst acute care in the country. Nursing home residents are treated by primary care personnel infrequently and too often superficially. Preventive health services, reviews of ongoing regimens, and even diagnoses of new conditions may be neglected. Although nursing home staff theoretically work on the basis of physician orders, communications between the nursing staff and physicians are frequently less than productive. Bad long-term care can accelerate the need for acute care. For example, poor skin care can lead to bedsores, and poorly managed incontinence can lead to urinary infections.

An acute episode is often the inciting event for a career in long-term care. Many nursing home residents enter from the hospital. The boundaries between acute and long-term care have become eroded. Many were artificially created by funding decisions, especially as they affect the jurisdictions of Medicare and Medicaid. The distinction between acute and long-term care is blurring as the service definitions and locations of care change. As Medicare has broadened its sphere of concern to encompass care that formerly was classified as chronic, the distinctions have become less clear. Patients that a decade ago were treated in hospitals are now found in nursing homes and under home health care.

Although the names imply some sort of transition, acute care does not stop when long-term care begins. Although one might imagine a frail person starting with acute services and making a transition to long-term care, the reality is quite different. Patients do not stop needing acute care when they enter the long-term care arena, and it is not always clear just when they enter it. Too often funding policies impede the effective delivery of acute care services, especially effective primary care (the term that refers to ongoing health care and preventative services). The blurring of the boundaries between the two is perhaps best illustrated by new types of care, like subacute care. In effect, subacute care represents hospital-level care in other settings. The pressure for earlier hospital discharges has created a market for care in less expensive settings to manage the recovery and rehabilitation of patients who are no longer deemed to require the expensive resources of a hospital but who have not reached a steady state in their healing. Nursing homes have leapt into this breech, seeing an opportunity for growth. It is not yet clear whether they are up to this challenge. Studies comparing such care in nursing homes and in traditional rehabilitative facilities reveal a mixed picture.[3]

Not only do many nursing home stays and home-health episodes begin with a discharge from a hospital, people receiving long-term care are often heavy users of acute care. The Medicare payment rate for capitated care, the Adjusted Average Per Capita Cost (AAPCC), uses nursing home status as one the multipliers for increased capitation for acute care. (See Chapter 9 for an elaboration of the AAPCC.) Patients in nursing homes are expected to generate more than twice as much expenditure for their acute care services as those who are not. This is because the same problems that led to an admission to the nursing home are also likely to require more intensive medical care. In the calculation, nursing home use is actually used as a proxy indicator of functional status. If a patient's actual functional status is taken directly into account, nursing home patients use *fewer* acute care services than people with equal impairments living in the community.

Conversely, residents in nursing homes are often sent to hospital emergency rooms for acute treatment when it is hard to get a physician to make a timely nursing home visit. Such actions are expensive and disruptive. Growing evidence suggests that more aggressive and responsive primary care for nursing home residents can reduce the use of hospitals. Moreover, many problems that traditionally result in hospitalizations can be managed in the nursing home (at a lower cost) if the nursing home personnel are prepared to render more intensive oversight and there is good coordination with primary care providers. One health maintenance organization (HMO), EverCare, relies heavily on nurse practitioners as primary care providers both to provide closer attention to daily health care needs and to mobilize more intensive care in the nursing home to reduce reliance on hospitals. (This program is described in greater detail in the next chapter, which deals with managed care.)

People getting long-term care at home also need acute care. Indeed, it is hard to say explicitly which services given at home should appropriately be labeled long-term and which should be called acute care. New technologies have made it possible to deliver sophisticated care at home including intravenous therapy and mechanical ventilation.[4] Almost every kind of care can be and is given at home it seems, except physician care, and even that may be changing (albeit very modestly). There is now even an Academy of Home Care Physicians. However, Medicare payment for physician home visits is still too limited to entice a groundswell of practice change. Even using nurse practitioners and physician assistants to deliver in a patients' home is not profitable at present.

Fragmenting Forces in Medical Care

American medical care has been shaped largely by payment practices rather than by service needs. These operating principles have become so ingrained into daily performance that it requires a deliberate effort to recognize and overcome the assumptions behind them. Before a more innovative and comprehensive approach to care can be created, these barriers to conceptualizing tasks and solutions must be addressed.

Programs are classified in part by who pays for various services. For example, Medicare and Medicaid cover different types of care with different rules for eligibility. These payment rules also dictate what kinds of persons can provide the services and under what circumstances. For example, Medicare pays for only skilled care in nursing homes or home care if provided by a certified home-health agency but Medicaid pays for a broad range of long-term care needs. Moreover, physicians visits are reimbursed by rule rather than by needs. Medicare both permits and requires physician visits to nursing home residents every 30 days (although every other visit can be done by a nurse practitioner or physician assistant) regardless of whether the residents require fewer or more visits.

In another vein, "medical necessity" as certified by a physician is usually the trigger for authorizing long-term care services under Medicare (e.g., home-health) and Medicaid, even although physicians receive no additional reimbursement for attending to such gatekeeper roles and may not be in the best position to determine what type of care is needed. Physician care is, thus, governed by reimbursement rules; yet at the same time, physicians have mandated roles that are not reimbursed at all. Both these conditions encourage perfunctory care.

The whole question of optimal physician services needs revisiting. Do reimbursement rules encourage too much service, too little, or the wrong service? What aspects of long-term care, if any, should require physician authorization? What aspects should require more active physician oversight? How can payment incentives and policy be realigned to keep physicians in the loop when they should be and removed from inappropriate roles? Sometimes the services of a physician are reimbursed when those of a nurse are not: When should this be changed?

Existing payment criteria may not be as unyielding as they first seem. For example, Medicare has changed its policies about coverage and payment considerably over its three decades. Medicare began explicitly as a program to cover acute care exclusively. Its benefits were directed at physician and hospital care and a set of other services that were intended to encourage recuperation in less expensive settings. It, therefore, covered limited stays in nursing homes, for patients needing skilled care, and home-health care targeted at the same group. As earlier chapters indicated, specific eligibility requirements for home-health care included being homebound (which significantly meant one had to stay at home except when traveling for medical reasons), needing at least one of a defined set of skilled services, and having a problem that was expected to change its course (either for better or worse). Custodial care was expressly prohibited. Over time, however, changes in the Medicare regulations and policies allowed Medicare home-health benefits to cover such services as "evaluation and management" of care. By 1992, a substantial portion of Medicare covered home-health care was going to persons who had been receiving it for more than 6 months, a duration that suggests chronic more than acute care.[5] However, physicians are still expected to authorize the need for home-health services and the actual amounts needed, even including the services of home health aides; this latter area is way beyond the physician's purview and expertise, and in practice aides are assigned and supervised by nurses.

As Medicare moves into prepaid managed care (see next chapter), the definition of specific benefits, such as home-health care, becomes especially important. When a Medicare managed care organization (MCO) offers a service, it is expected to provide the type and amount of services that would have been available to the Medicare beneficiary under the fee-for-service Medicare program. For those patients who are also covered by Medicaid, the greater the amount of home care paid for under Medicare, the less the demand for Medicaid. MCOs, which receive a fixed payment for Medicare services and could charge Medicaid for any additional care, thus have an incentive to try to minimize their Medicare-covered services. Conversely, the states have an incentive to maximize such care. New programs of managed care for so-called "dually eligibles" (i.e., those covered by both Medicare and Medicaid) offer a hope for better integrated care with an absence of cost shifting. These programs should provide a context for more innovative approaches to addressing the whole patient rather than subdividing on the basis of fiscal responsibility.

Payment regulations influence how services are provided and what they are called. Different payers emphasize the medical or social side of a problem. Driven by fears of Medicare "mills," where physicians would overbill for perfunctory care, payment policies for physician care in the nursing home make nursing home practice much less attractive than hospital or office practice. Despite the broad recognition of the phenomenon that hospital patients are being discharged sicker and quicker,[6] patients discharged from a hospital to a nursing home are determined to need much less intense medical management merely by virtue of where they have been placed. The same patient may be deemed to need daily physician attention in the hospital, but a day later each physician visit to the same patient discharged to a nursing home must be justified.

Conversely, there are strong incentives to transfer patients from nursing homes to hospitals at the first sign of illness. Nursing homes do not tie up nursing personnel, physicians are better paid for their care, and overall reimbursement is increased. It comes as no surprise that programs designed specifically to maintain patients in nursing homes can show enormous effects by changing the location of care. When these programs operate under a capitated arrangement that covers primary care and hospital care costs, there is every incentive to invest more effort in more intense primary care in order to prevent hospital admissions and to create a receptive climate in the nursing home to take back these patients as soon as possible after a hospitalization.[7]

As indicated, access to nursing homes and home-health care, under Medicare and Medicaid requires a physician's prescription. This artificial barrier, based on the notion that physicians are especially insightful in assessing the need for such services, often leads to pro forma activity. Physicians passively sign forms prepared by others. Rather than serving to involve medical practitioners more centrally in long-term care activity, these regulations have created a cadre of often reluctant participants. Ironically, however, when faced with an opportunity to discharge their responsibilities by delegating the tasks to others, some of these same reluctant practitioners are loathe to give up the control that comes with it. Nor is the situation so one sided. Newly energized groups of medical practitioners are emerging, who are committed to improving long-term care and who want to be actively involved in the solution. The transformation of organizations like the American Medical Directors Association, which represents the medical directors of nursing homes, into a more scientific and progressive force bears witness to the growth of geriatric expertise and commitment to this field.

Physician services are also fragmented by their location. Hospital care is distinguished from ambulatory or outpatient care. Home care is separated from institutionally based care. In fact, many of the same fundamental services can be provided in multiple settings. The definitions continue to change as more technology is moved out of institutions. Care that used to require a hospital stay can now be offered as an outpatient service, or even at home. In some cases, technologically intense care can be arranged easier at home than in a nursing home.

Professional definitions of service, based on who performs them, can create inefficiency. Numerous tasks essential to care of frail elderly persons can be performed by several different disciplines—for example, assessing activities of daily living. Nurses, physical therapists, physicians, and social workers may each carry out such assessments, sometimes on the same clients. Although each discipline may address the procedure slightly differently, there is a large degree of overlap in the information collected. It does not make sense to collect redundant information simply because data collection is part of each agency's customary procedures.

As more responsibility for medical care is placed in the hands of primary care providers (PCPs), they need to understand more about the management of frail older persons. Unfortunately, most PCPs have received little training in geriatrics. Their caseloads are often quite mixed, offering less incentive for them to become adept in geriatric care. The challenge then is to find ways to increase their sensitivity to the special problems involved in managing their clientele who also receive long-term care. Medical conditions may present quite differently in older persons. Typical symptoms may be absent, making diagnosis more subtle.[8]

The subtle way that diseases of older people present themselves can be illustrated by the *I's of Geriatrics*; which depict some major functional problems of older people.

immobility	isolation (depression)	infection
instability	inanition (malnutrition)	iatrogenesis
incontinence	impecunity	immune deficiency
intellectual impairment	impairment of hearing	impotence
irritable colon	and vision	insomnia

Each of the conditions listed can be caused by a variety of underlying factors. Careful evaluation is needed to elucidate the actual cause of the problem.

Much of geriatric lore focuses on the centrality of patient functioning. The traditional diagnostically based approach to care is necessary but not sufficient. While it is appropriate to make the correct diagnosis to initiate the correct treatment, care also needs to address the interrelated functional problems of the long-term care consumer. One solution used in some managed care programs concentrates the care of older persons, especially those receiving long-term care, in the hands of a few PCPs who express a special interest in such care. In some cases these PCPs work closely with geriatric nurse practitioners (GNPs).

It is also difficult for physicians to remain current about the range of long-term care settings, their capabilities, and the way physicians need to communicate and interact with their long-term care staff. As Chapter 6 indicated, a wide range of living situations with services are now appearing in the market with a welter of names attached. PCPs cannot readily know what, if any, internal capacity the organization has for nursing care, including administration of medications and treatments and monitoring of conditions. They may expect too much of some settings and too little of others. Yet, it is often the physician who advises patients and families of optional care arrangements, and it is certainly the physician and his or her team who carry forward ongoing preventive and primary care and make decisions about whether to hospitalize.

Care Management

Care management, a hallmark of social long-term care programs, is another area of role overlap and role confusion. PCPs often perceive care management as their own particular contribution, one that is reinforced by their roles as gatekeepers and authorizers for Medicare and Medicaid services for their patients. They may not take kindly to other care managers (more often called case managers in the long-term care arena) who impose themselves into this arrangement. Meanwhile hospital discharge planners, who are sometimes delegated the care-management role when the patient is hospitalized, are charged with the responsibility of facilitating the patients' discharges from hospitals. Especially under the pressure of prospective payment for Medicare services, they feel a real urgency to move patients out expeditiously. Representing the interests of the hospital may come into conflict with maximizing the preferences of the patients and their families. Hospital discharge planners may look upon other case managers as just another impediment they must confront rather than an ally in achieving a common goal.

Although there is usually some common core, care management means different things to different groups. From a medical perspective, care management addresses patients at high risk of medical complications or under poor control to intervene to reduce these risks. This intervention may include identifying the problems with adhering to the regimen or directly intervening to remind patients or suggest behavior that will yield a more positive result. Aggressive follow-up and close attention have been shown to reduce subsequent use of hospitals.[9] A social perspective would be more likely to emphasize obtaining needed services and assisting with the adjustment to those services.

Almost every proposal for new long-term care programs includes some capacity for care management. Some now prefer other names for the service, such as *care coordination*, to suggest a more equal distribution of power between client and professional, but the intent is still to assist patients to use services that will best accomplish the therapeutic or supportive goals. The enthusiasm for care management rests on a belief that some direction is needed. Its logic may block adequate acknowledgment of another critical factor: Care management per se is not enough; there must be real services to be managed. When care managers are given leeway to use available resources creatively, there is evidence that improvements in meaningful outcomes are possible.[10] To do their jobs effectively, care managers must be able to communicate meaningfully with PCPs. They must develop shared goals and integrated plans of care.

The potential for conflict arises when the goals of care management differ. In some contexts, care management is primarily concerned with utilization management. Its task is to reduce use of expensive care. This reduction can be achieved positively, by active intervention to reduce complications and avoid iatrogenic problems; or it can be more negative, by demanding oversight and prior approval. Thus, the utilization control function can conflict with the resource mobilization role of a case manager trying to obtain all needed services for her client. The confusion is exacerbated because few programs actively announce that care managers are involved in resource-constraining activities. Rather, they prefer to portray the care managers as facilitators only.

Integrating Care

Acute care is fragmented both within its own boundaries and in relationship to long-term care. Yet fragmented care giving need not be the dominant model. There are good reasons to believe that coordinated care would be more satisfying to patients and more effective. It also should be more efficient. Models of care coordination are most likely to be found in programs that emphasize geriatric care. Geriatrics is fundamentally an interdisciplinary pursuit.

Perhaps the strongest body of evidence about the effectiveness of the geriatric approach can be found in work concerning comprehensive geriatric assessment.[11] Comprehensive assessment and short-term management have been combined into what are now called *geriatric evaluation and management* (GEM) units. Careful assessment by geriatric teams on well-targeted patients who are at risk for long-term care has been shown to improve function and to reduce the subsequent use of nursing homes.[12] More surprising, simply assessing and reassessing unselected older persons living in the community and bringing the problems uncovered to the attention of their doctors has been associated with substantially the same basic outcomes: reductions in nursing home use and improved function.[13] Likewise, comprehensive assessments of persons who fell frequently did not lead to specific reductions in rates of falling or their sequelae, but those assessed did seem to enjoy benefits associated with a greater clinical attention.[14]

Growing experience with geriatric assessment indicates that assessment per se is not sufficient. There must be associated therapeutic action. Often providing this clinical action requires maintaining contact with the patient for some extended period until the new therapeutic regimen has stabilized.

The need to balance assessment with action applies to all of care. Often excessive effort is focused on developing careful assessment procedures, but insufficient thought is given to what actions these assessments should stimulate. Few people are helped by an assessment alone. Just as a diagnosis is not an end in itself, assessment's value lies in the positive actions it spawns. Whether we talk about care management or geriatrics, there is no great benefit from uncovering a problem, however precisely or comprehensively, unless something can be done to improve the situation. Especially in chronic care, ongoing monitoring is needed to ensure that the plan of care is implemented and to assure that changes in patients' status are detected and addressed.

Interdisciplinary Teams

The ideal method of integrating care is through teamwork. The idea of teams is very appealing but conducting them in a cost-effective manner is quite challenging. Working as a team requires several prerequisites:

1. A shared goal or objective
2. A clear sense of individual roles and responsibilities
3. Individual competencies
4. A common language
5. Common rules
6. An effective communication system

The goals of care may differ among disciplines in large and small ways. Consistent with their training and concerns, different professionals may focus on different aspects of a client's functioning. This role differentiation can be useful if the sum of the pieces equals the whole and the various actors are working in concert toward the same goal. However, much of the care of frail older persons involves trade-offs. Improvement in one area may come at the cost of loss in another. For example, mobilization may cause pain. These trade-offs must be anticipated and addressed.

Larger schisms in goals occur. Historically, long-term care has been operated under the general auspices of social programs, whereas medical care has been seen in a more aggressive therapeutic context. The social service approach has emphasized compensatory care, wherein a client's needs were assessed and a plan of care was developed to compensate for the deficiencies identified. Good care is defined as a service package that fits the profile of needs. Good outcomes are judged by the goodness of fit and the absence of untoward events, such as pressure sores or infections. By contrast, a therapeutic approach holds that good care should lead to some positive outcome, even if it is identified as simply slowing the rate of decline. Good care should produce a result that is as good as or better than would be expected.

These two models of care define a tension in the way long-term care has been approached by health personnel. The dominant compensatory philosophy has meant that long-term care has been viewed as an intervention process with generally little to show for its investment beyond staying out of trouble. It is small wonder that long-term care has failed to arouse much passion. Attention has instead focused on minimizing costs to the point where many now conclude that the costs of long-term care under Medicaid cannot be any further reduced without doing substantial harm to the beneficiaries.[15]

A more therapeutic approach shifts attention from concentrating exclusively on costs toward greater concerns about the outcomes of care. These outcomes need not be restricted to medical measures, or even function. Quality of life issues and satisfaction are equally salient. Thus, as we argued from the other perspective in Chapter 1, therapeutic and compensatory approaches are mutually compatible. Both are needed.

Closely related to common objectives are well-defined roles. Duplication of effort is inefficient and may place heavy burdens on clients, who are asked the same questions by multiple professionals. Similarly, having several professionals give a client either different or varying versions of the same messages can be quite confusing. Identifying areas of common interests and developing coordinated ways to collecting needed information are central to productive team function. Team members must be able to trust other members to collect needed information. All members should actively contribute to defining the database, but the data collection task can be apportioned.

Trusting another person to collect information or to dispense advice requires confidence in that person's professional abilities. One cannot have an effective interdisciplinary team unless each member is a competent representative of her discipline. Sometimes special education is needed to make others aware of just what each discipline can actually do. Professional education rarely offers insights into the perspectives and capabilities of other professions.

Each profession speaks in its own tongue. Different terms are used to describe the same thing, and each profession brings its own prism to view the world. Disciplinary constructs may affect the way different professions view the situation. Emphases may vary, with some disciplines more focused on positive well-being and others more concerned with reducing illness burden.

The communication gap may be exacerbated by needing to operate under different rules. Some of these may be imposed by professional practice and others externally. For example, medicine is comfortable directing and prescribing, whereas nursing or social work may prefer to suggest and educate. In some professions physical contact is a central feature of treatment. In others, it is generally discouraged. Some professionals feel very comfortable probing into clients' personal affairs; others do not.

Once a common goal and a common language have been established, it is possible to communicate. Communication can prove the undoing of teamwork. If teams members require frequent face-to-face contact to process information and to share ideas, teamwork will be prohibitively costly. Team members must be able to share ideas in a common record, or at least a linked information system. Ideally, the information system would serve not only as a place to exchange observations and conclusions but as a way to identify clients at high risk and to indicate when adequate progress has not been achieved.

A first step in establishing a common communications system is getting everyone to keep records the same way and in the same place. Computerization offers a great advantage by allowing people to be linked even when they are not geographically proximal. Computerization also represents the means to use information more actively. Specific protocols can drive data collection and can monitor client progress by requiring regular reporting on certain parameters. Information can be harnessed to create flags that identify patients at high risk and direct attention to them. Pertinent data collected by one person can be brought to the attention of other involved professionals.

One of the benefits of developing an integrated communications system is the need to define specific variables and the protocols that will be used to deal with them. In effect, this exercise clarifies the relationships among the players and forces them to utilize a common language.

New Primary Care Personnel

Many of the tasks that were the traditional purview of one discipline can be performed by others. The press for greater efficiency can be met, in part, by downward delegation. Historical physician services are now performed by nurse practitioners and former nursing tasks can be readily taught to personnel with less formal training.

Nurse practitioners have proven capable of filling many of the primary care roles traditionally played by physicians. Geriatric nurse practitioners (GNPs) have been shown to be effective in providing primary care to nursing home residents.[16] One managed care organization has used GNPs as a core element in establishing a system to provide aggressive primary care to patients in nursing homes, which seems to be cost-effective in reducing the subsequent amount of hospital care.[17]

The move toward managed care has produced a renaissance of enthusiasm for primary care. Primary care providers are more attractive than specialists in the managed care environment because they use fewer services and hence may be less expensive.[18] Indeed, a case can be made for even more dramatic downward substitution—for example, using nurse practitioners in lieu of physicians to deliver much of this care.[19] This type of delegation is much more feasible in the context of managed care, where each activity is not separately billed.

As the demand for primary care has grown, geriatrics has wavered in its self-definition. What began as a specialty designed to see complex patients on referral became a primary care enterprise when it appeared that the tide was turning toward primary care.[20] Yet the numbers of geriatricians being produced are far too small to make even a dent in the need for chronic care. Were there enough geriatricians, one might envision much of the care of older persons divided such that geriatricians would manage the most complex cases while geriatric nurse practitioners provided the basic primary care.

But care of older patients is being hotly contested. As chronic care has assumed a more dominant position on the medical care map, new interest has surfaced about what constitutes the most effective way to provide such care. Given the long history of specialty domination in American medicine, much of primary care has been given by specialists.[21] There is at least some reason to believe that managed care's rush to embrace primary care by generalists may have been too zealous. For at least a selected subset of patients, care from specialists may prove more cost-effective. Some patients with chronic illnesses may be too complicated to be managed by the average generalist, who has rarely, if ever, confronted such a case. For example, a patient with multiple sclerosis may be better managed by a neurologist who has the expertise in the dominant disease and its complications. Likewise, a cardiologist may do a better job with a patient with unstable congestive heart failure or unstable angina. Certainly many disability activists who reach age 65 with an impairment acquired when they were much younger, such as spinal cord injuries or cerebral palsy, complain that the average general physician does not know how to treat their specific conditions.

The evidence to support greater activity by specialists in delivering primary care is mixed.[22] The Medical Outcomes Study showed little difference in the outcomes of care for hypertension and non-insulin-dependent diabetes based on whether that care was given by specialists or generalists. In contrast, an earlier British study found better outcomes associated with specialist care for type II diabetes. Other studies showed that subspecialist care by rheumatologists was associated with better outcomes in treating rheumatoid arthritis. Allergists were more effective than generalists in reducing the complications of at-risk asthmatics. Cardiologists had better results with acute myocardial infarction (i.e., heart attacks) than did generalists.

If specialists assume primary care roles, they will need to change their modus operandi. They will have to address the needs of the whole person, paying closer attention to the functional aspects of care rather than addressing only the clinical parameters. Not all specialists, however, will be comfortable with this broadened mandate.[23]

Moving from physicians to the other end of the educational chronic care continuum, the frontline workers, one can make a stronger case for merging roles by creating a generalist function. In the case of home care, for example, the current practice of distinguishing between a homemaker and a home health aide may prove an anachronism. It should be much more efficient to use a single person to provide both types of care. Similarly, in a nursing home the role of nurse's aides could be recast as assistants to all the professionals who contribute to the resident's plan of care and, of course, to the residents themselves. They could, for example, assist the goals of physical therapists through range of motion exercises and assist the goals of social workers through facilitating residents in social interactions inside and outside the nursing home. The distinctions in roles of frontline workers have been reinforced by regulations and payment policies. As more long-term care programs come under the auspices of managed care organizations, the topic of the next chapter, the pressure to maintain such distinctions may abate.

Aggressive Chronic Care

Evidence is accumulating to demonstrate that more aggressive efforts to detect problems early and address them actively can improve outcomes and save money in chronic care. This shift in attitude began with the results from geriatric assessment trials. Although all were not effective, literature now suggests that active evaluation and management can produce substantial benefits, including reducing mortality rates and lowering admissions to nursing homes.[24] Although there is still a strong case in favor of careful targeting to identify those most likely to benefit, some benefits are found even when unselected older populations are addressed.[25]

The assessment and active intervention strategies have converged in the evolution of geriatric evaluation and management, whereby responsibility for managing patents is maintained beyond the initial assessment period to assure that the revised treatment regimen is followed and is effective. Following patients with unstable conditions closely to assess their condition and their compliance with medical regimens can also pay dividends. For example, when nurse practitioners worked with patients with congestive heart failure recently discharged from hospitals to assess patients' understanding of their medications and to respond quickly to identified minor problems, they were able to keep these patients functioning and reduce the need for subsequent hospitalizations.[26] The Kaiser Permanente Colorado Region addressed a similar problem of managing complex, high-risk geriatric cases better by instituting a Cooperative Health Care Clinic, which provides a comprehensive package of services in group settings for extended periods and emphasizes education and prevention. The initial results suggest both improved patient satisfaction and reduced use of clinics and emergency rooms.[27] Group Health Cooperative of Puget Sound is testing a similar concept of active patient education that emphasizes self-management, supervised exercise, and involvement in social activities.[28]

Providing chronic care is much more challenging than is usually appreciated. In the space of a brief encounter the clinicians must obtain and organize a substantial body of information. They must identify the clinical (and social) goals for this particular patient. They must recall the patient's clinical course and what has been the previous treatment regimen. They must assess the patient's present status and identify any changes since the previous encounter. They must establish a prognosis and modify their treatment in response to changing circumstances, to say nothing of educating the patients and acknowledging their immediate concerns.

The recognition of inconsistency in clinical practice has prompted a state of activity to create various forms of guidelines, pathways, and protocols. These tools are designed to provide a best practices approach to care, but they have several severe limitations. First, they are more often based on clinical consensus than on strong empirical data.[29] Second, they are designed to fit the usual case, but most geriatric chronic care is composed of atypical situations with patients who manifest multiple simultaneous problems.

Information Systems

Providing effective and efficient chronic care will require the use of emerging information technologies. The components of an adequate information system would cover the spectrum of care and would be easier to achieve under the rubric of managed care, where a single organization, at least in theory, is responsible for all acute care. Because managed care is based on the enrollment of a population, it is possible to assess the health status of the entire group rather than relying on only those who present themselves for care. Annual screening questionnaires can be used to identify those at potential risk. Filtered through clinical triggers, this information can indicate those who should benefit from more complete assessments to determine if a problem truly exists and what might be done to ameliorate it. Comprehensive assessments should lead to care plans, which in turn should lead to actions. The information system should track the actions taken, indicating if referrals have been carried out and what actions are indicated from them. Likewise, systematic tracking of pertinent patient parameters can allow clinicians to quickly see what progress the patients are making and to identify early signs of deterioration as indications for early intervention.

Even in the absence of managed care, clinical information can be better organized and used. Electronics permits sharing data with many members of the health care team, even those who may be geographically distant. Unlike the paper record, the electronic record can be shared without losing access to the original. The goal of computerized records is not to maintain the current style of unstructured note-taking but to use branching logic and other approaches to focus clinician attention on salient material.

In most instances the clinicians are poorly served by the present medical record system. Pertinent information is either not recorded or not readily accessible. A better information system could go a long way to improving the way chronic care is delivered. A chronic care information system would help to structure and facilitate the multiple tasks necessary. It would identify pertinent information and assure that it was collected at each encounter. The determination of what is pertinent will vary with each patient and their unique cluster of conditions. It would display information in such a way as to help clinicians recognize when clinically significant changes are taking place, preferably as early as possible.

Efforts to design computerized medical records typically try to capture all of the complexity of modern medical care. Just as in other situations that underwent computerization, the first instincts to capture the traditional approach in the new vehicle must give way to the ability of the new medium to organize and simplify information. The goal of a computerized medical record should be to provide structure that leads to clinical insight. Feedback should be simple rather than complex. Clinicians should be facilitated in focusing on pertinent information and prompted to take needed action. Summaries that indicate prognoses and progress should be available to assist in sharing information with other members of the clinical team. Graphic presentation of data can be used to demonstrate change in a patient's condition and even to flag the need to intervene.[30]

Concluding Comment

The challenge in defining the appropriate role for acute care in long-term care is to find the proper level of integration is to find the proper level of integration between social and health care, and acute care and long-term care. Long-term care clients need good medical care, but that service cannot come at the cost of dominating their lives. Although some people with severely disabling chronic conditions live lives overwhelmed by their medical care and health needs, most long-term care clients seek care in order to be free to enjoy their lives. There may be episodes of acute exacerbations in which illness becomes the preeminent concern, but most days medical care should play a supportive role only.

The unresolved question is how to effect that integration in a way that will preserve the close attention from primary care needed to prevent exacerbations without making such care a preoccupation. The social and medical providers will need to find a common language, a long-term care Esperanto, that can capture the nuances of both disciplines. Long-term care providers need to become sufficiently knowledgeable in the nuances of disease to recognize changes in status early and make appropriate calls for help. Primary care providers need to broaden their view to recognize that metabolic balance is hardly the ultimate goal of care. The emerging role for geriatric nurse practitioners offers one promising vehicle to create emissaries who may be able to bridge both worlds.

As in any collaborative effort, the first step lies in examining the goals that each side addresses. As these are made more overt, more common ground can be identified. Where philosophical differences remain, active discussion is needed to reconcile them. In most cases, the parties will discover that the client's preferences are the ultimate trump card in establishing the predominance of views.

Information management should be proactive. While it is valuable to identify mistakes after they occur, it is preferable to avoid them. Structuring data collection and drawing attention to early changes can facilitate midcourse corrections before serious problems arise. For example, detecting the inability to control congestive heart failure can stimulate a reappraisal of the treatment regimen before the patient needs a dramatic and expensive hospital intervention.

Despite the historic philosophical gulf represented by the so-called social and medical models of care, the future lies in finding the common cause between them. Good long-term care requires an effective synthesis of both acute and long-term care. The solutions created will have even wider applicability with the growing appreciation that most of the health care today addresses chronic disease. The traditional connotation of a medical model implies a loss of client sovereignty, a situation inimicable to the models of long-term care espoused here. But such a price need not, and should not, be paid. It is perfectly reasonable to provide attentive and competent medical care without demanding patient subservience. Indeed, most modern thinking about primary care encourages patients to play an active role in their care, making decisions and taking responsibility for implementing necessary behavioral changes.

Frail older persons generally need more than average medical care and attention from other health care providers. In good long-term care, health care needs are met through an integration of long-term care and acute-care efforts. Long-term care providers, be they staff of congregate living settings, staff of home-care agencies, or independently employed PAS workers, need to learn what to look for as signs of medical problems, construed broadly, and when and how to summon help. By assuming a proactive, data-driven approach, they can become colleagues in monitoring clients' progress and intervening in a timely way. Such partnerships are forged when all parties share a common philosophy. In this case, that approach to care is based on the premise that good care will make a difference in clients' outcomes. To be appreciated, that difference must be seen in comparison with what might be reasonably expected in the absence of good care. People receiving long-term care need more, not less medical attention, but that care should not compromise the desired lifestyle that their long-term care experience supports.

Notes

1. See Hoffman C & Rice DP (1996). *Chronic Care in America: A 21st Century Challenge.* Princeton, NJ: The Robert Wood Johnson Foundation. This report, based largely on the 1987 National Medical Expenditure Survey supplemented by other sources, provides exhaustive information about the prevalence and cost of chronic care for people of all ages.

2. Hoffman C & Rice DP (1993). *Strengthening Training in Geriatrics for Physicians.* Washington, DC: National Academy Press; Reuben DB & Beck J C (1994). *Training Physicians to Care for Older Americans: Progress, Obstacles, and Future Directions* (A background paper prepared for the Committee on Strengthening the Geriatric Content of Medical Education, Division of Health Care Services, Institute of Medicine). Washington, DC: National Academy Press.

3. See Kane, RL, Chen Q, Blewett LA, & Sangl J (1996). Do rehabilitative nursing homes improve the outcomes of care? *Journal of the American Geriatrics Society* 44:545–554; Kramer AM, Steiner JF, Schlenker RE, Eilertsen TB, Hrincevich CA, Tropea DA, Ahmad LA, & Eckhoff DG (1997). Outcomes and costs after hip fracture and stroke: a comparison of rehabilitation settings. *JAMA* 277(5):396–404.

4. See Arras JD (Ed.) (1995). *Bringing the Hospital Home: Ethical and Social Implications of High-Tech Care,* Baltimore, MD: Johns Hopkins Press; Mehlman, M & Younger SJ (1991). *Delivering High Technology Home Care.* New York: Springer.

5. Mauser E & Miller NA (1994). A profile of home health users in 1992. *Health Care Financing Review* 16(1):17–34.

6. Kosecoff J, Kahn KL, Rogers WH, Reinisch EJ, Sherwood MJ, Rubenstein LV, Draper D, Roth CP, Chew C, & Brook RH (1990). Prospective payment system and impairment at discharge. The 'quicker-and-sicker' story revisited. *Journal of the American Medical Association* 264(15):1980–1983.

7. See Malone JK, Chase D, & Bayard JL (1993). Caring for nursing home residents. *Journal of Health Care Benefits*, January/February: 51–54; Polich CL, Bayard J, Jacobson RA, & Parker M (1990). A nurse-run business to improve health care for nursing home residents. *Nursing Economics* 8(2):96–101.

8. Kane RL, Ouslander JG, & Abrass IB (1994). *Essentials of Clinical Geriatrics* (3rd ed.). New York: McGraw-Hill Information Services Company.

9. Rich MW, Beckham V, Wittenberg C, Leven CL, Freedland KE, & Carney RM (1995). A multidisciplinary intervention to prevent the readmission of elderly patients with congestive heart failure. *New England Journal of Medicine* 333(18):1190–1195.

10. Challis D (1993). Case management in social and health care: lessons from a United Kingdom program. *Journal of Case Management* 2(3):79–90.

11. Rubenstein LZ, Wieland D, & Bernabei R (1995). *Geriatric Assessment Technology: The State of the Art.* Milan, Italy: Editrice Kurtis.

12. Rubenstein LZ, Josephson KR, Wieland GD, English PA, Sayre JA, & Kane RA (1984). Effectiveness of a geriatric evaluation unit: a randomized clinical trial. *New England Journal of Medicine* 311(26):1664–1670.

13. Hendricksen C, Lund E, & Stromgard E (1984). Consequences of assessment and intervention among elderly people: Three-year randomized controlled trial. *British Medical Journal* 289:1522–1524; Stuck AE, Aronow HU, Steiner A, Alessi CA, Bula CJ, Gold MN, Yuhas KE, Nisenbaum R, Rubenstein LZ, & Beck JC (1995). A trial of annual in-home comprehensive geriatric assessments for elderly people living in the community. *New England Journal of Medicine* 333(18):1184–1189.

14. Rubenstein LZ, Robbins AS, Josephson KR, Schulman BL, & Osterweil D (1990). The

value of assessing falls in an elderly population. *Annals of Internal Medicine* 113:308–316.

15. Wiener JK, Lui K, & Schiedber G (1996). Case-mix difference betweenA. hospital-based and freestanding skilled nursing facilities. *Medical Care* 24(12):1173–1182.

16. Kane RL, Garrard J, Buchanan JCL, Rosenfeld A, Skay C, & McDermott S (1991). Improving primary care in nursing homes. *Journal of the American Geriatrics Society* 39:359–367.

17. Malone et al. (1993). See note 7.

18. Greenfield S, Rogers W, Mangoitch M (1995). Outcomes of patients with hypertension and non-insulin-dependent diabetes mellitus treated by different systems and specialties: results from the medical outcomes study. *Journal of the American Medical Association* 274(18):1436–1444; Carey TS, Garrett J, Jackman A, McLaughlin DBA, Fryer J & Smucker DR (1995). Outcomes and costs of care for acute low back pain among patients seen by primary care practitioners, chiropractors, and orthopedic surgeons. *New England Journal of Medicine* 333(14):913–917.

19. Mundinger MO (1994). Advance-practice nursing—good medicine for physicians? *New England Journal of Medicine* 330(3):211–214.

20. To dramatize the change, see Kane RL, Solomon DH, Beck JC, Keeler E, & Kane RA. (1981). *Geriatrics in the United States: Manpower Projections and Training Considerations.* Lexington, MA: D.C. Heath and compare this to Burton J & Solomon D (1993). Geriatric medicine: a true primary care discipline. *Journal of the American Geriatrics Society* 41(4):459–461.

21. Aiken LH, Lewis CE, Craig J, et al. (1979). The contribution of specialists to the delivery of primary care. *New England Journal of Medicine* 300(24):1363–1370; Mottur-Pilson C (1995). Primary care as form nursing-good medicine for physicians? *New England Journal of Medicine* 30(3):221–214.

22. For reports of the conflicting evidence on the effectiveness of specialists versus general physicians, see Gabriel SE (1996). Primary care: specialists or generalists. *Mayo Clinic Proceedings* 71:415–419; Greenfield S, Rogers W, Mangoitch M, Carney, MF & Tarlov, AR (1995). Outcomes of patients with hypertension and non-insulin-dependent diabetes mellitus treated by different systems and specialties: results from the medical outcomes study. *Journal of the American Medical Association* 274(18):1436–1444; Hayes TM (1984). Randomized controlled trial of routine hospital clinic care versus routine general practice care for type II diabetics. *British Medical Journal* 289:728–730; Ward MM, Leigh JP, & Fries JP (1993). Progression of functional disability in patients with rheumatoid arthritis: Associations with rheumatology subspeciality care. *Archives of Internal Medicine* 153:2229–2237; Zeiger RS, Heller S, Mellon MH, Ward J, Falkoff R, & Schatz, M. (1991). Facilitated referral to asthma specialist reduced relapses in asthma emergency room visits. *Journal of Allergy and Clinical Immunology* 87(6):1160–1168; Jollis JG, DeLong ER, Peterson ED, Muhlbaier LH, Fortin DF, Califf RM, & Mark DB. (1996). Outcome of acute myocardial infarction according to the specialty of the admitting physician. *New England Journal of Medicine* 325(25):1880–1887.

23. Speight JD & Blixt SL (1995). Heart specialists' art of care. *Social Science and Medicine* 40(4):451–457.

24. Stuck AE, Siu AL, Wieland GD, Adams J, & Rubenstein LZ (1993). Comprehensive geriatric assessment: A meta-analysis of controlled trials. *The Lancet* 342:1032–1036.

25. See Stuck AE, Wieland D, Rubenstein LZ, Siu AL, & Adams J (1995). Comprehensive geriatric assessment: meta-analysis of main effects and elements enhancing effectiveness. In LZ Rubenstein, D Wieland, & R Bernabei (Eds.), *Geriatric Assessment Technology: The State of the Art* (pp. 11–26). Milan, Italy: Editrice Kurtis for a meta-analysis of a large number of controlled studies of geriatric assessment in different contexts. For

a report of effectiveness even with an untargeted approach see Hendricksen C, Lund E, & Stromgard E (1984). Consequences of assessment and intervention among elderly people: three-year randomized controlled trial. *British Medical Journal* 289:1522–1524.

26. Rich et al. (1995). See note 9.
27. Scott J & Robertson B (1996). Kaiser's Colorado cooperative health clinic: a group approach to patient care. *Managed Care Quarterly* 4(3):41–45.
28. Wagner EH, Austin BT, & Von Korff M (1996). Organizing care for patients with chronic illness. *The Milbank Quarterly* 74(4):511–543.
29. Institute of Medicine (1992). *Guidelines for Clinical Practice: From Development to Use*. Washington, DC: National Academy Press.
30. Kane RL (in press) Managed care as a vehicle for delivering more effective chronic care for older persons. *Journal of the American Geriatrics Society*.

9.

Managed Care and Long-Term Care

Managed care is discussed more often than it is defined, perhaps because the term is used so variously and widely that it eludes clear definition. Some sort of management is, after all, part of any health or human service endeavor. In some ways, we have been talking about managing long-term care throughout this book. But managed care, as the new watchword of health care reform, and as a movement that has been sweeping the country, deserves a more precise definition.

Too often any sort of general management and rationalization of health care (e.g., requirements that patients be filtered through primary care gatekeepers before seeing specialists) is confused with a capitated system where managed care organizations (MCOs) receive a fixed sum of money per person enrolled as an operating budget and are at financial risk for providing all necessary care within that sum of money. Therefore, we offer two definitions to anchor our discussion: a general definition of managed care and a definition of *risk-based managed care.*

Managed care, in general, refers to efforts to coordinate, rationalize, and channel the use of services to achieve desired access, services, and outcomes while controlling cost.

Risk-based managed care describes care from MCOs that provide or contract to provide health care in broad but specified areas for a defined population for a fixed prepaid price. The MCOs are at financial risk to deliver the services within the fixed price, and they use various strategies to control costs.[1]

In some ways managed care can be thought of as hands-on health insurance. As this chapter illustrates, health insurance companies historically have used a variety of cost-control strategies in the way they construct their benefits, in the payments required of consumers, and in the prices paid to providers. MCOs similarly use a variety of strategies to hold down costs, but they are also directly responsible for the delivery of care.

Detractors sometimes say that managed care is a misnomer—the true term should be *managed costs*. This criticism is somewhat unfair, however; good managed care involves cost-effective care with equal emphasis on both components—the costs and the effectiveness. The original appeal of managed care, particularly the at-risk, capitated forms of managed care, lay in its potential to change the incentives for health care providers. Incomes would be based on achieving health rather than responding to illness. Within a payment system that presumably was sufficient to allow MCOs to stay in business by providing all necessary care, the incomes of the providers would increase if fewer services were used. This is the exact opposite of the purer versions of fee-for-service medicine, where the more hospitalizations, surgeries, physician visits, and all other kinds of services offered, the more money the providers make.

A particular form of managed care—managed competition—was the hallmark of the failed 1995 health reform efforts proposed by the Clinton administration. The idea here was that all working-age Americans and their families would have been covered by health insurance under some managed care arrangement required to meet minimum regulatory standards. Competition among competing plans in the marketplace would serve to control the costs and improve the quality of the product. This strategy for concluding an almost century-long effort to guarantee health insurance for all Americans conformed to the fundamental belief in the values of the marketplace that prevails in the United States. Although the reforms failed to achieve universal health insurance, the evolution of managed care and managed competition was catalyzed. Most Americans are insured through the workplace, and employers perceive advantages in offering various kinds of managed care plans rather than indemnity insurance. In 1997, more than 65 million Americans were covered in such work-related managed care. There is a trend: Fewer workers can rely on health insurance from the workplace (partly because of the growth of "contract" jobs that do not carry benefits, and partly because smaller companies are finding they cannot offer health insurance), but those who do receive insurance are likely to be in managed care.[2]

The broad enthusiasm of this strategy for cost control has already begun to affect the care of people with disabilities and the functional impairments of old age. This is a population largely insured through Medicare (which was largely left out of the proposed 1995 reforms) and Medicaid (for long-term care and for acute care for those who are poor, usually under 65, and not qualified for Medicare disability coverage). Managed care is fast becoming the dominant modality for all Americans. It is no longer creditable to expect these publicly financed programs to achieve the access provided under classic indemnity plans by "buying in" to fee-for-service medicine.

Public payers for health care, that is, federal and state governments, are attracted to using managed care mechanisms for several reasons. At a minimum, managed care serves a useful political role, seemingly distancing the policy makers from the responsibility for unpopular rationing decisions. It also limits government's liability

to fixed amounts. When operational responsibility is turned over to separate contracted organizations, governments can claim to have met public needs. Managed
care has been increasingly used in the Medicare and the Medicaid programs in the
last decades of the twentieth century; these developments are described in some
detail in the rest of this chapter.

Managed care's impact on long-term care is still modest. The large majority of
managed care, including within Medicare, is directed toward acute care. The dominant acute care activities have some limited implications for long-term care. MCOs
have incentives to use nursing homes and home-health care more actively as vehicles for subacute care to allow for early hospital discharges and outpatient procedures. Nursing home residents who are enrolled in managed care under Medicare
and develop complications are more likely to be treated in the nursing home,
thereby avoiding costly hospital admissions. This could be considered a good result
if its effect is to avoid disruptive and almost cruel hospitalizations at the end of
life, allowing people to receive care, including terminal care, in the place that has
become their home. It will be a bad result however, if it means that older nursing
home residents fail to receive care from which they could benefit.

Moreover, managed care is expanding. If trends persist, managed care will affect
more and more of long-term care. The present course of policy development supports efforts at the intersection of acute care and long-term care with programs
designed to merge both types of care under a single auspice and a single payment.
State policies for long-term care largely involve the Medicaid program, but the
nature of Medicaid, especially for older persons, is shaped heavily by Medicare.
Therefore attention has been directed at the so-called dually eligible group (i.e.,
those people eligible for both Medicare and Medicaid coverage). Obtaining federal
waivers to implement special capitated programs for the dually eligible population
can be cumbersome; it is necessary for states making these proposals to establish
eligibility criteria, service coverage, rates, and payment structures for both the Medicare and Medicaid components, and to establish a way of coordinating and integrating benefits. Therefore, some states have elected to convert into managed care
only the Medicaid component of coverage. For dually eligible people, the state
Medicaid programs still must cover the premiums, deductibles, and coinsurance
that individuals of private means pay as their share of the Medicare program. As
indicated in Chapter 2, state Medicaid programs also tend to cover health-related
services that other Medicare beneficiaries pay out of pocket, with outpatient prescription drugs being a notable component. However, many Medicare managed
care programs offer drug coverage benefits as an inducement to enroll. Finally, of
course, Medicaid covers long-term care. It takes creative planning for states to use
a managed care plan to cover the Medicaid expenses that are secondary to acute
care while the beneficiaries use the Medicare fee-for-service system with its emphasis on free choice of providers for their acute care.

It is also possible to envision managed care for long-term care only. For example,
in the 1980s Arizona established such a plan for its frail Medicaid recipients. To

receive the Medicaid benefits dually eligible people in Arizona must receive their Medicare benefits from the same sources that provide their Medicaid benefits. At present the Medicare services are paid for under traditional fee-for-service arrangements, but efforts are underway to develop merged capitated rates.

In theory, combining programs under Medicaid and Medicare could eliminate duplicated effort and enhance coordination, but the benefits need to be weighed against the risks. Such an alliance seems likely to put long-term care even more strongly in the health camp. MCOs and health insurance companies, which tend to know little about long-term care, have the track record, administrative structure, and capital to dominate this arena. So far, these organizations have emphasized cost control over innovation. On the other hand, managed care may be the best route to serious reform in long-term care. Because they have no strong ties to past arrangements and are interested in finding service packages that achieve the best results for the least cost, MCOs may encourage more innovation.

Managed care has a number of features that should make it attractive for those interested in improving long-term care and geriatric medicine. In theory, it should encourage a strategy of investment in primary care and comprehensive assessment, whenever such activities can be expected to lower the risk of subsequent expensive events like hospitalizations. It encourages the use of less expensive alternative services to hospital care in the community and in nursing homes, and it may encourage use of less expensive alternative residential services instead of nursing homes. Under enlightened clinical leadership, managed care could also make investments in rehabilitation for long-term care clientele, not only in formal rehabilitation programs but also in nursing homes.

There are, of course, pitfalls to avoid, many related to the orthodoxy of MCOs and their general lack of interest and experience with long-term care populations. MCOs could, for example, assume the nursing home is the only step-down setting of choice without realizing the danger of setting clientele on this trajectory or exploring use of other settings. MCOs could also devalue the labor-intensive activities in geriatrics and rehabilitation medicine. With the overriding tendency toward under-service in managed care, the burden of proof is placed on the proposed more intensive long-term care or geriatric services to show their value. Yet, there is often a dearth of empirical data and some of the value must be seen in the more amorphous area of quality of life issues, discussed in Chapter 7. In the absence of strong evidence for cost-effectiveness, MCOs may place their emphasis on cost controls without adding any new services. It is not yet clear just how acute and LTC can be packaged in a single managed care product, although there is active experimentation underway.

Historical Background

As we suggested, managed care has evolved out of health insurance. It combines the responsibility for paying for a defined set of services with an active program to control the costs associated with providing those services. Historically, health insurance was a method of redistributing the risk associated with paying for health services. Insurance companies would receive funds from individuals or others paying for their care and pool that money to be used as demands for payment were made. In effect, the insurance company had capitated the persons enrolled in the program, to the extent that they were responsible for the costs of their care toward meeting a defined set of health services benefits.

In practice, health insurance companies thus served as conduits. They would take in a predetermined amount of money per person covered and pay it out as costs were incurred. If at the end of the year the actuarial calculations of expected outlays proved an underestimate, rates for the subsequent year would have to be raised to make up the deficit and prevent such an error from recurring. Different insurance companies established alternative arrangements with health care providers. Some paid the rates charged; others negotiated special rates, sometimes a discounted rate, sometimes rates based on fixed payment schedules.

Health insurance began by charging a fixed premium for all insured people. A major shift in health insurance philosophy occurred just after World War II, when health insurance became an important component of employee benefit packages. As the competition for the health insurance business became more intense, insurance companies recognized that they could charge different rates for different parts of the population. In effect, because employed persons tended to be healthy, the companies could offer coverage for them at lower rates than those paid by the rest of the population. This shift from community rating (one rate for the whole community at risk) to risk rating (rates based on likely usage) eventually led to the exclusion of many older persons from the private insurance market, because their care was too expensive when its cost was isolated. This disproportionate burden, combined with the large numbers of older persons who were impoverished, provided the rationale for the passage of Medicare.

The availability of health insurance has been seen as a major contributor to the rapid escalation in health care costs. Financial barriers to obtaining care were removed, and the idea that someone else was paying the bill encouraged both providers and consumers to take full advantage of the growing array of technological advances becoming available.[3] As the costs of health care continued to rise much more rapidly than inflation and health care consumed an ever larger share of the gross domestic product, policy attention shifted to ways to curtail health care spending. Two basic strategies emerged, one aimed at consumers and one at providers.

The consumer strategy was to impose some barriers to use by levying various forms of copayments. The most common approaches used either deductibles (where the consumer paid the first portion of the bill—a technique familiar in other types of insurance) or copayments (where the consumer paid a portion of the bill and the insurance company the rest) or combinations of both. A major health insurance study conducted by the RAND Corporation showed that when these copayments were applied utilization declined dramatically.[4] An unexpected corollary was that for the entire insured population studied there were few differences in the health status of the groups with and without the copayments.[5] The obvious explanation for this finding was that, at any time, most insured persons are not very sick. Indeed, if they were, health insurance would not work, because the actuarial component that allows for spreading the risk would be absent. When the results of this RAND study were reanalyzed to look specifically at the health status of those who were sick, a different pattern of results emerged. Those who were poor and sick were especially disadvantaged by the copayments, even though these payments had been adjusted for differences in people's incomes.[6]

The provider-based strategies of cost control largely are directed toward changing the price paid for services. Perhaps the best known technique was applied to hospitals under Medicare. The Prospective Payment System changed the way hospitals were paid from a reimbursement for the actual costs incurred to reimbursement of a fixed amount per admission (or discharge), with that amount established on the basis of expected length of stay. Some 470 Diagnosis-Related Groups (DRGs) were created from available data that used diagnoses, patient age, and the presence of complications as the basis for estimating lengths of hospital stays.[7]

Although insurance companies did alter their payment methods, they at first played a fairly noninvasive role in the way care was delivered. But gradually information became available to show substantial differences in the way that care was given, including the numbers of procedures done, the length of hospital stays, and the cost of care from one area of the country to another. This body of literature, called *small-area variation studies*, seemed to show no discernable differences in the outcomes for patients despite the variation in inputs.[8] As payers learned that the substantial differences in the amounts and costs of services received from one location to another were not associated with concomitant differences in outcomes, the stage was set for a more active approach on the part of insurers.

Managed care, in effect, takes the insurance approach one step further. For a fixed fee, the MCO agrees to provide a package of services. Having accepted a fixed amount of money for the task, its incentives are to conserve these funds. Its strategies are similar to those used by insurance companies, but its motivation to contain costs is much stronger because its market advantage lies in offering lower costs than do more conventional insurers in exchange for more restricted options.

In theory, managed care can succeed in its cost-cutting agenda in two ways. It can lower costs for individual services or it can improve the efficiency of service across the full spectrum of an individual's illness. It can save money by restricting access to expensive forms of care or restricting services to providers who agree to accept lower payments. By providing more effective care early, it may avoid more costly care subsequently; or by substituting less costly modes of care, it may achieve the same ends less expensively. These two generic approaches are not mutually incompatible. In order to consider the likelihood of MCOs achieving these goals for the population of long-term care consumers, it is necessary to consider the various types of MCOs in today's medical marketplace and the incentives that they create for the health care providers and consumers alike.

Forms of Managed Care

HMOs, IPAs, PPOs, and POS

"Managed care organization" (MCO) is the general term used to describe the variety of organizations that have arisen to offer various forms of managed care. The name Health Maintenance Organization (HMO) was given to prepaid group practice around 1970 as a way of making it more attractive by emphasizing health promotion. The federal government was looking for a way to make health care more affordable. At the time, prepaid group practices were actively opposed by the medical profession as socialistic.

In 1970 a federal law was passed supporting the development of HMOs. Not only were funds made available to support the creation of such organizations and accredit them, but also every business with more than fifty employees was required to offer enrollment in such certified HMOs if they existed in the market area. The original concept was a "staff model" HMO, where doctors worked as salaried employees of the organization, which also owned the hospitals and all major parts of the delivery system. Indeed, when most people think of managed care, they think of variations of staff models such as Kaiser Permanente on the West Coast or New York City's Health Insurance Plan.

Reliance on staff models, however, did not permit HMOs to expand as quickly as policy-makers desired. Rather quickly the structure of the HMO was modified to include several different models. In addition to medical groups where all the doctors were on salary or shared in the profits, other models developed more akin to variations on insurance schemes. For example, a central company could sell coverage as an HMO (and accept the capitation) but then contract with independent providers (physicians, other health professionals, hospitals, nursing homes, laboratories, and so on) to meet the service needs. Such providers formed Independent Practice Associations (IPAs) to negotiate with the central MCOs. Physicians and hospitals could belong to several different IPAs. The providers in turn were asked to offer special rates to these MCOs in exchange for an anticipated high volume of business. Those that agreed became part of Preferred Providers Organizations (PPOs). MCOs would then ordinarily limit their enrollees to receiving services from members of the PPOs under contract to them.

Pure staff-model HMOs are now relatively rare, having been overtaken by these hybrid forms. Two general issues about this deserve comment. First, depending on the arrangements made with providers, the incentives for efficiency may not be pertinent at the level of the people and organizations who actually give the services. Some arrangements may be based on capitation and genuine financial risk sharing for providers, or at least offer economic incentives for less service. Other arrangements may strictly be on a fee-for-service basis with the usual incentive to do more. Second, in many communities the competition that was envisaged among MCOs has not really transpired. This is because most of the care providers in the community may be eligible to be paid by most of the MCOs.

242

Despite the active efforts to introduce them, MCOs did not catch on quickly. Few were prepared to mount all the services and reporting required to be officially accredited, fearing that such regulation and oversight would render them unprofitable. Instead, they set about to make themselves attractive on their own merits. One way was to offer services that would appeal to people who were not sick. Preventive services, active prenatal services, and expanded mental health coverage, for example, would be sought by young people who were unlikely to have high health risks. Plans could offer this sort of coverage for this population at very competitive prices.

One of the major reasons people resisted joining HMOs despite their lower costs was the limitations on choice of physicians. To attract more customers, the HMOs created another hybrid program, called Point of Service (POS). Under this arrangement, a subscriber, for an additional premium, can opt to use either an authorized HMO provider or to go outside the plan's "network" and use any provider. Typically, the amount of the bill covered in a POS option is less than when network providers are used. Nonetheless, POS has appeal to consumers because it hedges their bets to get the best possible care if they develop serious or specialized needs.

Medicare and Medicaid MCOs
The earliest MCOs operated exclusively in the private sector. Gradually, as their popularity grew, the Medicare program became interested. If such a competitive approach was seen as controlling costs for younger workers, why could it not work for Medicare beneficiaries as well? In the early 1980s a set of demonstrations was initiated to test the feasibility of enrolling Medicare beneficiaries in HMOs. By 1982, before the results of the demonstrations were analyzed, legislation was passed establishing a program of risk-based Medicare HMOs. Because the enabling legislation was called the Tax Equity and Fiscal Responsibility Act of 1982, the Medicare HMOs were known as *TEFRA HMOs.*

Care under Medicare is different from care provided as part of workers' benefit packages. With the latter, the employer can simply decide which type of health care benefits to offer or it can agree to cover the cost equivalent to only the least expensive. Medicare, in contrast, provides a similar set of minimal benefits to all beneficiaries. The TEFRA HMOs were required to provide at least the same package of benefits as would be available to Medicare beneficiaries. TEFRA HMOs can offer a broader set of benefits for an additional premium (or in some cases for the basic premium.)

The payment formula for TEFRA HMOs is also different. Whereas MCOs in the private market negotiate costs in relation to benefits and fix their rates to enrollees or their employers, the Health Care Finance Administration (HCFA) sets the rates for Medicare managed care. The amount paid was fixed as a sum equal to 95% of the Adjusted Average Per Capita Costs (AAPCC) under Medicare fee-for-service in each county. The adjustments took into account beneficiaries' age, gender, Medicaid status, and residence in a nursing home. Essentially the philosophy was to create a payment system linked to fee-for-service so that organizations in places where fee-for-service costs were high would have an incentive to form a TEFRA HMO. But given the enormous variation in health care costs from county to county, this payment system froze the inequities in place. At present, capitated payments are more than twice as high in the highest paid counties compared to the lowest paid counties. Differences are also found within states. (Recent modifications of this approach mandated by the 1997 Balanced Budget Act will gradually shift rates to a more natural basis to reduce this variation.)

Many potential MCOs balked at the idea of assuming so much risk for Medicare clients who would be likely heavy users of care. A bad year, they thought, could mean bankruptcy. The industry's initial response to the government's offer to market to Medicare beneficiaries was less than had been hoped. To make the opportunity more attractive, Medicare created some new programs. It allowed organizations that could not qualify for full HMO status to apply under special terms. In particular, it created a program that covered only Part B of Medicare (i.e., physician and other special services) as a risk product while the regular Medicare program continued to pay for Part A (hospital care) under the traditional fee-for-service arrangements. These programs were called Competitive Medical Programs (CMPs).

As the competitive climate has grown more intense, hospitals and their medical staffs formed joint venture companies to create new managed care products. These are often referred to as Physician-Hospital Organizations (PHOs). Under these arrangements resources are pooled to create a range of services that can be either marketed directly as an HMO or offered as a package to existing HMOs. New laws in the 1997 Balanced Budget Act package will gradually permit a wider variety of managed care entities to offer services to Medicare beneficiaries and will reduce some of the current protections. On the benefit side, they will be able to join other kinds of insurance programs such as PPOs and POS plans under a new "Choices+" program rather than be restricted to TEFRA HMOs.

Initially Medicare beneficiaries received an unusual protection. They were allowed to disenroll from MCOs at any time. Medicare enrollees will lose this protection when the plan is fully operational. Similar to other managed care participants, Medicare beneficiaries will be locked into their choices and, except for annual open enrollment periods, will not be permitted to "disenroll" and return to fee-for-service at will. (People in employment-based programs already must function with limited open enrollment periods, but most of them are well people with less at stake if their care is insufficient.) MCOs claim that they cannot plan adequately or reap the benefits of efficiency under current Medicare rules when the members can disenroll at will. But, some consumer advocates take the position that Medicare clients should not be locked into plans with dubious track records in serving people with chronic illnesses because too often they will be unable either to escape or to fight for better care. Even among Medicare recipients, most of the health care costs are incurred by a small fraction of the beneficiaries. Arguably, these are the people whose care matters most because these are the people who are sick. Disproportionately, they will also be the people receiving long-term care. Again, some advocates for the elderly fear that these high-risk beneficiaries will be lured into managed care with the promise of extra benefits and no out-of-pocket payments only to be disappointed when they seek care. Also of concern is whether such individuals could get back their Medigap insurance—the private insurance many Medicare beneficiaries depend upon to cover their out-of-pocket expenses. Once given up, such insurance may be prohibitively expensive to buy because of the beneficiary's more advanced age and preexisting conditions.

Meanwhile states have been extremely active in enrolling their Medicaid recipients in managed care, beginning with their younger populations such as women and children receiving income support and following with other recipient populations such as people with developmental disabilities, people with mental illnesses, people with physical disabilities, and the elderly. Managed care for groups like younger "workfare" recipients is very different from that for older persons. The former are more likely to have modest health care needs centered largely around childbirth and preventive care. Elderly persons, by contrast, have high rates of use. However, most of these costs are tied to Medicare. Few states have yet tried to bring the full range of long-term costs (notably nursing homes) under managed care.

Some Medicaid MCOs have been structured largely as primary care gatekeeper programs, whereas others involve full capitation. Sometimes the state makes special capitations for mental health programs, which are an expensive item for state Medicaid programs; in other instances the contracting MCOs make arrangements with a specialized firm to provide mental health care under a separate subcapitation known as a "carve-out." We have already described the complications that arise when states attempt to enroll people who are dually eligible for Medicaid and Medicare into their managed care programs, but several demonstration projects, described below, are underway to test the feasibility of such dually eligible programs. The carve-out mechanism described for mental health services may also be a mechanism that states use to grapple with long-term care under their managed care programs.

The dually eligible population is an important component of the Medicare program because they tend to be high utilizers of services. In 1995 approximately 6 million people were dually enrolled in Medicare and Medicaid at some point during the year. Although this group represents about 16% of the Medicare beneficiaries, they account for about 30% of Medicare's expenditures. Conversely, this group represents about 17% of Medicaid beneficiaries but uses about 35% of that program's expenditures. In 1995, about $106 billion was spent on dually eligible people, about evenly split between the two programs.

Analysts at the Health Care Financing Administration (HCFA) have used data from a national survey (the Medicare Current Beneficiary Survey) to compare the characteristics of the persons enrolled in dually eligible programs with those who are not. The dually eligibles are both older and younger. (Fourteen percent, com-

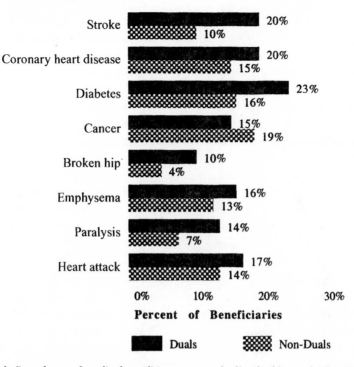

Figure 9.1. Prevalence of medical conditions among dually eligibles and other Medicare beneficiaries [Source: Health Care Financing Administration—Data from the Medicare Current Beneficiary Survey].

pared to 2% of nonduals, are under age 44; and 17% compared to 10% are 85 and older). Duals are much more likely to reside in an institution (24% versus 2%). Duals are more disabled; 36% have at least one ADL dependency compared to 19% of non-duals; they are twice as likely to have IADL limitations (62% versus 30%).

The health status for duals is worse than for nonduals. Almost half of duals (49%) rate their health status as fair or poor compared to 26% of nonduals. As shown in Figure 9.1, duals have higher rates of most of the common medical conditions that produce disability. Duals are much more likely to suffer from dementia (22% versus 5%). Almost half of all Medicare beneficiaries with cognitive impairment are duals.

Duals are less likely to be enrolled in HMOs. In 1995 only 3% of duals compared to 10% of nonduals were enrolled in an HMO. Duals constitute 7% of all Medicare beneficiaries enrolled in HMOs.

The Growth of Managed Care

Membership in Medicare HMOs grew from 4% at the end of 1989 to 6% at the end of 1994 to 11% in December 1996 and was expected to reach 15% by the beginning of 1998. Initially Medicare beneficiaries in MCOs were clustered on the West Coast (California, Oregon, and Washington), Arizona, Nevada, New Mexico, Colorado, Minnesota, and Florida, a combination of some states with a strong tradition of HMOs and other states taking advantage of very high AAPCC rates in some of their cities. Although the proportion of Medicare beneficiaries involved is still rather slight, the annual growth rate has been high and growing. From 1990 through 1992 enrollment grew at a rate of 13% annually, which increased to 23% between 1993 and 1994 and 30% between 1994 and 1995.[9] With that growth, Medicare MCOs are rapidly spreading to states and localities previously not well represented.

Managed care has been slow to develop in rural areas, especially with regard to Medicare patients. Of thirty-eight HMOs with Medicare risk contracts and offering coverage to commercial clients in 1990, only seventeen served Medicare beneficiaries in rural areas. The reasons given for such poor coverage often related to the low or erratic AAPCCs, the sparseness of the Medicare population, and the difficulties negotiating with providers.[10] The 1997 budget bill provided for floor payments for the AAPCC in an effort to make managed care a more attractive option for rural areas.

Cost Containment Strategies

Most observers agree that the early experience with managed care has emphasized the cost reduction strategy much more than the increased efficiency approach to saving money, but some are hopeful that as the programs mature the transition will occur. Costs can be controlled in a variety of ways, each of which has implications for consumers. In general, the trade-off from the consumer perspective is lower costs for more restricted choices.

Some managed care companies own their own services (e.g., hospitals and doctors). They use their ownership to create an environment that operates with more consistent rules and encourages efficient practice. They can control use of expensive services by establishing rules that govern their access. But the majority of managed care firms are predominantly contractors rather than owners. In one sense, these managed care companies can be compared to retailers that use their buying power to negotiate discounts. They buy large quantities of often brand-name merchandise at greatly reduced prices and sell it at a lower price than traditional retailers. Often these discounts come at the price of reduced amenities, such as selection, knowledgeable salespersons, or other services.

Managed care firms have used a variety of devices to obtain lower prices from providers. Some will contract with only those providers who offer them a discount. They monitor the use of both basic and ancillary services by providers and punish excessive (more than average) use. They require the use of restricted lists of tests or drugs. They require that access to specialty care be granted by a primary care provider, who serves as a gatekeeper (and is held responsible for the use of such specialty care). They provide financial rewards for using fewer or less expensive services in the form of bonuses (or penalties in the form of withheld payments if heavy usage is made). They may encourage or even require that the providers share the risk of the costs of elements of care under their direct or indirect control, often by imposing some form of subcapitation whereby individual aspects of care are provided on a capitated basis. In the worst case, a managed care organization may be nothing more than a front company charging a high rate for marketing and subcapitating all of the services to various providers.

Effects on Consumers

From the consumers' perspective, managed care usually means less choice and restricted access. People paying for their own care may opt to suffer these inconveniences because managed care is less expensive or less bureaucratic. The myriad of forms often associated with traditional fee-for-service care and its payment are no longer necessary, although the appeals process if one is dissatisfied with a judgment about eligibility may be even more complex. Many consumers have not been given a choice. When their care is paid by a third party, that organization may opt for managed care as a means of controlling its outlay.

The specific negative implications of entering a managed care program for the average consumer may include the following:

- *Loss of one's own doctor.* If the person's doctor is not a participant in the managed care program, the person will have to choose one who is. Because managed care programs want to grow, they will often attempt to enroll as many physicians as possible in the hopes of attracting their patients, but some of these physicians may be weeded out subsequently on the basis of their practice patterns. In all fairness, although many people attach great importance to continuity of care, there is little evidence to support its centrality to good quality. If patients have to choose a new doctor, and if they can choose among competent practitioners, there may not necessarily be a diminution in quality of care, although they will have to form new interpersonal bonds.
- *Restricted access to hospitals.* The managed care plan may not contract with the hospital a patient prefers. Some older patients have surprisingly strong emotional ties to specific hospitals. Also, admission to hospitals may be restricted through shortening stays or replacing them with outpatient procedures. For older people, however, hospital stays have already become short as a result of prospective hospital payment under Medicare, so they are unlikely to become much shorter. Nursing home residents may have less access to hospital care, which, as Chapter 8 pointed out, could even be an advantage depending on the circumstances.

- *Restricted access to specialty care.* Many managed care programs require that patients see specialists only on the referral on a primary care practitioner (PCP). The PCP role as a gatekeeper may be enforced by the payment system. PCPs may be held to a fixed budget for services they authorize or they may be required to share the costs of these services above a fixed threshold. This mandate may be simply a minor inconvenience, or it could become a major impediment if the PCP feels pressure to restrict access to specialists. (If the PCPs do not feel this pressure, there is little rationale for requiring the gatekeeper role.) In some cases, managed care firms may restrict the number of specialists with whom they contract, causing queues to form.
- *Restricted access to tests.* Once again, if the PCPs (or specialists) are judged or paid on the basis of their parsimonious use of laboratory testing or X-rays, they will be pressured to avoid such tests in marginal situations. Many managed care programs use clinical protocols to establish norms for ordering tests. Practitioners often complain that these protocols are too restrictive.
- *Restricted access to medications.* When the benefit package includes drug coverage, consumers may find that certain expensive medications are not included on the plan's formulary. Similarly, the plan may require that less expensive medications with greater side effects be tried first.

In general, most practitioners who have worked under the aegis of managed care note that the predominate way this payment system affects their clinical behavior is in the gray areas of decision-making. When there is no clear evidence that a given course of action is indicated, the balance may swing to less intensive care under capitation, the opposite effect from under fee-for-service. The problem is that much of medicine, especially that involving the care of frail older people, lies in this gray zone where no single approach has been proven most efficacious. With complicated cases that are influenced by many factors, simple algorithms to decide whether a certain action should be pursued do not apply easily. There is not enough evidence yet to state clearly whether managed care is associated with any significant diminution in the quality of care. Indeed, it is not clear whether it is even associated with less patient satisfaction.

There are offsetting advantages for consumers who receive care in managed care settings. The underlying quality of the traditional fee-for-service, individually based practitioner situation has been questioned for some time. Having an organization that feels both professional and legal responsibility for the quality of care it provides may offer greater protection for consumers. As we become more sensitive to the importance of system factors in determining the outcomes of care, the role of structured decision making and oversight becomes better appreciated.

- Managed care organizations should be more willing to think in terms of episodes of care rather than simple incidents. They should be more anxious to treat problems more aggressively early if such treatment can avoid costly care subsequently. In the arena of geriatric care, they should be prepared to underwrite the costs of appropriately targeted geriatric assessments because such actions have been shown to save money in the long run.[11]

- Managed care organizations can afford to establish information systems that can track patients over time and can provide information to PCPs about patients at risk. They can employ additional personnel to work at keeping patients healthy, or at least facilitate their compliance with therapeutic regimens. They can develop programs that offer patients better information about how to care for themselves, in terms of both improving individual health habits to reduce risks and monitoring their own health and treatment.
- Managed care offers a way to coordinate care. A central administration and common working systems should reduce fragmentation. A common record system should improve the flow of communication about a client.
- Managed care has the opportunity to be more creative in developing ways to meet its service obligations. Less expensive forms of care can be used where they are shown to be as effective. Nonphysicians can perform tasks normally assigned to physicians, and the chain of delegation can continue. Subacute care can be substituted for hospital care. In the sphere of LTC, new forms of care, such as assisted living, can be utilized in lieu of the constrictions of nursing homes.
- Case management can take on a more aggressive approach. Growing evidence suggests that aggressive monitoring of high-risk patients can reduce the subsequent use of expensive hospital care.[12] Case management by nurse practitioners working with congestive heart failure patients discharged from hospital has been shown to be quite cost-effective.
- Managed care typically offers seniors the inducement of lower out-of-pocket costs and no bureaucratic hassles in terms of claims processing. Sometimes premiums, deductibles, and coinsurance under regular Medicare are waived. Often additional benefits are included. In theory, consumers can give up the expense of carrying Medigap insurance, though, as already noted, some consumers are afraid to give up that insurance lest they be unable to get reinstated.

Evidence of Effectiveness

The primary expectation for managed care is increased efficiency. In the short run that efficiency should come from saving money. In the private sector, MCOs offer their products at competitive prices, usually enticing customers with prices lower than those available under traditional indemnity coverage. In effect, most buyers are trading off restricted choice for lower costs.

The situation with public programs is different. The Medicare program elected to set the price for managed care instead permitting price competition. With government programs, MCOs contract to serve a population at some proportion of the expected cost. In the case of Medicare, the rate was set at 95% of AAPCC. This rate creates two serious problems: It includes factors that are part of the Medicare program for political convenience, but have little to do with care of older persons (i.e., graduate medical education and service to poor persons). Indeed, few MCOs are actively involved in either. Including these costs in the AAPCC provides a "gift" to the MCOs. Second, by using a fixed rate based on an average, Medicare allows MCOs that recruit healthier than average enrollees to make a greater profit. In order to be truly cost-saving, managed care must serve a population at least comparable to that used for the calculation. If the population served is less expensive than average to care for, then paying the average cost will actually cost the government money. This phenomenon of enrolling consumers with less than average need is called *favorable selection.* Studies of early TEFRA risk contracts suggest that just this sort of favorable selection occurred. Additional evidence of favorable selection can be seen in an analysis done by HCFA based on data from the Medicare Current Beneficiary Survey. Figure 9.2 compares the rates of specific ADL and IADL dependencies for Medicare beneficiaries enrolled in HMOs and fee-for-service. In each instance the dependency rate is higher for those in fee-for-service, suggesting that the managed care enrolled group is substantially less impaired.

When the selection effect is considered, Medicare was paying 95% of approximately 110% of the costs. In essence, it was losing money, not saving any.[13] When one considers that these calculations ignored the fact that about 10% of the AAPCC went to the two programs that MCOs had little to do with (i.e., graduate medical education and disproportionate share of poor patients), the size of the "savings" from managed care is in even more doubt.

Favorable selection can occur for many reasons. Medicare is especially vulnerable to this problem because beneficiaries must opt to join an HMO; they cannot be forced to join. (Medicaid beneficiaries do not enjoy this same privilege. Although they may be given the choice of which HMO to join, they may have to join one; those that do not elect an HMO are assigned to one.) All things being equal, one might expect that those with the most serious health problems would be least willing to change the way they receive their care for fear of disrupting the present equilibrium. They would be less willing to join a program that saves money by controlling access to at least some types of expensive care. Some evidence, in fact, suggests that older persons may be joining managed care to obtain savings in costs and then moving out of managed care when they use up the benefits allowed. Conversely, the MCOs may be encouraging these high cost clients to disenroll.[14] If the HMO then launches a marketing campaign designed to attract healthier enrollees, the favorable selection bias will be even greater.

In effect, managed care's ability to save money for public programs is dependent on the way the payment rates are established in relation to the people actually enrolled. The capacity for selection bias is greater under Medicare, where enroll-

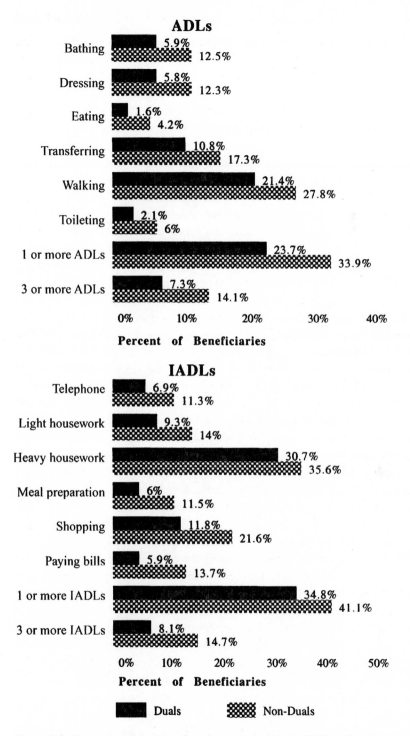

ADLs

Bathing — 5.9% / 12.5%
Dressing — 5.8% / 12.3%
Eating — 1.6% / 4.2%
Transferring — 10.8% / 17.3%
Walking — 21.4% / 27.8%
Toileting — 2.1% / 6%
1 or more ADLs — 23.7% / 33.9%
3 or more ADLs — 7.3% / 14.1%

Percent of Beneficiaries

IADLs

Telephone — 6.9% / 11.3%
Light housework — 9.3% / 14%
Heavy housework — 30.7% / 35.6%
Meal preparation — 6% / 11.5%
Shopping — 11.8% / 21.6%
Paying bills — 5.9% / 13.7%
1 or more IADLs — 34.8% / 41.1%
3 or more IADLs — 8.1% / 14.7%

Percent of Beneficiaries

Duals   Non-Duals

Figure 9.2. Proportion of medicine beneficiaries enrolled in HMOs in free form service with various types of dependencies [Source: Health Care Financing Administration—Data from the Medicare Current Beneficiary Survey].

ment is voluntary, than under Medicaid, which can mandate enrollment in managed care.

Looked at another way, to determine the overall benefit of managed care, one must consider what happens to the money invested. Most MCOs charge at least 15% for administrative costs. These costs do not displace the other administrative costs in the health system (e.g., for doctors or hospitals) or the governmental administrative costs. Thus, for an MCO to provide the same level of service that could presumably be purchased in the fee-for-service market, it must be initially 15% more efficient. When this amount is added to the 5% discount usually applied to encourage governments to purchase managed care, the MCOs must achieve a 20% saving to provide the same value of services or they are actually providing fewer services. If the latter is true the question becomes, What is the impact on quality?

Thus, the other major criterion by which to judge the effectiveness of managed care is quality. Capitation provides an a priori incentive to underserve their enrollees. Conversely, fee-for-service has an incentive to overtreat. Neither too little care or too much care is necessarily good for quality of care; too much care can be especially bad for older persons who are more susceptible to iatrogenic side effects of treatment. There has not yet been extensive research on aspects of quality in MCOs compare to fee-for-service. Most of the studies that have examined quality for older persons do not show any impressive difference between the two types of care.

Table 9.1 summarizes major studies examining the effects of managed care on quality. A 1985 study of seventeen Medicare risk HMOs in ten communities, which was designed to evaluate the early Medicare HMO demonstration project, compared their care to that for a sample in ten matched communities without Medicare risk HMOs. Overall, fewer HMO patients experienced functional decline, but after adjusting for initial differences in the two groups the difference was not statistically significant, nor were there any differences in measures of access or quality.[15] Other studies with this same population showed that outpatient hypertension management in the HMOs was equal or better to that in fee-for-service.[16] Also, comparing ambulatory care for diabetic patients, the investigators found the care at least as good for HMO patients as for fee-for-service patients. HMO patients were more likely to have their eyes checked for diabetic changes and to have their urine examined than were fee-for-service controls. HMO diabetic patients in poor control were more likely to be referred to an ophthalmologist for more extensive eye examinations. On the other hand, fee-for-service patients were more likely to receive an influenza vaccination.[17] Another study done as part of the same evaluation looked at care for patients with congestive heart failure.[18] The sample was identified from hospital records but the study examined both ambulatory and hospital care. No differences in the quality of outpatient care for HMO and fee-for-service patients were found. The hospital management of these patients was comparable.

Table 9.1. Summary of Studies on Quality of Medicare Managed Care

Study	Sample	Findings	Reference
National Medicare competition evaluation, 1985	17 Medicare risk HMOs in 10 communities; matched FFS controls in 10 similar communities	Less functional decline in HMO patients; no significant differences after case-mix adjustment	Retchin et al., 1992, note 15
	Elderly diabetics in 8 HMOs and FFS patients in the same area	HMO patients more likely to have fundoscopic exam and be referred to ophthalmologist if in poor control; HMO patients less likely to get flu vaccine	Retchin & Preston, 1991, note 17
	Elderly congestive heart failure patients in 8 HMOs and FFS patients in same area	Ambulatory management and hospital management comparable; HMO patients more likely to get follow-up visit in 1 week after discharge from hospital	Retchin & Brown, 1991, note 18
	Hypertensive patients of 8 HMOs and FFS patients in same area	HMO patients got equal or better care	Preston & Retchin, 1991, note 16
Medicare Risk contract evaluation, 1990	Medicare patients from 75 HMOS and FFS patients from the same areas	HMO patients with joint pain more likely to see MD but not to get specialist referral; more likely to get treatment including PT; less likely to report improved symptoms; HMO patients with chest pain less likely to see MD or be referred but no differences in quality or outcomes	Clement et al., 1994, note 19
RAND, 1986	AMI patients admitted to hospitals from 3 HMOs compared to previous national FFS sample	No mortality differences at 30 or 180 days. HMOs better on process measures	Carlisle et al., 1992, note 20
HCFA, 1987	National data on HMO and FFS	HMO enrollees had lower adjusted mortality rates	Riley et al., 1991, note 21
Home health care, 1990	Patients from HHAs: 9 HMO-owned, 15 FFS and 14 mixed	Patients from HMO-owned HHAs got less service and had worse outcomes	Shaughnessy et al., 1994, note 22

HMO patients were more likely to have a follow-up visit within a week of discharge from the hospital.

A 1990 study looked at Medicare patients in seventy-five HMOs and compared them to matched persons in the same communities who were not enrolled in HMOs.[19] The study focused on persons with joint pain and chest pain. The fee-for-service group again were sicker and more disabled. The HMO enrollees with joint pain were more likely to see a physician, but less likely to be referred to a specialist than were the fee-for-service controls. More of the HMO patients got medications and other treatments (including physical therapy) for their joint pain, but they were less likely to report improvement in their symptoms. The differences for chest pain were much less. HMO patients were less likely to get a referral to a specialist, but there were no significant differences in the quality indicators.

A study of hospital care for patients with heart attacks compared a sample of 1986 hospital admissions from three HMOs with data from a national sample from around the same time.[20] There were no death rate differences at 30 or 180 days after admission. The HMOs had better scores on the process criteria for quality used.

A large national analysis of mortality compared death rates for Medicare beneficiaries enrolled in HMOs and those in fee-for-service.[21] The HMO death rates were lower even after adjustments for age, gender, and institutional status, but other factors associated with favorable selection could not be eliminated. For example, fewer HMOs may attract people with illness or better health behaviors.

Taken together, these studies suggest that managed care for Medicare enrollees seems to be at least as good as that offered under fee-for-service arrangements. There are no indications of extensive underservice. A study of home health care offers quite a different picture, however.[22] HMO-funded clients received less home health care and had poorer outcomes than did fee-for-service controls. However, another study that followed Medicare patients through their post acute care phase and beyond found no evidence that patients enrolled in HMOs were less likely to receive home care or that they suffered poorer outcomes.[23]

Information on Medicaid managed care for older persons is more scant. A randomized controlled trial in Minnesota found no differences in the outcomes of care for older Medicaid recipients with hypertension or diabetes assigned to managed care or fee-for-service.[24] However, it must be recognized that Medicaid is not the primary payer for these dually eligible persons. Most of them were not enrolled in an HMO for the Medicare portion of their care. To obtain the greatest effect, Medicare and Medicaid funding need to be coordinated.

Managed Long-Term Care

Most managed care activity to date has been directed at acute care, but there have been some developments that involve long-term care as well. As enthusiasm for managed care as a cost-saving device has grown, several states have introduced it for their Medicaid populations, or have begun steps to implement this strategy. Although most have begun their efforts around the simpler situation of the welfare mothers, some have included long-term care in their plans.

Coverage of older persons becomes more complicated because of the dual eligibility status. Because Medicaid benefits for older persons are defined to complement those provided under Medicare, Medicaid effectively covers services not paid for by Medicare (i.e., copayments and deductibles, drugs, most nursing home care, and some home care)—a coordinated program must include both sources of payment. However, Medicare rules require that beneficiaries cannot be forced to choose managed care. Hence, although older Medicaid clients can be required to use managed care for their Medicaid coverage, they must voluntarily elect such care for the Medicare portion.

Two of the best known programs that combine Medicare and Medicaid on a capitated basis are the SHMO and the PACE programs (identified below). Both are demonstration projects, initiated by partnerships between the federal government and the private sector; negotiations for the applicable state portions of the capitations were then negotiated with each state involved. In contrast, two other programs, one in Arizona and one being initiated in 1997 in Minnesota, are the result of state initiative for a statewide program. Another program with popular appeal is EverCare, a program that provides capitation for Medicare only but is often grouped with long-term care capitation programs because it serves long-term nursing home residents only. In fact, it capitates acute care (hospitals and physician services) to benefit people living in nursing homes. The nursing home costs themselves are covered privately or under Medicaid.

Table 9.2 summarizes these five major models, which are described below. Commentators readily can become confused about the major distinctions among these programs.

Social HMOs (SHMOs)

The Social Health Maintenance Organizations grew out of a theoretical belief that enrollees would benefit and overall costs would be reduced if some of the expenditures spent on acute care for older people could be spent on long-term care and if some of the expenditures on health-oriented services could be spent on socially oriented services. On a demonstration basis beginning in 1982, four organizations received extra Medicare capitation and enrollees paid extra premiums in order to be eligible for an expanded array of long-term care benefits not usually found under Medicare. This expanded benefit included some long-term care services, mostly community-based, up to a set dollar limit with vigorous case management for those needing the long-term care component.[25] Note that the SHMOs were not really designed for Medicaid clientele, though they did negotiate rates with their separate states to include some Medicaid people; rather the idea was to enroll a population of people who largely did not need long-term care and to redistribute the enhanced

Table 9.2. Comparison of Major Managed Care Programs Involving Long-Term Care*

	PACE/On Lok	S/HMO	ALTCS	MSHO	EverCare
Population served	–Dual eligibles –Medicare-only –community-based NHC only at enrollment	–Medicare-only (community and limited NHC) –Dual eligibles (may be served under separate state contract)	–Medicaid only –Elderly, physically disabled, or developmentally disabled	Dual eligibles only (NF and community based)	–Medicare-only (NF only) –Dual eligibles (NF only—may be served under separate state contract)
Benefit package	Medicare A & B Medicaid: all HCBS, all NF care	Medicare A&B Medicaid: limited HCBS, limited NF care, private costs limited	Medicaid coverage for acute care, HCBS, NF	Medicare A&B Medicaid: HCBS, NF care 6 months	Medicare A&B –Medicaid copays & deductibles –May include Medicaid ancillaries
Funding model	–Medicare capitated at 100% AAPCC; insti. Cell with 2.39 modifier for NHCs –Medicaid costs capitated per state arrangements	–Medicare capitated at 100% AAPCC; insti. cell AAPCC for NHCs –Private premiums (approx. $85 per month) –Medicaid costs may be capitated per state arrangements	–Medicaid capitated –Medicare pays FFS	–Medicare capitated at 95% AAPCC; insti. Cell for NHCs & conversions –Medicaid ancillary (95% of Medicaid cell; insti. Cell for NHCs & conversions) –Medicaid HCBS-ave. EW payments & 2x ave. EW payments for conversions	–Medicare capitated at 95% AAPCC –Medicaid ancillaries may be capitated if under state contract
Funding sources	–Public (Medicare, Medicaid) –Private premiums (rare)	–Public (Medicare, Medicaid) –Private (premiums)	Public (AHCCCS-Medicaid)	–Public (Medicare, Medicaid)	–Public (Medicare, Medicaid) –Private (premiums)

*NF = nursing facility; NHC = nursing home certifiable; HCBS = home- and community-based services; EW = elderly waiver; conversions = relevant to residents who have been in a nursing facility for greater than 5 months (i.e., excludes short-term residents); FFS = fee-for-services.

service dollars to benefit those with the greatest needs. The first four SHMO sites represented two different models. Two were based in existing HMOs, which expanded their activities in long-term care, one of which formed a partnership with a large long-term care organization. The other two began in long-term care organizations and had to find hospital and physician partners.

The first set of SHMOs used a complicated stratified enrollment scheme to balance their actuarial risk. Fearing adverse selection by frailer older persons who would be attracted to the program because it offered a wider range of covered services, they set a limit on what proportion of the enrollees could be frail equal to that found in the general elderly population. The results of the evaluation of this first round of SHMO experience are shrouded in controversy but seem to indicate that the SHMO did not produce the expected levels of benefit its name suggests.[26]

The demonstration was judged to have established the feasibility of this approach but further work was felt to be needed to establish its effectiveness. It was also noted that the added SHMO benefits tended to be overlaid on the benefits covered under Medicare without much genuine integration at the clinical level. Furthermore, physicians were often unaware that some of their patients were participating in the SHMO, especially when they had many more non-SHMO patients than those in the program.

A second generation of SHMO demonstrations has been developed which will test whether a more deliberately geriatric strategy will yield more promising results. The second generation will not use a stratified enrollment structure. Rather, all eligible enrollees will be accepted. A more complex rate cell adjustment to the AAPCC has been developed to acknowledge the associated variation in risk. Likewise, geriatric and case-management efforts will be directed at all high-risk clients, not just those who are judged to be nursing home eligible. Special devices such as geriatric protocols and case-management protocols have been developed to encourage PCPs to address geriatric issues more competently and consistently.[27]

Program for All-Inclusive Care of the Elderly (PACE)

In some ways PACE is the mirror-opposite to SHMO. In SHMO only the minority of the enrollees are poor and only the minority need long-term care. The PACE program is specifically targeted to Medicaid clients residing in the community at the time of enrollment whose needs for long-term care are deemed to be at the nursing home level. This is a restricted group because most frail Medicaid recipients are already in nursing homes and hence are not eligible for PACE. The program's objective is to manage the care of its enrollees with minimal reliance on either hospitals or nursing homes. Intended to replicate the highly regarded On Lok program, which began in San Francisco's Chinatown, PACE programs use a coordinated set of services that include both medical and social care services delivered at a day health center. Interdisciplinary teamwork is a key component, and the programs have their own staff physicians. PACE programs may also purchase a variety of in-home services, and some have been quite creative in developing housing settings with services (e.g., the program might pay attendants to live in an apartment with two or three PACE members and provide services).[28]

In contrast to SHMOs, most of the financial support for PACE enrollees comes from Medicaid. PACE sites receive the regular AAPCC payment from the Medicare program except that they are paid for at the nursing home rate even when the enrollees are in the community. In addition, about two-thirds of a PACE client's funding is paid by the state Medicaid programs. Because its combined capitation rate is very high, befitting the frail nature of the persons served and the coverage of all acute and LTC, the program is essentially dependent on coverage under Medicaid. Few individuals have been willing or able to pay the Medicaid capitation rate out of private resources. Also, because the capitation is sufficient for the actual care of a group already in need, no insurance principle is at stake, and PACE programs can survive with relatively small enrollments of 200 or 300 people.

Although the PACE model is widely sought to be replicated, its formal evaluation has been difficult. A small-scale evaluation study suggests that PACE has been able to reduce hospital and nursing home use without adverse effects on outcomes or satisfaction. It is not clear whether the rates established for PACE correspond to real costs or are too favorable.[29] Despite the lack of clear evaluation data, the PACE program was established as a permanent waiver alternative rather than a demonstration project in 1997.

Arizona Long Term Care System (ALTCS)

The most well-developed managed care system for a statewide low-income population (Medicaid equivalent) began with the Arizona Health Care Cost System (AHCCS) program in 1982. AHCCS contracts with managed care organizations for the coverage of all Medicaid enrollees. AHCCS enrollees who also need LTC are covered by a special arm of this program, Arizona Long Term Care System (ALTCS), which contracts with managed care organizations for both acute and chronic care. In the two most populous counties, where Phoenix and Tucson are located, ALTCS services are managed by the existing county-operated long-term care programs. In other counties, contracts were made to private vendors. In each instance client care is coordinated to provide both acute care and long-term care. However, at present this program covers only Medicaid costs; Medicare costs are still paid on a fee-for-service basis. Negotiations are underway to include Medicare in the managed care arrangement. There is some concern about the quality of care offered under this program. An evaluation study found the quality in some areas of care to be less than in a comparable population treated in New Mexico.[30]

Minnesota Senior Health Options (MSHO)

After several years of intensive planning, Minnesota received a waiver from HCFA to implement a managed care program for dually eligible persons, called Minnesota Senior Health Options (MSHO). Under this program, the state is contracting with organizations that can offer both acute care and long-term care on a capitated basis.

Medicare and Medicaid funds are pooled at the programmatic level to permit integrated care. All Medicaid benefits will be included except for a portion of nursing home care. The first 180 days of nursing home care each year will be covered under the capitation, with longer stays to be paid under the existing Medicaid program. The program uses financial incentives to encourage early discharge from nursing homes and efforts to keep potentially eligible clients out of such institutions. High-risk patients receive case management. Case managers have the authority to use resources to develop effective interventions to maximize clients' independent status. At present, most of the enrollees are already in nursing homes. From the patient's perspective the benefits of MSHO lie in the potential for receiving more coordinated care. Yet dually eligible clients should fare well in the fee-for-service arena because they have broad coverage from the combined resources of Medicare and Medicaid, and thus, they have little incentive to give up their benefits to accept managed care.

EverCare

EverCare is an example of a Medicare HMO targeted at a special long-term care population. It enrolls nursing home residents under the conventional risk-based HMO program allowed by Medicare. This project appears to have shown that it is feasible to provide more intensive primary care to nursing home patients (in this case, by active use of nurse practitioners) and thereby to reduce the use of hospitals. In effect, the program succeeds financially by investing more effort in primary care and reaping its benefits from lower hospital costs. Although no formal evaluation of EverCare's effectiveness is yet available, it appears to save most of its money by shortening length of stay (presumably because nursing homes are willing to receive back unstable patients knowing that they will receive close attention from PCPs. EverCare pays the nursing homes for the additional costs associated with caring for patients who would otherwise be in the hospital).[31] Interestingly, EverCare relies on the cooperation of nursing homes and succeeds only if a critical mass of residents of participating nursing homes wish to participate in the program. EverCare, therefore, is marketed in selected nursing homes. Nursing homes themselves have no financial incentives to participate other than any marketing advantage that may accrue from the better coordinated and managed health care that is provided.

Issues and Challenges

Some parts of the long-term care industry have responded to the national enthusiasm for managed care by developing their own strategies. Nursing homes have increased their horizontal integration with other nursing homes and their vertical integration with assisted living, foster care, and home care to be better positioned to negotiate with MCOs. Some large home care agencies have also responded by developing partnerships with managed care organizations. Managed care is high on the agenda of all the provider trade organizations, most of which have had summit meetings on the subject and provided briefing papers for their members.

In some geographic areas, long-term care providers have created their own networks to negotiate with MCOs on a larger basis, providing a single entity to deal with and gaining broader control of the market. An example is Optage, a newly incorporated Minnesota-based firm that is providing services to several of the vendors that have contracted with the state as providers under the MSHO program for the dually eligible. For a subcapitation, Optage can provide both case management and a full range of medical, hospital, home-based, and nursing home services for those dually eligible enrollees who indeed require long-term care.

Some of the more socially oriented long-term care agencies, especially those that provide case-management and Medicaid-waiver services are alarmed by the advent of managed care, though they too are attempting to organize to become vendors, holders of capitation, or both. In some ways, a power struggle has arisen over which organizations should manage long-term care if long-term care is to be capitated. If large MCOs that provide acute care and long-term care are at financial risk for the services, they reasonably wish to be in charge of their management. But when states have already developed community-based local networks with the competence to organize, manage, and purchase inexpensive long-term care services, these agencies argue that it would be a disservice to the clientele to disband their services for the untried and theoretical advantages of having vertically organized competing firms that manage both long-term care and acute care. In Florida and in Massachusetts, proposals have been made to declare the agencies in the Medicaid waiver case-management system to be essential providers and to require MCOs to contract with them for long-term care case management. Some of these same issues have arisen in the MSHO program, where the county-based case-management agencies are struggling to articulate a unique role for themselves.

Some of these power struggles are survival struggles for community agencies growing out of vested interests and resistance to change. But some are also born of the conviction that MCOs are not the right entities to manage long-term care. When acute care and long-term funding is combined under the same entity, difficult questions are inevitably raised about the locus of care management. Many advocates for long-term care consumers fear that such a merged authority will be dominated by a medical mentality and that important attributes of long-term care will receive short shrift.

In truth, acute care and long-term care do respond to somewhat different goals. Much of long-term care can be said to be based on a compensatory approach, wherein functional deficits are met by providing services that clients can no longer provide for themselves. Acute care has historically had a more curative bent, seeking to change a client's status rather than cope with it. However, as emphasis in medical care has shifted from infectious disease to chronic disease, there has been a growing appreciation of the need to address the patient in a larger life context.

Increasingly health authorities speak and write about quality of life and consumer control. But long-term care leaders fear that these terms have a different and narrower meaning to acute care providers. For example, some clinical pathways developed for meeting the chronic care needs of older patients specify the best care setting for various levels of need. To some long-term care authorities, it is anathema that the place where the consumer is to live is specified in a clinical protocol rather than remaining a matter for highly personal choice.

The alliance of these acute care and long-term care forces is bound to be uneasy. Each brings a distinct perspective, and even a separate language to the merger. Acute care providers are accustomed to more aggressive action and concomitant spending and bring more resources to the table, though managed care organizations have endeavored to constrain these impulses to action. Long-term care providers at their best bring detailed experience with how to make do with limited resources, how to build on client and family strengths, and how to rally voluntary assistance from local community leaders. Increasingly, they have endeavored to respect consumer choice. They are uncertain whether these functions will translate well to the world of large for-profit, national-scale organizations.

There should be a substantial middle ground. The present lack of coordination between acute and chronic care suggests that there are attractive opportunities for better liaison and actual integration. Fragmented funding based on source has led to parallel and redundant efforts. It is feasible to consider managed care for only the acute-care portion, or even to develop two separate managed care entities, one responsible for acute care and the other for long-term care, although it would seem likely that numerous boundary disputes would erupt. Especially in areas like home health care, the Medicare program has increasingly been used to provide chronic-care services. As Medicare's coverage extends into areas that at least overlap with long-term care responsibilities, jurisdictional questions and efforts at cost shifting seem imminent.

Capitating long-term alone would, in effect, mean giving an organization responsibility for creating a set of services to meet clients' long-term care needs. Arrangements for providing medical care could be made separately or subcontracted. The clients' long-term care needs could be met in more innovative ways, including greater use of community-based care, perhaps in new hybrid settings. Where needs were identified to consolidate or coordinate medical care, the long-term care MCOs could negotiate appropriate contracts for such services or make mutually satisfactory cooperative arrangements. Of course, the clock is ticking and many older long-term care consumers are already enrolled in Medicare MCOs that impose specific requirements. For example, some nursing homes with exemplary health care services have found that some of the consumers seeking admission are required by prior arrangement to use some other medical service instead of the one in the nursing home.

It is not yet clear how many long-term care organizations currently have the capital and skills to undertake capitated arrangements for long-term care (either as holders of a subcapitation in an integrated system or in a long-term-care-only system). But if past experience is any guide, it is safe to predict that a market would quickly develop. It is also not clear how public agencies such as case-management organizations housed in state or local government can participate in such a program. They would need to build up capital or accumulate surpluses at a time when many state governors prefer to hand such money back to the taxpayers. The most important challenge in developing this capability is to avoid repeating the patterns of earlier times when exploitation was a key feature of development.

One of the challenges to managed care is establishing a workable system of accountability. If vulnerable long-term care consumers are to flourish in this ever-thickening alphabet soup of health care and long-term care organizations, they and their family members will need to be well armed with information. As already noted, the primary incentives favor underservice. Public funds can be exploited in several ways. If the actuarial calculations are weak (and because there are few data bases available that link client characteristics with expenditures, this seems likely), it is very possible to overpay MCOs, especially if enrollment is voluntary. Early experience with Medicare capitation found that the government was paying average costs for populations that were healthier than average.

Monitoring quality will be an even more difficult task. The more providing specifically prescribed services is mandated, the less opportunity exists for meaningful innovation. But consumers will need to be protected against inadequate care. At the very least, active vehicles for quick response to complaints will be needed. Active monitoring of outcomes, including satisfaction, with careful adjustments for case-mix differences, will be needed.

Concluding Comment

To conclude, managed care represents both an opportunity and a threat to improving long-term care. On the one hand, managed care with capitation offers a virtual clean slate under which one could design and implement a system that makes sense. Such a system would integrate social and medical care, taking full advantage of modern information systems to facilitate coordination and focus attention on salient objectives. Because managed care organizations have no stake in the existing structures, they will seek the most efficient approaches. On the other hand, the track record of managed care fails to inspire confidence. The current environment encourages quick-fix solutions. The rewards favor discount purchasing and favorable selection of enrollees. Cost cutting takes precedence over investments. Restricting access and options seems more likely than innovation.

The future for managed care in general is uncertain. Various purchasers, including governments, have embraced the concept as a way to control the costs of care; but public programs have benefited little because of the way capitation rates are calculated. As managed care becomes more like health insurance, the advantages seem to diminish. Some observers see an optimistic future where competition will be based on quality and MCOs can indeed do well by doing good, but the foundations for such a rosy scenario are hard to discern from the present patterns of practice. Apropos of long-term care, the challenge is at the practice level: to effect a comfortable merger with acute care in a capitated system that builds on the lessons learned through decades of experience with HCBS. To serve long-term care consumers well, MCOs must incorporate considerable individualization into their protocols, develop ways to purchase services from numerous vendors—even individual PAS workers—and refrain from applying guidelines about where people live that run rough-shod over individual preferences.

Notes

1. These definitions and some of the material in this chapter were first presented in a manual designed to acquaint aging-services organizations with managed care and used as the basis for a conference sponsored by the Administration on Aging on February 28–March 1, 1996. See Starr L, Kane RA & Baker MO (Eds.) (1996). *Managed Care: Handbook for the Aging Network.* Minneapolis, MN: National LTC Resource Center, Institute for Health Service Research, School of Public Health, University of Minnesota.
2. See Institute for the Future (1997). *Piecing Together the Puzzle: The Future of Health and Health Care in America.* Menlo Park, CA: Institute for the Future. In this report submitted to the Robert Wood Johnson Foundation on its twenty-fifth anniversary, the authors describe the trends in private insurance, Medicare, Medicaid, and health care-delivery systems in the past decade and develop scenarios for the future. All scenarios call for the continuation of managed care arrangements.
3. Newhouse JP (1993). *Free for All? Lessons From the RAND Health Insurance Experiment.* Cambridge, MA: Harvard University Press.
4. Newhouse JP, Manning WG, Morris CN, Orr LL, Duan N, & Keeler EB (1981). Some interim results from a controlled trial of cost sharing in health insurance. *New England Journal of Medicine* 305:1501–1507.
5. Brook RH, Ware JE, Rogers WH, Keeler EB, Davies AR, Donald CA, Goldberg GA, Lohr,KN, Masthay PC, & Newhouse JP (1983). Does free care improve adults' health? Results from a randomized controlled trial. *New England Journal of Medicine* 309(23): 1426–1434.
6. Keeler EB, Brook RH, Goldberg GA, Kamberg CJ, & Newhouse JP (1985). How free care reduced hypertension in the health insurance experiment. *Journal of the American Medical Association* 254(14):1926–1931.
7. For a description of the DRGs, see St. Anthony Publishing (1995). *St. Anthony's DRG Guidebook, 1995.* Washington, DC: Lorenz, EW.
8. See for example, Chassin MR, Kosecoff J, Park RE, Winslow CM, Kahn KL, Merrick NJ, Kessey J, Fink A, Solomon DH, & Brook RH (1987). Does inappropriate use explain geographic variations in the use of health care services? A study of three procedures. *Journal of the American Medical Association* 258:2533–2537; Leape LL, Park RE, Solomon DH, Chassin MR, Kosecoff J, & Brook RH (1990). Does inappropriate use explain small-area variations in the use of health care services. *Journal of the American Medical Association* 263:669–672; Wennberg JE, Freeman JL, Shelton RM, & Bubolz TA (1989). Hospital use and mortality among Medicare beneficiaries in Boston and New Haven. *New England Journal of Medicine* 321:1168–1173.

9. United States General Accounting Office (1995). *Medicare Managed Care: Growing Enrollment Adds Urgency to Fixing HMO Problem* (GASO/HEHS-96-21). Washington, DC: Government Printing Office.

10. Serrato C, Brown R, & Bergeron J (1995). Why do so few HMOs offer Medicare risk plans in rural areas? *Health Care Financing Review* 17(1):85–97.

11. Stuck AE, Siu AL, Wieland GD, Adams J, & Rubenstein LZ (1993). Comprehensive geriatric assessment: a meta-analysis of controlled trials. *The Lancet* 342:1032–1036.

12. Brooten D, Naylor M, York R, Brown L, Roncoli M, Hollingworth A, Cohen S, Arnold L, Finkler S, Munro B, & Jacobson B (1995). Effects of nurse specialist transitional care on patient outcomes and cost: results of five randomized trials. *American Journal of Managed Care* 1(1):45–51.

13. Brown RS, Clement DG, Hill JW, Retchin SM, & Bergeron JW (1993). Do health maintenance organizations work for Medicare? *Health Care Financing Review* 15 (1): 7–23.

14. Morgan RO, Virnig BA, DeVito CA, Persily NA (1997). The Medicare-HMO revolving door—the healthy go in and the sick go out. *New England Journal of Medicine* 337: 169–175

15. Retchin SM, Clement DG, Rossiter LF, Brown B, Brown R, & Nelson L (1992). How the elderly fare in HMOs: outcomes from the Medicare competition demonstrations. *Health Services Research* 27(5):651–669.

16. Preston JA, & Retchin SM (1991). The management of geriatric hypertension in health maintenance organizations. *Journal of the American Geriatrics Society* 39(7):683–690.

17. Retchin SM & Preston J (1991). Effects of cost containment on the care of elderly diabetics. *Archives of Internal Medicine* 151: 2244–2248.

18. Retchin SM & Brown B (1991). Elderly patients with congestive heart failure under prepaid care. *The American Journal of Medicine* 90: 236–242.

19. Clement DG, Retchin SM, Brown RS, & Stegall MH (1994). Access and outcomes of elderly patients enrolled in managed care. *Journal of the American Medical Association* 271(19):1487–1492.

20. Carlisle DM, Siu AL, Keeler EB, McGlynn EA, Kahn KL, Rubenstein LV, & Brook RH (1992). HMO vs fee-for-service care of older persons with acute myocardial infarction. *American Journal of Public Health* 82(12):1626–1630.

21. Riley G, Lubitz J, & Rabey E (1991). Enrollee health status under Medicare risk contracts: an analysis of mortality rates. *Health Services Research* 26(2):137–163.

22. Shaughnessy PW, Schlenker RE, & Hittle DF (1994). Home health outcomes under capitated and fee-for-service payment. *Health Care Financing Review* 16(1):187–222.

23. Holtzman J, Chen Q, Kane, RL (in press). The effect of HMO status on the outcomes of home-care following hospitalization in a Medicare Population. *Journal of the American Geriatrics Society.*

24. Coffey E, Moscovice I, Finch M, Christianson JB, & Lurie N (1995). Capitated Medicaid and the process of care of elderly hypertensives and diabetics: results from a randomized trial. *The American Journal of Medicine* 98:531–536.

25. For the theoretical basis of the first four SHMOs and early startup experiences see Leutz WN, Greenberg JN, Abrahams R, Prottteas J, Diamond LM, & Gruenberg L (1985). *Changing Health Care for an Aging Society.* Lexington, MA: DC Heath; Morris R (1974). The development of parallel services for the elderly and disabled. *The Gerontologist* 14:14–19; Morris R (1980). Designing care for the long-term patient: how much change is necessary in the pattern of health provision. *American Journal of Public Health* 70:471–472.

26. The evaluation of these first Social HMOs has produced a large literature, including: Harrington C, Lynch M,& Newcomer RJ (1993). Medical services in social health main-

tenance organizations. *Gerontologist* 3(6):790–800; Harrington C, & Newcomer RJ (1991). Social health maintenance organizations' service use and costs, 1985–89.*Health Care Financing Review,* 12(3):37–52; Harrington C, Newcomer RJ, & Moore TG (1988). Factors that contribute to Medicare HMO risk contract success. *Inquiry* 25:251–262; Harrington C, Newcomer RJ, & Preston S (1993). A comparison of SHMO disenrollees and continuing members. *Inquiry* 30(4):429–440; Leutz W, Greenlick MR, Ripley J, Ervin S, & Feldman E (1995). Medical services in Social HMOs: A reply to Harrington et al. *The Gerontologist* 35(1):6–8; Manton KG, Newcomer R, Lowrimore GR, Vertrees JC, & Harrington C (1993). Social/Health Maintenance Organization and fee-for-service health outcomes over time. *Health Care Financing Review* 15(2):173–202; Manton KG, Newcomer R, Vertrees JC, Lowrimore GR, & Harrington C(1994). A method for adjusting capitation payments to managed care plans using multivariate patterns of health and functioning: the experience of Social/Health Maintenance Organizations. *Medical Care* 32(3):277–297; Newcomer R, Harrington C, & Friedlob A (1990a). Awareness and enrollment in the Social/HMO. *The Gerontologist* 30(1):86–93; Newcomer R, Harrington C, Priboth B, Pendergrass F, & Yordi C (1992). *The Evaluation Design and its Implementation. Second Interim Report to Congress: Evaluation of the Social Health Maintenance Organization Demonstrations.* Baltimore, MD: U.S. Department of Health and Human Services, Health Care Financing Administration; Newcomer R, Manton K, Harrington C, Yordi C, & Vertrees J (1995). Case mix controlled service use and expenditures in the social/health maintenance organization demonstration. *Journal of Gerontology: Medical Sciences* 50A(1):M35–M44; Newcomer RJ, Harrington C, & Friedlob A (1990b). Social Health Maintenance organizations: Assessing their initial experience. *Health Services Research* 25(3):425–454.

27. Kane RL, Kane RA, Finch MD, Harrington C, Newomer R, Miller N, & Hulbert M (1997). SHMOs: the second generation: building on the experience of the first social health maintenance organization demonstration. *Journal of American Geriatrics Society* 45 (1):101–107.

28. See Branch LG, Coulam RF, & Zimmerman YA (1995). The PACE evaluation: initial findings. *The Gerontologist* 35(3):349–359.Also see Kane RL, Illston LH, & Miller NA (1992). Qualitative analysis of the Program of All-inclusive Care for the Elderly (PACE). *The Gerontologist* 32:771–780 for a study of the early start-up experience of the PACE projects.

29. Branch et al. (1995). See note 28.

30. McCall N, Kor J, Porringer L, Balaban D, Wrightson C, Wilkin J, Wade A, & Watkins M (1993). *Evaluation of Arizona's Health Care Cost Containment System Demonstration.* San Francisco: Laguna Research.

31. Malone JK, Chase D, & Bayard JL (1993). Caring for nursing home residents. *Journal of Health Care Benefits* January/February: 51–54; Polich CL, Bayard J, Jacobson RA, & Parker M (1990). A nurse-run business to improve health care for nursing home residents. *Nursing Economics,* 8(2):96–101.

10.

International Perspectives on Long-Term Care

Aging is a global affair. Virtually every country faces, or will soon face, societal needs to respond to the aging and disability of its population. Even developing countries face serious questions about how to care for their rapidly aging populations. In regard to aging in the developing world, 1980 can be seen as a demographic watershed. In that year the number of older people in developing countries outnumbered those in the so-called developed world. Although most developing countries have a smaller percentage of older people than developed nations (through a combination of higher birth rates and earlier death rates), the absolute numbers of older persons in these often populous areas demand attention. Developing nations simply cannot afford the patterns of long-term care that have been established by their wealthier counterparts. One hopes they can learn from the experience of those that have already passed through this demographic revolution and avoid some of the mistakes that predecessors have made. In countries where total expenditures on health care amount to only a small fraction of what is spent in affluent nations, the approach to long-term care cannot rely on expensive institutions. Natural community systems must form the bulwark of the approach to providing long-term care.

Among developing countries, the first steps in creating long-term care programs entail putting societal aging on the political agenda. This involves symbolic activities such as compiling demographic data, identifying problems, and articulating goals for elderly citizens. Typically, physicians are heavily involved as leaders in these efforts. A second phase of development is often the establishment of a few geriatric practice sites as models for care and as training sites for health personnel. Actual formal long-term care service options tend to be minimal. The articulation of a service system is a later development, and is more characteristic of developed countries. A commentator who formerly was an official with the Global Aging

Program of the World Health Organization pointed out that countries seem to move from a stage of having only a few services for older people to a stage of turf battles among health and social service authorities, national and local authorities, and various provider and case-management organizations.[1] These kinds of tensions, which we have discussed in earlier chapters, seem to be in the nature of long-term care. As soon as services are available, the dilemmas of who should organize them, who should be in charge, and how they should get distributed inevitably arise.

Despite or perhaps because of these jurisdictional struggles, the most salient global lessons for the United States can be drawn from developing countries where national wealth and industrialization are more comparable. Even these must be regarded cautiously. International comparisons often provide valuable lessons, but the specific data used to compare services across countries must be viewed with some tolerance. Even when special efforts are made to collect comparable statistics, the projects are typical thwarted by varying definitions of services, institutions, and even disabilities. Phenomena with the same name may not be similar, and those with different names may be more alike than it appears. This problem is especially true with regard to institutional care, where some countries make active use of housing arrangements that are not necessarily comparable across nations despite similar terms being used to describe them. Thus, cross-national comparisons of rates of institutional care use must be interpreted particularly carefully.[2]

The focus of this chapter is on the lessons that can be applied in the United States. A number of countries have already faced serious aging of their populations. Their ability to cope economically and socially offers some hope to those who view the demographic forecasts for aging in the United States with panic. It is worthwhile to examine how various developed countries have gone about the task of developing a long-term care infrastructure. Although each country must respond to its own cultural norms, resources, and values, the experience elsewhere can offer new insights into the developments in the United States.

Common Themes

Some common themes resonate among the countries of the developed world as they cope with aging populations and the concomitant increased disability.

- Most try to establish and then build on a base of income support through public and private pensions. They then must grapple with determining when the solution to a long-term care need is best expressed through augmenting the income of the long-term care consumer and when it should be expressed through services.
- Most try to establish health policies suited to a population with chronic health problems and disabilities. In so doing, they build on their existing health entitlements. (The United States is almost alone among industrialized countries

in its lack of a universal system for health care coverage for all its citizens, though the Medicare program fills that role for people over 65.) When building on a health program, they face the problem of determining what belongs in a health service and what is more properly a social service.

- Family care and other so-called informal care are central to each nation's planning. The expectation is that any paid long-term care services will supplement rather than supplant family care. In many countries, a stream of research and policy attention is now directed toward family caregivers. Some countries are also grappling with equity considerations for family caregivers, attempting to determine whether and under what circumstances family caregivers should receive financial compensation for their services.

- Community care is being emphasized over institutional care. For some countries that invested heavily in institutional care at an earlier period, this represents a shift. For others, the effort is to avoid building institutions. However, the preoccupation with avoiding institutional care leads to a consideration of adequate housing. Some countries are better than others in planning for the best use of their existing housing stock and trying to develop housing arrangements to support people needing long-term care.

- Cost is a concern everywhere. The efforts to substitute less expensive forms of care for more expensive ones is widespread. There is considerable interest in developing systems to rationalize the inputs of long-term care, and, therefore, many countries are looking at arrangements such as the case-mix adjusted payment systems developed in the United States.

- Some consolidation or, at least, coordination of the administrative locus for long-term care programs is occurring. Along those lines, health and social programs are beginning to converge for aging and disabled consumers who need long-term care.

- Care provision is devolving from central to local governments. Nongovernmental agencies and private organizations are also often involved. Local control and decision making are emphasized. In countries much smaller than the United States, very small political units in terms of population and area serve as decision-making entities for long-term care programs. For example, each Swiss canton has its own variation of long-term care policies.

- At the level of individual service, some countries are pursuing the idea of providing consumers with a budget and using case managers to assist them in making purchasing decisions within that budget.

- Consumer activism is on the rise, especially among younger people with disabilities.

The proliferation of approaches and the convergence on central tendencies suggest that no country has found the answer to the long-term care conundrum. Countries with liberal policies seem to be becoming somewhat more conservative, while those that have been more conservative (e.g., loath to establish benefits that might replace family care) are moving in the opposite direction. None of the these shifts is happening quickly, but there is a universal air of searching.[3]

Illustrative Countries

Although few countries have been able to establish a fully publicly supported long-term care system, many have made important inroads. We turn now to a brief examination of five countries that together may prove relevant to the United States: Denmark, Canada, Germany, Japan, and the United Kingdom. Each has an affluent society. Each has pursued a different approach to addressing the social issues of long-term care. In this chapter, we examine some of the differences in how long-term care programs have been established in these countries and the policy issues that underlie the choices made. From time to time, we will make reference to developments in other countries as well.

The relative investment in institutional and community care varies from country to country around the developed world. Some countries are high in both; some are low in both; others show a mixed pattern. Table 10.1 uses the best data available from the Organization for Economic Co-Operation and Development (OECD) to illustrate the extent of coverage for institutional and community care for elderly people in our five selected countries. The data were obtained for the year closest to 1990. As the table shows, no pattern of relationship can be discerned between the use of institutions and extent of community care.

Denmark
Denmark stands at once as a symbol of the Nordic countries, which have historically offered progressive programs for the care of older persons, and as an outlier among them. It has consistently had more generous welfare-state programs than even its neighbors in Sweden and Norway. The Danish system has traditionally

Table 10.1. Proportion of Elderly People in Selected Countries Receiving Long-Term Care in Institutions and Home Help in the Community

Country	% elderly people in institutions	% elderly people receiving home help
United States	5.2	4
Denmark	5.6	17
Germany	5.3	1–3
Japan	6.4	1
United Kingdom	5.1	9

Source note: OECD (1996). *Caring for Frail Elderly People: Policies in Evolution* (Social Policy Studies, Number 19). Paris, France: OECD, tables 3.1 and 3.6, p.50 & p.62.

provided ample health and long-term care benefits, including comfortable private quarters in nursing homes. Since the early 1970s the policy has been to provide care in a person's home for as long as possible. This policy was supported by a dramatic expansion in home help services.

A 1982 commission report to the Danish government reemphasized the importance of commitment to community care and the need to avoid forcing citizens to make catastrophic moves. The principle of older persons' rights to self-determination was underscored, including self-determination over what services they would receive and where. The role of public support was defined as facilitating older persons in the use of their own resources. In an effort to avoid institutionalization, an extensive system of 24-hour care and quick response teams were established to assure older persons that they could live in the community and get needed assistance, either in an emergency or on a scheduled basis.

These expansive Danish home care services are the responsibility of the almost 300 municipalities (called *communes*). Communes are also responsible for providing residential care including nursing homes and service flats, but most have emphasized domiciliary care (that is, home care). Domiciliary care includes nursing visits, and equipment, but the backbone of the service is home helpers, who offer personal care, medication assistance, and housekeeping. According to Holstein and colleagues, the prevalence of home help is so great in Denmark that 17% of the population over 65 and 38% of the population over 85 received some home help from the local authorities in 1984.[4] As of 1989 home help became completely free to elderly users. As soon as an application for home care is made, the service begins; assessment and formal allocation and planning come later, so no waiting lists act as a deterrent to services. In recent years, there have been collaborative efforts between communes and hospitals have collaborated to facilitate better discharge-planning to the home.

The move away from nursing homes included the construction of special housing designed to afford frail older persons more autonomy. For many people, except the frailest, this special housing was deemed more desirable and appropriate than hospital-style nursing homes. The boundaries between residential living and nursing homes are less clear than in many other countries. Even in nursing homes, all cognitively intact residents are treated primarily as renters, with control over their space. Single rooms are the norm. Residents retain all their rights.

Payment for nursing home care recognizes the board-and-care components. Residents who subsist only on a state pension pay all of their pension less a small monthly personal allowance, toward the cost of the nursing home accommodations, board, and care. Persons with incomes above the pension level are required to contribute 60% of their additional income up to the level of the actual cost of the nursing home care.

Several municipalities are experimenting with a payment scheme that overtly separates the room-and-board costs from those for services. In these models, rent is pegged at up to 15% of a person's pension. Services are charged as they are used. Under this arrangement the financial structure for nursing home care is indistinguishable from that for residential care.

Japan

Japan faces several demographic challenges at once. Its population is aging rapidly, spurred by both increased life expectancy and a falling birth rate. The tradition of children caring for parents in their homes has been threatened by the press for urbanization and the high cost of housing. Smaller dwelling units have made personal parental care less feasible. But until recently Japan had no strategy for long-term care. Instead the country relied on filial responsibility for care in the community and on heavy use of hospitals for prolonged stays. Average lengths of stay on the order of 40 or 50 days suggest that hospitals sometimes were serving as nursing homes. Nursing homes have been available since the 1960s but have not been heavily used.

All Japanese citizens are enrolled in health insurance programs. These are of two major types: the Employees' Health Insurance System, which covers salaried workers, and the National Health Insurance System, which covers the self-employed, the retired, and the uninsured. Each of these systems encompasses many separate plans.

The Gold Plan, introduced in 1989, provides support for frail older persons at several levels, from active rehabilitation, to the construction of nursing homes, to supporting more home care. The Japanese system does not provide direct cash payments for family care, but it does offer services and some tax credits for such family care. Funding for these activities regardless of site of service comes from a mixture of state, prefecture, insurer, and municipality. User fees are levied for virtually all forms of care. The size of these fees varies with the type of service. A range of alternatives is available, including residential care (in *care houses*), health services facilities for the elderly (nursing homes that emphasize rehabilitation), special nursing homes for the elderly (providing more chronic care), home help, and visiting nursing. Some of these programs (namely, hospitals and visiting nurses) operate under a medical mandate; others (e.g., special homes for the elderly) are seen as more related to long-term care. All these services are provided by governmental and private nonprofit organizations. In addition, a private market exists for personal care services that are not covered by insurance but are regulated by governmental guidelines.[5]

As noted earlier, Japanese hospitals have historically been used for long-term care. The situation was exacerbated when the 50% copayment for health care for older persons was removed in 1973. Some sense of the effect of this change can be seen in the observation that the number of persons aged 65 and older in a hospital at any one time increased tenfold between 1963 and 1993.[6]

The overall pattern has featured tremendous growth. From 1990 to 1995 home helpers expanded from 36,000 to 92,000. Short-stay hospital beds increased from 7,700 to 31,000. Whereas special nursing home beds for the elderly increased from 172,000 to 232,000, beds in health services facilities for the elderly grew from 48,000 to 140,000. By contrast beds in care houses rose from 1,700 to 31,000. Japan has embarked on a tremendous growth program in institutional care, while the rest of the developed world seems to be reining in its institutional commitments. Partly this investment is designed to catch up and partly it is responding to strong social pressures to serve the growing numbers of frail older persons in a context that will not place too much strain on the nuclear families often living in cramped quarters.

A new public long-term care insurance program scheduled to take effect in the year 2000 has been enacted for Japan. It represents an enormous financial investment in long-term care at the national level, but programs will be administered by the municipalities. The money to fund the program will come from two sources. Half will come from mandatory premiums. The other half will come from general taxation, divided among the central government (one-fourth) and the municipalities and prefectures (one-eighth each). The program will provide institutional care in geriatric hospitals and units of general hospitals designed for older persons; special health facilities for the elderly (a more skilled version of a nursing home); and nursing homes and group homes for persons with dementia. Community care covered would include home helps, visiting nurses, and day care. Other provisions include the loan of durable medical equipment and money for home modifications. Physicians' services related to this care would also be covered.

Although all persons over the age of 40 who have paid the premiums are eligible, the eligibility criteria will differ with age. Eligibility is automatic for those 65 and older, but those younger must have an "age-related disease" (likely to be limited to dementia and stroke). Six levels of community long-term care will be established, each with a corresponding insurance benefit cap. (Levels proposed are remarkably generous.) Care managers will provide assistance and advice in developing a plan of care, but all such plans must be agreed to by the consumer and his/her family. Anticipating a need for about 40,000 case managers, Japan has developed a licensure examination and expects that newly qualified case managers will be attached to provider agencies.

Germany

Germany has a long tradition of social insurance. In January 1995, the country expanded its programs of universal health insurance to encompass long-term care. Ironically, this expansion came close upon the heels of the major financial investment necessary as a result of reunification, placing a considerable strain on the social financing structure. The German sickness insurance scheme has historically made a sharp distinction between curable illness and incurable illness, covering only the former. This distinction was eased because the sickness scheme covered limited amounts of disability care (primarily as respite care). Basically, the sickness insurance covered only professional services and some community care, leaving the costs of institutional care to be borne privately. For those unable to pay, means-tested welfare programs were available.

Universal health care is provided through a variety of sickness funds. Many of these are privately operated, but there is a statutory fund for those not covered by the private systems. The core benefits are the same regardless of sponsorship. In 1994, the sickness fund approach was expanded to include long-term care. Mandatory payments from both workers and employers were used to create the resource pool. The threshold for eligibility for benefits was set at needing care at least once each day. The program was being phased in, with initial coverage being limited to people living in the community. By April 1996 all institutionalized citizens were also phased into the program. As of 1997, 2.75 million people had applied for the home care program and 654,00 people for the nursing home program. Four levels of need (from 0 to 3) are determined as a result of an assessment, and three levels of benefits are set depending on the extent of disability and the intensity of care needed. To qualify at all, users must be at Level 1, requiring at least 90 minutes of care a day. Questions have been raised about the reliability of the assessment process used to establish a client's disability level.

Germany (in common with other European countries such as Austria and France) has begun offering its home care benefit in two forms: as formal home care services allocated by local care manager, or in the form of cash to support informal care-givers. Those who opt for cash receive cash sums that substantially discount the value of the service; the sums vary by level of care but never exceed 53% of the assumed value of the formal home care services, and the discrepancy widens as disabilities increase. For example, consumers at the third and highest level of need would receive 1,300 deutsche Marks (D-Marks) per month in cash, which is 43% of the $2,800 D-Marks worth of formal home care services they may receive at that level. Despite this discounting, 66% of the community-dwelling clients chose the cash in the first year of the program, 15% chose a mix of formal services and cash, and only 10% applied for formal care only.[8] The payment levels, even for services themselves, are not estimated to cover the full costs. In essence, this approach represents first dollar coverage. The room-and-board charges for institutional care are expected to be paid privately. For low-income people, additional financial support is available through a welfare scheme. (Note that Japan considered and, at least for now, has rejected a cash benefit plan for fear that the already strong social obligations of the wife of the oldest son toward her in-laws would be increased.)

Some of the boundary issues remain to be worked out between the long-term care insurance scheme and the sickness funds. Some services may appear as responsibilities of both, and there is a potential for some cost shifting. This problem is accentuated when families opt for the cash payment.

Canada

Canada is one of the more slowly aging countries in the developed world. It is of particular interest to the United States because many aspects of culture, geography, politics (e.g., a federal system), and health care organization are held in common. Yet Canada has had a system of universal health insurance covering hospitals, physician services, and a range of other services since 1972. The approach is essentially run by each province under the umbrella of broad national policies and federal cost sharing. The caveats for receipt of the federal contribution are that the provincial programs must be comprehensive, universal, portable from province to province, publicly administered, and without charges to the consumer at the point of service use.

Since 1977 when the federal government exchanged a plan to pay half the costs for a plan to transfer some taxing authority to provinces, the federal government's financial role in the health insurance schemes has gradually diminished. In effect, the federal government has fixed the growth of its contribution, leaving the provincial governments to finance any shortfalls through various tax mechanisms. Although the health insurance programs were fundamentally directed toward supporting acute care, they have been expanded in almost every province to cover at least some elements of long-term care. Some provinces began covering long-term care at the time that federal per-capita grants became available to each province to fund more flexible health provisions. By 1985 all but two of the ten provinces had some universal long-term care entitlements, including both community-based care and institutional care.[9] Nursing home coverage, although a universal entitlement not based on income, is far from free. Although the details vary a bit from province to province, the consumer cost sharing for basic double-room service equals about one-third of the price, a sum that is keyed to the minimum public pension. Thus, a consumer whose only income was a public pension could afford this service and also had a modestly generous monthly spending income (keyed to the Consumer Price Index and about three times greater than the needs allowances permitted in the United States for Medicaid clients in nursing homes). Consumers with more funds can purchase other amenities, including private rooms. As in Germany, the public provision covers the first dollar or the floor, and people with greater incomes are free to supplement services. (This contrasts with the system in the United States where the consumers pay the first dollars for nursing home care until they have reached a poverty level.)

Home-health care, thought to replace or shorten hospital stays, has been covered by the provincial health insurance programs since 1972 and tends to be provided at no charge by health department nurses and other health-related personnel or by nonprofit agencies. In contrast, personal care (what has sometimes been called "chronic home care") and even more socially oriented services (such as homemaking only) became available more gradually, often with copayments based on income. In recent years, there has been growing pressure in Canada to shift care from institutions to the community as much as possible, largely because of a belief that such a course would save money. This strategy has worked best when it is part of a deliberate political effort to redirect support to community care by restricting the growth of nursing homes. In some cases clients with the least amount of disability have been excluded from at least routine nursing home eligibility and managed at home, thereby increasing the case-mix severity of nursing homes. Yet, although Canadian provinces have been encouraged to expand home care provisions, the home care budgets are vulnerable to political chopping in a way that nursing home budgets seem not to be. In some provinces the official policy is to refrain from public provision of any HCBS component if an agency in the community is available to provide the service.[10]

In some provinces the responsibility for nursing homes has rested in two different ministries, one charged with social programs and the other responsible for health. This separation has created several political and programmatic problems with different rules for eligibility for coverage and payment. Increasingly, uniform standards are being introduced to permit both types of institutions to compete more equitably. Long-term care has also been provided in acute care hospitals, where there are designated beds for extended care. These patients vary in the intensity of care they receive. Some benefit from close management; other simply linger while awaiting more permanent placement. Although there are frequent complaints about these so-called "bed blockers," some observers have pointed out that these cases play an important role in the hospitals' economy. Canadian hospitals have been paid on a fixed-rate global budget, based in part on utilization levels. These long-stay patients use relatively few resources and thereby prevent the admission of patients who might make much greater demands on the hospital. From a larger systems perspective such an arrangement is very inefficient. Provincial governments are actively reconsidering the role of extended-care units in their overall long-term care strategy.

In many provinces the payment from nursing home care and for community care comes from the same tax pool that supports acute care. The nursing home occupies an indeterminate place. It is viewed as a medical establishment but its board-and-care function represents more social services. As indicated, the relevant Canadian strategy to address this dilemma has been to charge the patients for the room and board by asking them to pay a fixed amount (set at a rate that would allow persons with only Canada Pensions to retain a reasonable living allowance).

United Kingdom

The history of long-term care in the United Kingdom reveals a shift over time in priorities and methods. The remnants of the Poor Laws vacillated from direct payments to institutional care. The legacy of this philosophy was the workhouse, which played a dominant role in early geriatric care. Responsibility for long-term care of older persons has been divided between the National Health Service, which addressed primarily acute care issues, but also managed long-stay hospital wards (sometimes literally located in very old poor house buildings), and the local social service authorities in each borough or county. The latter oversaw social programs that included home help, sheltered housing schemes, day care, and old people's homes (known as Part III accommodations), which provided shelter and supervision for frail older people. The relationship between the social agency and the medical service varied with time and region. In some areas there was close coordination, with local authority social workers being based in the hospital to help plan access to services; in other areas coordination was less close.

Many changes in both the National Health Service and the local authority programs came about in the wake of an overall effort during the 1980s to reduce the dependence on governmentally provided services. Much of the change was ideologically based, stimulated by the conservative Thatcher administration and concerns about the pressures of societal aging.[11] Opportunities to purchase "council housing" previously rented from the local authorities gave more older people a permanent dwelling and a greater stake in remaining at home. The establishment of a means-tested Supplementary Benefit payment in 1980 provided the financial resources to allow for coverage of private nursing home care. Long-stay beds covered under the National Health Service dramatically reduced. As the number of long-stay beds in hospitals shrank, those in nursing homes increased. Between 1980 and 1990 the proportion of geriatrically oriented beds in nursing homes rose from 6% to 22%. The numbers of private nursing home beds increased by 400% during this period. Residential beds also grew but much less (about 48%). Almost all of this growth was in the private sector. This shift to direct payments for poor older persons increased the use of institutional care much more than community care. In effect, the British system moved to more closely resemble the American approach, with public subsidies linked to income used to purchase private care. Community care provided under the health banner was universally available at no charge, while socially sponsored (through the local authorities) home help was offered under a form of means testing. Changes in funding priorities left local authorities with more fiscal responsibility for community care.

Studies of the community care program found great inequities in funding and scope. The home help program was seen as delivering small aliquots of services to many clients rather than responding differentially to those who needed more care. Institutional care was no longer seen as a last resort. In the 1980s, the pressure, fueled by cost concerns, was to divert care from the institutions back to the community. But no commensurate increase in community services was seen over that decade. About 6% of elderly persons saw a visiting nurse and 9% got home help during both 1980 and 1991. Some critics of the changes allege that "care in the community" actually had come to mean "care by the community," with family members and charitable organizations being obliged to pick up the slack left by the withdrawal of local authority programs.

More recent changes have pushed toward more coordination of care. The locus of responsibility is vested in the local authorities, who are supposed to make better use of the national health service programs. Financial support for privately provided care in both nursing homes and in the community over and above the Supplementary Benefit comes from the budgets of the local authorities, who increasingly have become purchasers and brokers, rather than major providers of services. At the same time, local authorities have been placed under global budgeting arrangements, which require that they allocate their resources on the basis of more careful assessments of need and financial status. Elaborate assessment processes have been developed and great stress has been placed on the role of case management.[12]

Social care for frail older people in the United Kingdom is poorly coordinated with medical care. Primary care is the responsibility of general practitioners (GPs) who are paid a fixed amount for each patient on their roster. These GPs are expected to provid care to nursing home residents, but have no incentive to assume this added role. Geriatricians, who formerly managed extensive rehabilitation and post-hospital resources, have now become largely acute-care physicians for a portion of hospitalized elderly patients. The multidisciplinary rounds, in-patient rehabilitation, and adult day health programs that used to be the hallmarks of geriatric care in the United Kingdom have all but disappeared under the pressure of offering the most cost-effective hospital care. This would be a less serious problem if rehabilitation services and specialized input from geriatrics were available in other settings. It seems that older people who are hospitalized in the United Kingdom may be prematurely relegated to a ''social model.''

Lessons for the United States

Long-Term Care Is Related to Health Coverage
All of the countries illustrated had in common some system of universal health coverage, although the approaches used vary widely. It is much easier to build long-term care benefits on a foundation of a national health care system. In the United States, of course, Medicare constitutes a universal health insurance system for older people, but older people stand out as the only citizens who really have access to this coverage. As a result, seniors have come to be viewed as a privileged group. Moreover, many of the provisions under Medicare afford older persons health benefits that are more generous than those available to younger persons, whose taxes are supporting the Medicare program.

Everywhere the boundaries between health care (such as should be covered by insurance) and long-term care are hard to identify. When services are provided in hospitals, regardless of the nature of those services, they seem to fall readily under the purview of medical authority and coverage as a health service. In countries such as the United Kingdom with a well-established history of geriatric medicine as a speciality, a variety of hospital and outpatient facilities have been encompassed as health services and at the disposal of geriatricians. However, the geriatric specialists are hospital-based and have become increasingly focused on providing acute care. Primary care for older people rests with general practitioners. In Canada, too, there is a tendency to protect some hospital-based rehabilitation and long-stay units as part of health programming, but this situation could change if the basis for hospital payment moves away from global budgeting.

Long-Term Care Involves Consumer Cost-Sharing
Usually some boundaries are drawn between health care and long-term care, although differently in different countries. Whereas health care is generally provided either free or at modest cost, in the countries we have examined long-term care is

never intended to be free. It is recognized everywhere that long-term care is as much a social service as a health service, and to the extent that it is a social service it involves private expenditures with discretion for the individual on how much he or she can or wants to spend. On the other hand, it is also recognized that long-term care is at least in part a service responding to health needs that fall erratically and unevenly on individuals in society. One part of this solution seems to be to establish a minimum set of services that can be treated as part of the universal health package. These services would be available to all on the same basis as other health benefits. Additional services could be made available under a broader long-term care mandate or might be expected to be paid for by recipients with some provisions for coverage for those who required it under a welfare arrangement. In the case of housing, individuals would be expected to pay for their own room and board as their incomes allowed, but some minimal benefit would be guaranteed for everyone.

Promoting Autonomy and Dignity

Much attention in this book has been devoted to developing long-term care options that promote individual autonomy, choice, dignity, and normal lifestyles. Our quick review of five international examples shows a similar preoccupation, though the goal of cost containment and (in the case of the UK) privatization also has force. Sometimes saving money and promoting autonomy can be pursued in tandem, as with the UK's efforts to allow consumers to choose from a menu how the local authorities purchase services on their behalves. The Danish system perhaps comes closest to our aspirations for a long-term care system. It is, therefore, of interest that in this idealized system personal care is widely available and institutions look very "uninstitutional"—more like an apartment complex. It would seem feasible for the United States to adopt many of the principles of the Danish system without incurring the high public costs characteristic of that social welfare state. Of course, the United States presents a much more massive scale than Denmark and a more heterogeneous population. The degree of local control even in relatively small Denmark underscores the importance of downsizing and refining long-term care programs in the United States at the state and even sub-state level.

The Changing Scene

It is instructive to look back at a pair of international studies conducted over two decades ago to appreciate how the international scene has changed in that time and what has remained constant. A study by Kahn and Kammerman[13] looked broadly at social policies, including aging and long-term care policies, in eight countries— Canada, the United Kingdom, Yugoslavia, Germany, Poland, France, Sweden, and Israel. A study by two of the present authors, Robert and Rosalie Kane,[14] specifically examined long-term care in six countries: Sweden, Norway, the Netherlands, England, Scotland, and Israel. Comparing the observations from these studies to the current situation, one cannot help by being struck with two major conclusions.

First, the same problems exist today as did two decades ago; and second, there has been substantial convergence in the approaches taken across countries, although national differences remain prominent. In essence, knowledge has been an actively traded commodity. Countries have become aware of what has been tried in other lands and have imported those ideas that fit their goals. Because most places have been dissatisfied with their long-term care arrangements, foreign ideas seem attractive. Thus, the United States has imported community care concepts developed in the United Kingdom while that country has embarked on an American-style nursing-home program. Similarly, the United States is testing cash benefits seen in Germany and elsewhere in Europe, whereas in Europe and Japan, authorities are adopting elements of the minimum data set developed for nursing homes in the United States.

Alfred Kahn and Sheila Kamerman observed in 1976 that the major models of living and care arrangements for the aged were remarkably similar across the countries they studied. There was general dissatisfaction with the adequacy of special housing and living arrangements. They noted several trends: *(1)* the expansion of long-term care facilities under medical auspices where such coverage is extremely inadequate; *(2)* the development of sheltered or congregate housing; *(3)* growing stress on providing physical and social service supports to allow older persons to remain in their own homes as long as possible; *(4)* development of multifacility living and care complexes with a range of separate facilities that respond to different levels of need; *(5)* development of comprehensive, community-based service centers, whether freestanding or attached to medical facilities; and *(6)* a mixture of medical and social services in the most heavily used community services. The relative emphasis on various aspects of programs varied across the countries studies. At that time, the United Kingdom emphasized community-based services the most, whereas Sweden emphasized housing. Germany was already using some cash benefits.

At the time of their book, they noted several unresolved issues, all of which are with us still today:

1. There was no clearly superior basis on which to determine the optimal ratio of services per impaired person.
2. The relative place of cash benefits as an alternative to services was not clearly established. However, Kahn and Kamerman strongly argue that cashing out all services is undesirable and, in fact, impossible.
3. Although each country had established some sort of family policy explicitly or by omission, these policies were not consistent or equitable within the particular countries.
4. The health, housing, and social services were poorly coordinated and lacked clear boundaries.
5. It was not clear whether long-term care belonged under medical or social auspices.

6. It was not clear whether the aged should have their own long-term care system or be part of a general program.

Writing at about the same time, Kane and Kane arrived at slightly different conclusions. Summarizing our examination of the long-term care services in six developed countries, we found a few areas of commonality: *(1)* Families played a central role, although this role was not always formally acknowledged; *(2)* there was a large disparity in services between rural and urban areas; *(3)* no single all-encompassing solution worked for all older persons; *(4)* in each country studied, the goal was keeping the older person at home as long as feasible; *(5)* separate facilities were preferred to manage physically and cognitively impaired persons; and *(6)* local administration of programs was the rule, albeit often with federal guidelines.

They identified several problems and issues to be addressed:

1. Problems with the coordination of health and social services left many lacunae.
2. Rising costs were a universal concern.
3. Management of the cognitively impaired was frustrating.

It is instructive to compare these observations with those made earlier in this volume. It appears that although we have amassed substantial experience in delivering long-term care and achieved both larger and more sophisticated investments in this area, many of the problems that plagued the systems two decades ago are still with us. The two most pronounced differences between the United States and the various countries examined several decades ago were that the United States relied more than other developed countries on for-profit providers of long-term care, and the United States was unable to build a long-term care system upon the base of a national universal system of health care. The United States still relies more on for-profit providers than do most other countries, including those we highlighted in this chapter, but the differences are narrowing somewhat. And the United States is still challenged to build a long-term care system without having first established some guarantees of acute care services for all its citizens.

Notes

1. Hermanova HM (1996). Global challenges in long-term care case management. Paper presented at the 3rd International Conference on Long Term Care Case Management, San Diego, CA, December 4, 1996.
2. A number of cross-national studies on aging and long-term have been undertaken in the period between 1970 and 1995. Among the available books are Jamieson A (Ed.) (1991). *Home Care for Older People in Europe: A Comparison of Policies and Practices.* Oxford, UK: Oxford University Press, which summarizes findings from a coop-

erative project involving nine developed countries; Kendig H, Hashimoto A, & Coppard LC (Eds.) (1992). *Family Support for the Elderly*. Oxford, UK: Oxford University Press, which began under World Health Organization auspices and summarizes family care policies in both developed and undeveloped countries. See also Schwab T (Ed.) (1989). *Caring for an Aging World: International Models for Long-Term Care Financing and Delivery*. New York: McGraw Hill Information Services Company; Lesemann F & Martin C (Eds.) (1993). *Home-Based Care, the Elderly, the Family and the Welfare State: An International Comparison*. Ottawa: University of Ottawa Press. Kahn AJ & Kamerman SB (1979). *Social Services in International Perspective: The Emergence of the Sixth System*. Washington, DC: USDHEW (SRS 76-05704); Kane RL & Kane RA (1991). Long-Term Care in Six Countries. Washington, DC: Government Printing Office (NIH Publication No. 80-1207)

3. Several documents of the Organization for Economic Cooperation and Development (OECD) illustrate these themes well. See OECD (1994). *Caring for Frail Elderly People: New Directions in Care*. (Social Policy Studies, No. 14). Paris, France: OECD; OECD (1996). *Caring For Frail Elderly People: Policies in Evolution*. (Social Policy Studies, No. 19). Paris, France: OECD.

4. Holstein BE, Due P, Almind G, & Holst E (1991). The home-help service in Denmark. In A Jamieson (Ed.), *Home Care for Older People in Europe: A Comparison of Policies and Practices*. Oxford, UK: Oxford University Press.

5. The entire double issue of the *Journal of Aging and Social Policy*, Volume 8 (2/3), 1996 was comprised of a series of articles on the topic "Public Policy and the Old Age Revolution in Japan." Masato Oka served as guest editor.

6. Ikegami N (1997). Public long-term care insurance in Japan. *Journal of the American Medical Association* 278:1310–1314.

7. Ikegami (1997). See note 6.

8. Becker C, Leistner K, & Nikolaus Th (in press). Long-term care insurance in Germany. *Facts, Research, and Intervention in Geriatrics*.

9. We conducted a book-length study of long-term care systems in Canada in 1985, concentrating on three provinces: Manitoba, British Columbia, and Ontario. Our focus was to examine how Canadian provinces dealt with pent-up demand and escalating costs when they switched long-term care from a means-tested program to a universal benefit, albeit with heavy consumer cost participation for the nursing home component. See Kane RL & Kane RA (1985). *A Will and A Way: What the United States Can Learn from Canada About Caring for the Elderly*. New York: Columbia University Press.

10. Kane RA & Kane RL (1991). Home and community-based care in Canada. In D Rowland & B Lyons (Eds.). *Financing home Care: Improving Protection for Disabled Elderly*. Baltimore: The Johns Hopkins University Press.

11. Walker A (Ed.) (1966). *The New Generational Contract*. London, UK: UCL Press.

12. See Davies B & Challis D (1986). *Matching Resources to Care*. Hants, UK: Gower.

13. Kahn & Kamerman (1997). See note 2.

14. Kane & Kane RA (1979). See note 2.

III
THE HEART OF
THE MATTER

11.

Conclusions: The Heart of the Matter

At the heart of long-term care are people living their lives with disabilities, people needing help with everyday matters. Long-term care, therefore, is inescapably intertwined with everyday life. The disabilities we describe as requiring long-term care may get better in time, but they will probably get worse. In any case, life will go on for the people needing the care, their family members, and other significant people in their lives. A good long-term care program will have the capacity to help people achieve their maximum functional capabilities, and it will be able to suggest ways to provide care that helps avoid future problems. The challenge is to manage this care without presuming to manage lives. Moving to a residential care facility or nursing home is a life decision that should not be casually "prescribed" to meet efficiency goals of a health care system. It should not be spoken of as a "placement." People who need care will make decisions with their care needs in mind, but their lives should not be held hostage to their need for care.

In the United States, long-term care policies are largely made at the state rather than the federal level, although federal money is expended through cost-shared and block-granted programs. Unlike health care services, which are insured publicly or privately, long-term care services are largely financed privately by individuals and families with public funding programs available for low-income people only. Over at least a 20-year period, long-term care policy makers have had the following laudable goals: *(1)* to make long-term care services available in the community so that people of all ages can, as much as possible, lead normal and dignified lives, pursuing age-appropriate pursuits, experiencing personal relationships, and enjoying privacy; *(2)* to introduce more user choice and control into long-term care; *(3)* to curb the growth of long-term care costs; *(4)* to assure that long-term care services meet acceptable quality standards; *(5)* to coordinate and integrate long-term care with acute care; and *(6)* to provide support and encouragement to family members who are giving long-term care to their relatives, usually without direct payment. The problem is that we can achieve some of these objectives some of the time, but not all of them all of the time. If we hope to have more community care and curb costs, we will not be able to subscribe to what everyone will agree is an adequate quality standard. Therefore, we need to place a high priority on widespread use of community care and fashion other standards with that emphasis in mind.

Some progress has been made toward the above goals. Although the bulk of government money spent on long-term care is still spent in nursing homes rather than in the community (84% in 1996), some of the most marked trends and developments in the last decades seem to be in the right direction. These include: great increases in the amount and type of in-home services available, emergence of new kinds of residential care in private homes (i.e., adult foster care) and in private apartments (i.e., some forms of assisted living) where severely disabled persons receive services without deeply compromising their quality of life; efforts to redesign nursing homes to achieve the same improvements in quality of life; some experimentation with providing long-term care consumers with additional income rather than providing them with in-kind services; some use of public money to compensate low-income family caregivers; and the growth of geriatric care and geriatric teams along with general improved understanding about health conditions in old age. Another trend, the advent of managed care organizations that are financed on a capitated basis, will undoubtedly have a major effect on long-term care, too, but it is not yet clear whether the direction will be positive or negative. In this chapter, we take stock of where we are now with long-term care and raise some issues for the next century of program development.

Taking Stock

Is the glass half empty or half full for long-term care? How far have we come, how far do we have to go, and is the road map clear? The past decade has seen some remarkable changes in the way long-term care is delivered. Medicare, the nation's only universal health care program, has broadened its coverage of long-term care substantially in terms of home health care and nursing home care, albeit with a reliance on an expensive mode of home care. A 30-year history of accelerating use of nursing homes has been halted and even reversed. Despite an aging population, the number of residents in nursing homes has begun to decline, although the cost of nursing home care continues to increase. The current investment in nursing homes (i.e., in the physical structures and capital) may prove one of the greatest impediments to changing the face of long-term care. Yet, new forms of congregate residential care have evolved. Assisted living facilities are springing up all across the country like fast-food chains. Many are targeted to the private market and to light care, but some states have shown that assisted living can be efficiently used for a Medicaid market and for people with substantial care needs.

Managed care promises to change thinking about long-term care. Although most of the current managed care effort has been directed toward acute care, it is just a matter of time until it extends more actively into long-term care. Because managed care has no history with long-term care, it may prove to be the new broom that sweeps clean. In the rosiest scenarios, managed care's search for the most efficient ways to deliver long-term care could open new opportunities for creativity. Even if they provide the capitation, governments will be distanced from some of the political decisions that affront existing providers and prevent sensitive state officials from acting. On the other hand, this possible advantage cuts both ways. The pressure for cost cutting may lead to a level of parsimony that will create new and greater threats to the less tangible but central aspects of quality of life so important to long-term care. Those state governments that have invested in case management capacity at the communitywide rather than the organizational level may find these organizations are the first to be deemed expendable, at considerable cost to the community infrastructure.

Changes in acute care have had effects on long-term care. Nursing homes and home health care have been catalyzed to develop more intensive services to manage patients being discharged from hospitals earlier in the wake of changed hospital payment systems under Medicare. It seems likely that managed care will extend that trend even further.

Models of innovative care, including consumer-directed care, are being tried in several states. Indeed, there is wide interstate variation in the way long-term care is handled. The types and amount of long-term care available and specifically what is covered under Medicare and Medicaid waivers vary extensively from state to state. State variation is another two-edged sword. Although states have been the laboratories for long-term care and social welfare programs for some time, the extent of variation means that at the same time as some states are developing innovative approaches, people in other states remain poorly covered.

Community-based long-term care has been a goal since the 1970s, but without everyone actually being aware of it, the paradigm has changed. Historically, long-term care policy has been heavily influenced by what we call the "alternatives paradigm." Community care was expected to displace nursing home care and, at the same time, save money. Substantial frustration grew out of the early studies that tried to prove but instead refuted this relationship. Closer examination reveals, however, that the alternatives paradigm is really composed of two different components: a prevention paradigm and a substitution paradigm. The preventive paradigm essentially argues that community care can be viewed as a form of prevention. It holds that if people with modest needs for care are actively assisted in the community, their conditions can be affected to the point where entrance into a nursing home can be delayed or averted. Advocates for this perspective are less vocal in arguing that the approach makes good economic sense in terms of producing enough savings to offset its costs. Skeptics question whether the preventive effects can even be demonstrated.

The substitution paradigm suggests that a person with a level of disability or other need that justifies admission to a nursing home can be treated more cheaply or at least at the same price, and certainly more happily, in the community. To us, this thought process makes the most sense. In acting on the substitution paradigm, one needs to be vigilant to keep the costs of community care from drifting upward. One must strive to provide the care, at least at public expense, to those with substantial needs. Families need to be recognized as largely willing but, nonetheless, conscripted labor, who are necessary to make HCBS affordable. And the services need to be heavy-duty long-term care services, the kind provided by personal assistants and attendants on a regular basis. A person who is deemed to need care twice a week to stay out of a nursing home probably really needs it much more—or else he or she was not destined for a nursing home in the first place.

Old ideas die hard. There are still care providers, policy-makers, and lawmakers who believe that an ounce of prevention is worth a pound of cure, that home-delivered meal programs and friendly visiting make the difference between being in or out of a nursing home. This thinking leads to wistful faith in voluntary and private solutions to the community's long-term care programs. Many commentators hope that the religious and philanthropic organizations of the country, combined with an army of individual volunteers, can solve the long-term care problems that governments prefer not to tackle. Of course, volunteers can be helpful in any long-term care endeavor. But they cannot be the main event. The work of long-term care is arduous; its time commitments are stringent; its hours are peculiar; and the people who do it (outside of family members who do it out of affection and duty) must be paid.

Consumer direction is an important goal. Continued attention needs to be paid to ways to put consumers in charge of their care and to develop the kinds of care consumers prefer. If money expended is a sign of preference, it is notable that many long-term care consumers are reluctant to pay for in-home services from their own funds. We also have noted that some consumers resist accepting even free services. Given that scenario, some would argue that care has little marginal value. Why should we publicly subsidize programs that consumers with money do not wish to purchase? Just as with acute care, this reluctance to use services seems greatest in the preventive mode. Faced with a catastrophe the same older people who did not buy help at home may impoverish themselves (although some will seek ways to preserve their assets) by entering a nursing home. But, based on the experience in those states offering real options, it is likely that many people would opt for some approach that allowed them to remain at home or to live in a more appealing alternative living environment, although some will still opt for the nursing home.

The definition of community, at least in the HCBS waivers, has been extended to include the new forms of housing with services as described in Chapter 6. We are delighted to see these new congregate settings appear and are enthusiastic about some of the models. That part of the glass is half full. Nevertheless, we need to worry about whether 10 or 20 years from now all or even most of the assisted living programs will really be conducive to the dignity, privacy, and choices that we want for long-term care consumers. The half-empty part of the glass concerns quality.

Apropos of that, we spent much of the early part of this book discussing the strong nursing home lobbies and their influence on long-term care systems. But assisted living programs are already emerging as a strong organized interest group. The industry is almost entirely proprietary, and stockholders have their usual priorities. We are hopeful about assisted living because, at its best, it is a better model for living than today's nursing home. But not all states require the positive features of assisted living—especially the full private apartments—in order to reimburse under Medicaid. Government officials will need to believe that what they perceive as necessary for themselves and their family members is also necessary for poor people and stick to those principles.

Trade-Offs

Those turning to this book for easy answers to the long-term care conundrums will be disappointed. Finding the right balance in long-term care is perplexing. Nor is one approach likely to fit all situations. It would be simplistic to argue that one form of care is all good or all bad, although harmful or disrespectful aspects of any type of care should be eliminated. Basically, much of the discussion about long-term care policy comes down to making trade-offs. When some elements of care are emphasized, others are given less priority. Having said that, however, we argue that some trade-offs should be unnecessary and, indeed, off limits. Responsible oversight and adequate physical protection should not entail loss of dignity and the invasion of privacy. It is feasible and practical to offer frail older persons safe and compassionate care in a setting where they can control their own lives and determine important elements of their own routines.

It should not be necessary to forgo needed medical care to receive long-term care, nor vice versa. Good primary care is an essential component of good long-term care. Long-term care and acute care can be provided from different sources, but the different providers must communicate effectively. Long-term care providers, including independently employed attendants and family members, need to know what to look for to detect important changes in a patient's status. Primary care providers need to understand how much and what kinds of care can be provided in the patient's current setting and to work with those care givers to maximize the benefits of total care.

A person needing assistance to meet the demands of long-term care faces some of the most important and difficult decisions in his or her life. Unfortunately, consumers seldom have the opportunity to make many of these crucial decisions deliberately and explicitly. Instead, providers or case managers infer or ignore consumer preferences in the belief that certain issues trump all others and that professionals must make judgments where safety is concerned. Especially when consumers rely on publicly supported services, concerns about their safety become preeminent, partly because of a strong sense of responsibility and partly for fear that a tragedy could lead to a scandal. Although the ability to purchase assistance privately usually creates more options, even then excessive protection or insufficient appreciation can lead to unnecessarily circumscribed decisions. Sometimes, family members have safety instincts that mirror those of state officials, and sometimes the state has defined and licensed programs in such a way that heavy service, strong protections, and extensive restrictions are inextricably linked.

The most basic trade-off seems to be between safety and freedom. Fears about a person's ability to function safely may catapult people into controlled environments where they are thought to be less likely to harm themselves or expose themselves to danger. A related trade-off involves the extent of oversight provided. A person may elect to live on his or her own, taking the chance that help may not be as readily available as if personnel were already at hand. Likewise, a person may prefer to live in his or her own home and do without some services because the travel costs associated with bringing the services to each consumer separately render them too expensive to distribute in large amounts. With the same level of dependence, a long-term care consumer living in close proximity to others needing care is likely to get more service.

Another trade-off issue relates to geographic equality. Is society obliged to provide equal availability of services to persons living in all locations? For example, should rural dwellers enjoy the same depth and variety of services as do those living in cities? Generally, we would say no; the choice to reside in remote areas carries with it (or should) the realization that some forms of care will not be as readily available. This doctrine does not mean that rural dwellers are ineligible to receive care, but simply that they must expect care to be somewhat less available, or to travel or even relocate to obtain it. If a service is designed to be delivered in their own homes, then they may have to forgo all or some of it, or it may be possible to develop an alternative approach that does not entail so much staff travel time. Likewise, people needing a substantial amount of service, especially spread out over multiple times during the day and night, might not be able to afford this care in his or her original home because of the travel–time costs involved. At some point that person would face a decision to either relocate to some type of congregate living situation where many people could be served by the same staff without incurring expensive travel time or receiving less care. Under this scenario, a person could opt to remain at home and accept the loss of care and the consequences that follow from it, as long as the decision was made overtly. Even here some choices are unconscionable. For example Native Alaskans in Western and Northern Alaska who need care and cannot remain in their homes face a 1,000- to 1,500-mile move to Seward or Anchorage, where they don't understand the language, hate the food, and don't know the culture. Some investment in an infrastructure is needed to prevent such wrenching dislocations.

Preferences

Closely linked to the concept of trade-offs is the element of preferences and values. Each of us holds certain ideas and actions dear. Some aspects of life take priority over others. Ideally, those making recommendations about long-term care should first elicit the client's preferences and emphasize the ends most desperately sought as the first step in identifying the activities that are most likely to achieve them.

Individuals will have their own preferred outcomes—maintaining a job, being in close contact with loved family members, promoting the goals and well-being of loved family members rather than their own well-being; having a "good death"; having a sense of contributing to society or to one's own family or community. Their emphasis will depend on many factors—their ages, interests, abilities, family structures, degrees of introspection, health status, and prognosis. At some points, they may articulate preferred trade-offs: for example, less life prolongation in exchange for living out their lives where and how they please; less costly care for themselves so that they can conserve resources for their family. Most people will develop their preferred outcomes in interaction with family members with whom their lives and aspirations are intertwined.

Thus, different people aspire to different goals for long-term care. Some reach the stage of needing such care with a sense that they are content to simply cope. They are looking for sufficient assistance to allow them to function as normally as possible, maintaining their life routines. Others want to do everything possible to hold on to their functional abilities, or even improve them. They may shun assistance, preferring to emphasize rehabilitative strategies that promote independence. For them, accepting help may be seen as sign of weakness. Some people place great stress on their privacy. Opening their affairs to the oversight of case managers and paid caregivers may be too exposing.

Ideally, each consumer should be able to identify the goals he or she wants to maximize. Several things stand in the way of maximizing individual preferences, however. It is not clear what views have priority, for example, when personal preferences are in conflict with societal norms. The debate over the future of assisted suicide offers a vivid example of the fallout from this conflict. When public funds pay for the programs the potential for overriding individual preferences is even greater. Also, preferences are not necessarily universally shared within a family unit. Clients may place much more emphasis on autonomy than do concerned family members, who fear for the person's safety. Opening up the issue may lead to conflict, but resolving this conflict is a necessary first step in arriving at a plan of care that has a reasonable chance of success.

In practice, providers rarely elicit consumer preferences and may even avoid them. Especially when a provider (or a case manager) suspects that the client's preferences may lead to an expectation that cannot be fulfilled, discussions are directed away from such dangerous topics. More commonly client preferences are simply ignored. Some may view them as the icing on the cake, believing that societal values should determine which outcomes are most favored, since society pays the bill.

Eliciting preferences is difficult. Clients are unaccustomed to thinking clearly about just what they hope to achieve, although many have strong feelings about what aspects of care they want to retain or avoid when specific options are afforded. It is, nonetheless, possible to train case managers and similar personnel to become more sensitive to the need to elicit client preferences and more skillful in obtaining them.

Preferences may apply at several levels. Clients have strong feelings about which aspects of the outcomes of care are most important. Theoretically, these priority outcomes would be used to determine what modes of care have the greatest like-lihood of achieving the desired ends, either unconstrained by cost or within some cost-constraint parameters. Preferences can also be expressed about the attributes of a care setting of a particular type. For example, one foster home may be better suited to a particular person than another because it emphasizes certain aspects of care or life. It may be a religious setting or it may cater to a particular cultural group. Similarly, for some people location may be a major concern because of a belief that proximity will encourage more visitors or allow the person to continue to participate in aspects of familiar community life.

Preferences are largely shaped by expectations. Although people can theorize about what they might like out of life, most of their visions are circumscribed by their beliefs about what is feasible. The further one moves away from what is construed as reality, the more difficult it becomes to extract statements of prefer-ence. Because frail older people often view their world has highly constrained, the options available to them need to be portrayed concretely if one hopes to expand their conceptions of what is possible. If not, they are likely to choose among a narrow range of alternatives and strive to adapt to these constrained circumstances as best they can. Making do and getting by are active components of their coping strategies.

Recommendations

It would be satisfying to conclude this book with a set of specific recommendations about what should be done, but that is impossible. It is highly unlikely that any single approach will work in all circumstances or even that there is a single best solution to this complex problem. Also, the nature of long-term care suggests that the best solutions are local and that multiple models will emerge. Thus, we conclude with some ideas to be kept in mind as new approaches are considered. Indeed, the one unqualified recommendation is that the search for new solutions should continue with even greater-intensity imagination.

Related to that, the policy-making environment must support reform. The currently heavily regulated approach, while justified by historical exploitation, casts a heavy pall over innovative efforts. It would be impolitic and foolhardy to propose eliminating all regulations, but they should be carefully considered in terms of their ultimate effects. Wherever possible, it will be better to emphasize outcomes (with appropriate corrections for case-mix) in order to permit greater flexibility in structural and process elements.

For-Profit Ownership

Although there is no convincing body of evidence to demonstrate that for-profit ownership produces a different level of quality from nonprofit, it seems reasonable to suggest that ownership will make a difference in the long run. Especially in an area like long-term care, where much of the service seems to relate to intangible elements, for-profit motivations may emphasize reducing costs to generate a return, whereas nonprofit programs may plow resources back into the programs themselves. Some have and will argue that for-profit operations are inherently more efficient and may perhaps be more sensitive to external pressures, especially from regulators and the market. But it is worth examining the underlying belief systems in the United States. The heavy reliance on proprietary vendors has been a hallmark of long-term care for some time, and the trend is expanding. This pattern of ownership distinguishes the United States from most other developed countries, especially those whose programs are often admired. If the specific course of long-term care remains uncharted, we may feel safer in a vessel owned by a nonprofit organizations. When the crisis comes, they may be better trusted to act in the community's interest, if only to avoid the opprobrium associated with poor performance.

The greatest danger to providing better care lies not so much in for-profit ownership as with ownership by publicly traded companies. It is likely that future historians of health care will look back on this era as a watershed period, when health and social care became a publicly traded commodity. We have, in effect, crossed a policy Rubicon with little hope of turning back. Once services become the purview of Wall Street, the situation becomes perilous. The bottom line is shareholder profits. Even when profits and good care are compatible, their timelines are often different. Building a new program takes time. It requires a philosophy of investment in the future, changing infrastructure. Publicly traded companies are driven by quarterly schedules with an emphasis placed on short-term returns. CEOs are under great pressure to show earnings that meet financial analysts' quarterly forecasts. Even a well motivated CEO will not last long if he or she fails to show returns at least as large as forecasted. If CEOs are called to account every quarter, few leaders will pursue approaches that require substantial time to implement, let alone harvest. Although we are aware of several companies in long-term care, both in the nursing-home and assisted living sector that are publicly traded and adhere to progressive, client-centered philosophies, we, nonetheless, think that systematic oversight and protection is needed to make sure that the public interest remains paramount.

Managing the Lobbies

Closely linked to issues of ownership is the power of the political lobbies that represent the currently enfranchised. Probabilities for effective reform will vary directly with the ability to develop sufficiently powerful countervailing forces to contend with those whose oxen are likely to be gored. Thus far the track record is discouraging. With a few remarkable exceptions, lobbies representing older persons have not taken up long-term care as a major cause. When they have, they have been at least as likely to argue on behalf of more support for extant structures. Arousing the interest of elderly consumer groups in the often complex issues of long-term care is a major undertaking. But without such support, reform seems hopeless.

It may also be feasible to seek areas where those in power, at the moment the nursing-home lobbies, can be convinced that change will favor them. Opportunities for growth can prove a strong enticement. At the very least, it may be possible to convince them that it is better to seize the initiative than to live with the consequences of programs developed solely by others. Given all the criticism of the nursing home in this book, it is appropriate to emphasize now that the nursing home industry is replete with owners, administrators, professionals, and line workers who want to make change, who mourn for the situation of the people they attend, who feel paralyzed by what the human predicament has wrought. Like any enterprise, the nursing home industry must protect its business interests. But the people involved for the most part are eager to apply their considerable skills to fashioning a system that works better for clients if they need not commit organizational suicide in the process.

Managing Dementia

Unless a major scientific breakthrough identifies the etiology of dementia and develops an effective medical treatment, this tragic affliction will continue to provide a major reason for long-term care. Better ways are needed to care for persons with dementia. More experimentation, including the effects of providing less, rather than more service, are desperately needed. Some reports suggest that even quite demented persons can sometimes live independently with well-thought-out efforts to create a safe environment and with care provided at intervals. This would certainly lead to less frustration among family members with a widowed parent with dementia.

Common sense, if not empirical data, suggests that severely cognitively impaired persons should be cared for in surroundings different from those used to house people who are cognitively intact but physically compromised. It may well prove to be that less is more. Aggressive management efforts may engender more resistance and rage reactions than leaving people with dementia somewhat on their own, and providing in-home services as needed for a longer time than is currently considered prudent.

The data from the various recent studies of special care units in nursing homes offer some insights into the best forms of management in congregate settings. Geographic segregation certainly makes special programming possible. It also theoretically assists those who are cognitively intact by separating them from disturbing aspects of close proximity to those who are confused. But, because few of the units are large enough to accommodate all of the demented residents in a given home, this protective effect is modest at best.

The greatest challenge in care for people with dementia is to determine what really constitutes a success story in the middle of personal and family tragedy. What is a good quality of life for a person with dementia? In actuality, this riddle cannot be definitely answered in the absence of the ability of the consumers to tell their own stories. However, it is not a mystery to identify a poor quality of life for the person with dementia. This poor quality of life is manifested by visible anxiety, frustration, and distress. It is present when the person is tied up or constantly sedated. Consumers describe a poor quality of life through weeping, screaming, and other overt signs. We would consider care for people with dementia to be good when these clear distress signals are minimal and when positive and obvious signs of well-being are present—smiles, energetic activity, and engagement with the environment.

Setting a Price for Care

Part of the interest in developing dementia special care units has been stimulated by providers' desires to increase payment for the care of cognitively impaired people in nursing homes. The predominant payment system used for nursing home care relies on extrapolating case-mix measures to the time spent caring for persons with these particular case-mix traits. Under such systems people with dementia fare poorly. This raises a more general question about all of long-term care. What is a fair way to price services so that providers are properly remunerated and public payment programs are not overcharged.

The data on which case-mix systems are calculated are derived from direct observations of the amount of time that actual care takes. They are based on the status quo rather than on any ideal models of care. Hence, the relative payments are based on extant practices rather than what is needed to produce good results. Historic patterns of neglect can thus become even more entrenched.

If payment is to be used as a means of changing the way care is delivered, it should be tied to effectiveness. This link can be established either indirectly by establishing how much of which care is associated with good results, or it can rely on actual achievement of outcomes, developing some form of incentive payments for better-than-expected results. Using outcomes as a basis for payment runs directly into the other major determinant of costs—namely, case mix; but payments that reflect case mix create an incentive to have clients become more dependent rather than to improve. An adequate payment system must address both the case mix and the outcomes components. It is impossible to escape this paradox. One potential compromise is to incorporate case mix on admission (and perhaps at infrequent intervals of reassessment) but to use outcomes as the basis for incentives on an ongoing basis.

Applying case-mix payment systems to newly emerging forms of residential care and to home care of various types may be a recipe for trouble. New databases must be created to time the inputs and the outcomes of care for various groups served, a laborious task. That done, it is likely that the status quo will be measured, without any evidence either that the care is done well or that it is even efficient. If states and insurers are to cover new forms of long-term care, they may be wisest to set what seems to them a fair price based on an understanding of necessary costs for the services rather than try to assess current costs and pay at some percentage of that distribution.

Labor Force Issues

Long-term care is often described as "low tech/high touch." Beyond family care providers, it relies heavily on minimum-wage workers. A perpetual problem is how to create jobs that can attract and retain the types of these personnel needed to provide competent and compassionate care. The problem is exacerbated by the low wage scale and the general absence of benefits. Given these facts, it seems inevitable that these workers will continue to be drawn from the lowest social strata. Many will be immigrants whose language and culture will be distinctly different from those they serve.

Although it is important to advocate a higher minimum wage, it is unlikely that this wage will ever be high enough to make such work attractive. Indeed, the very nature of the work involves dealing with several types of unpleasantness. Intimate bodily functions are involved. Many of the clients may be confused and resistant. Some are abusive. Many cannot respond with the gratitude that might be experienced from other types of clientele.

A number of solutions have been proposed to address the long-term care personnel puzzle. Some have advocated various forms of career ladders, by which personnel may obtain education and training to advance from aide to licensed practical nurse and even higher. However, the career ladder concept rarely works as planned. Many of these workers have precarious living situations and limited education. Sustaining the effort required for training, especially in the face of full-time employment, is a tall order.

Instead, it may be more fruitful to seek ways to make the work more personally rewarding. Studies of the people who perform these jobs suggest that a specific subset of the minimum wage workers concentrate their employment in the personal service sector. Although they may migrate from nursing home to home care to hospital, they are much less likely to move into fast foods or other comparable work. These people have sense of service. They enjoy helping others. Building on this intrinsic motivation, one could enhance the working environments by supplying more information and better sense of accomplishment. The training needs to explain not only what needs to be done but why. Understanding the rationale behind the routines may make it easier to adhere to them and render personnel more sensitive to the changes they should be looking for in the clients' status.

Long-term caring can be very demanding and very frustrating. From the providers' perspective, many consumers seem to be constantly deteriorating. It is hard to see what difference good care makes. Not seeing the results of one's efforts can be extremely disheartening. In the main, the major effects of caring must be seen as the difference between what is achieved and what would have otherwise occurred. Because the overall trend is a decline in function, good care can be interpreted as slowing the rate of decline, but without some point of reference all that is seen is decline. Developing simple but sensitive measures of outcomes and presenting the longitudinal data in the context of expected results without such care can provide the necessary feedback to line workers to demonstrate the value of their efforts.

Given that the preponderance of future personal care workers will be immigrants (a worldwide pattern), cultural as well as language problems arise. Some of these people may bring with them belief systems quite different from those in this country. The challenge is how to adapt workers to the culture of the consumers. The first step is recognizing the discrepancies. Long-term care professionals will need to become more culturally sensitive even to appreciate the problems.

Separating Living Situation and Services
One of the basic conflicts in long-term care arises over the historical linkage represented by the nursing home. Drawing on the hospital model and tempered by the almshouse, the nursing home has combined under a single roof the care for disabled persons in the context of an institution. Although many may seek the safety and shelter of a caring environment, few would voluntarily elect to live in an institution. Nonetheless, because the nursing home is such a dominant a part of the long-term care landscape, it shapes almost everyone's image of the terrain. Few have the vision to see how the barren ground can be reshaped to provide more hospitable living circumstances.

In reality, the combination of housing and services is artificial. The acute hospital model, which organizes patients' lives to meet the needs of the staff in the belief that greater efficiency in the life-saving goals justifies the temporary impositions, makes much less sense in the context of chronic care, where the life experience is a major component of the total value of the care. It is neither necessary nor desirable to link institutional clustering with the availability of services. Likewise, the payment for care should not foster such a linkage.

Because the nursing-home payment structure operates on a different principle from that for community care, it is difficult to make meaningful comparisons. At a time when the present and future costs of long-term care are a cause for concern, it seems especially useful to focus those costs on those that relate most directly to long-term care services. Both therapeutic and compensatory care can be provided in a variety of settings. Although there are some efficiencies to be gained from combining functions associated with room and board with those for compensatory services, it is quite feasible to look on these as separable activities and to pay for them accordingly. Separating the payment would have several immediate advantages: *(1)* It would maximize the funds available for services and thus allow the same dollar pool to cover more people. *(2)* It would create a climate that would encourage better living conditions for persons needing long-term care. *(3)* It would classify recipients of care not as patients on whom work is done but foremost as tenants of a specified living space.*(4)* It could empower consumers to become more self-assertive about expressing their preferences, even to the point of refusing care because they would retain control over their living space and hence over a central aspect of their lives. *(5)* It would facilitate fairer competition between nursing homes and other forms of long-term care, perhaps encouraging nursing homes that could not reconfigure themselves as assisted living programs to provide better living situations.

Separating the payment for housing from that for services would mean that people could live in distinctly different levels of surroundings and still be entitled to the same services based on their dependency needs. It would still be necessary to provide housing subsidies for those who otherwise could not afford adequate housing, just as is done for the rest of the population. Some provision needs to be made for post acute care. Implementing such a program might involve limiting payments for service-related housing for those on inactive convalescence or rehabilitation to no more than some arbitrary amount, say 30 days (to recognize the continuation of a hospital-like situation). That period would be needed to cover the care associated with post-hospital recovery, when the hospital paradigm would be applicable. But after the specified time of care, housing costs would be calculated separately.

Under such an arrangement nursing homes would undoubtedly be motivated to compete by upgrading their living situations. Although single rooms with full baths need not be mandatory, it seems very likely that they would be widely available because consumers would prefer them. The tradition of a fixed routine to which the resident must accede would give way to more individualized approaches to care.

The transition would likely involve some increase in overall costs. Clients would be expected to pay more out of pocket for their room and board, although these persons are currently expected to provide the first dollar coverage under the current Medicaid arrangement. The sum of the new housing allowances for poor persons and the new service costs could exceed the current amount spent under Medicaid depending on how the service pricing structure was established. Theoretically, the portion of Medicaid payments now going to cover room-and-board costs in nursing homes could possibly be redirected to offset housing costs, although some skeptics may despair of ever recovering these funds.

Financing

There is general concern about where the money will come from to support long-term care in the future. Straight-line extrapolations of current expenditure patterns on forecasted populations suggest that the demands will require a substantial proportion of available public dollars. Responses to these forecasts have gone in both directions. Some have proposed various incentives for people to take out private long-term care insurance in the hopes that such coverage would prevent dependence on Medicaid. Others have urged that all long-term care be brought under a universal publicly supported program.

As noted earlier, the demand for private long-term care insurance has grown substantially but most observers see strong limitations to its role in solving the cost crisis. Some states have tried to foster purchase of such insurance coverage. They hope to thus prevent demands on their Medicaid programs by offering credit for the amount covered. This would be applied toward the size of the purchaser's assets excluded from the eligibility calculation.

One way to increase the number of persons covered under a public financing program would be to cover only services and not housing, as suggested above. Another approach would be to cover only part of a long-term care episode. In effect, this strategy would create a public–private partnership by default, leaving individuals to address the uncovered portion on their own or to buy newly created insurance packages.

The two basic models for covering costs can be thought of as front-end and back-end coverage. Under the former, public funds would pay for a fixed amount of care, after which each individual would be expected to cover the rest. (Presumably, poor persons would continue coverage under some type of welfare model similar to the present Medicaid program.) Back-end coverage would entail a substantial deductible. In essence, public support would take over only after individuals had first expended significant resources to meet the costs of long-term care. The back-end financing would affected fewer people (because many people would likely need less long-term care than would be covered by the deductible) but would prevent financial catastrophe. (The financial impact and proportion of the population served would depend on the size of the mandatory deductible.) This approach could potentially create an attractive opportunity for the insurance industry. Just as Medicare's requirements for copayments spawned Medigap insurance, so too might a ready market for private gap-filling, long-term insurance develop. Because the upper limit of risk would be set by the threshold for public coverage, the insurance companies' risk would be capped. The costs for such coverage might be quite affordable and would not require that someone purchase the policy at a very young age to obtain a favorable rate.

The implementation of long-term care insurance can be accomplished through either a service benefit or a cash benefit (that is, an indemnity payment). More stringent eligibility criteria will be needed if a cash benefit is used than with a service benefit because of the increased risk of induced demand. With a service benefit the threshold for use can be relaxed if one requires a substantial copayment. In effect, people will get coverage only if they think the service (or a substantial portion of it) is worth paying for themselves.

We believe in a public responsibility for long-term care just as we believe in a public responsibility for acute health care. To say otherwise is to perpetuate vast horizontal inequities—for example, the family that draws high acute care expenses is financially relatively unscathed compared to those who draw high long-term care expenses. Distinctions about what care is a right also encourage expensive cost-shifting from long-term care to acute care. But long-term care is difficult to fashion as an entitlement because of its essential nature as a social program. Because long-term care is so intertwined with everyday life, discretionary standards exist.

We will need to forge some blend of universal programs and means-tested programs. The universal programs could include much of what is now in Medicaid waivers and should include residentially based services, including nursing home services. Universal programs, however, are not free programs. A hefty copayment (such as for nursing homes in Canada) is much more appealing and fairer than a spend-down policy. There is considerable evidence that the current spend-down policies to become eligible for Medicaid cause hardship. As these policies have been applied to HCBS services under the waivers, some states report that financially eligible citizens are unwilling to accept services. The psychological price of having to impoverish themselves and allow their homes to revert to the state after their deaths (and the deaths of their spouses) is too high for many people.

Managed Care

Managed care seems destined to shape the evolving long-term care system. States have looked to this approach to funding as a potential panacea for solvency, but they should be wary. Although most of the current effort is directed at acute care, initial forays into long-term care have already begun and more can be expected. Managed care has the potential to serve as a potent vehicle for positive change, Because it effectively has no institutional memory and is interested only in finding the most efficient way to deliver care, it may avoid the baggage that more established programs bring. Many of the ultimate goals of managed care may be achieved by more effective integration of social and medical approaches to care, by implementing a philosophy of making investments in more thorough assessments and more aggressive approaches to caring for patients' chronic problems in the hopes of preventing later complications. Information infrastructures can support better clinical decision-making, track patient progress, and help to focus clinician attention on pertinent elements of care. Better information will improve communication among the various players and increase their ability to identify when their goals are discrepant.

For those pressing an agenda that champions more social care with more attention to the everyday aspects of life, managed care is at best a mixed blessing. Its entry is a little like the 400-pound gorilla. Although it may pave the way for more innovation and a search for less professionally dominated, expensive modes of long-term care, it also reenforces the dominance of the medical model. It will be less feasible to think in terms of managed care for Medicaid only when programs are addressed to older persons. Integration with Medicare will be the norm and that merger will likely be based on some variant of a medical model.

The United States is in one of its perennial transformations on health care and the right to such care. With the failure of the 1993 Clinton reforms, we are now witnessing radical (though somewhat concealed) health care reform through private sector changes. Assuming that the managed care movement does not fizzle, long-term care may become part of what is capitated or may remain outside of it. In the latter case, long-term care will still be very influenced by the acute care changes. If long-term care is capitated, decisions are still necessary about who holds the capitation (the larger MCO, a subcapitation of that MCO, or a separate long-term care organization), who collects the money, and whether the program is voluntary or mandatory.

Because managed care organizations may run roughshod over many of the fragile elements of long-term care, states should carefully consider the potential consequences of leaping too enthusiastically into this option. The promise of quick saving should be weighed against the possible sequel. Once control is lost, it will be hard to regain. The current system is flawed, but the managed care remedy may prove worse than the disease.

Family Care

The backbone of long-term care is the informal support system. Especially as the demographic pressures grow, no one wants to see this critical source of support diminish. But the same demographic and economic pressures are threatening to do just that. Women's roles are becoming untenable. However unfair they may have been in the past, the demands placed on some women are now insupportable. Although most family care comes from spouses, children (an ironic term to describe aging adults) also play a crucial part. Simultaneously meeting the demands of multiple roles (which could include wife, mother, daughter, wage earner) may exact too great a price. Some have suggested that the working adults will do for their parents what they do for their children—hire people to assume the caregiving responsibilities their busy schedules no longer allow. Such a step should create a new market for personal care akin to that for children's day care.

Although public policy should encourage family care when it is mutually desired by long-term care consumers and family members, policies must not be built on expectations of family labor. They must also be predicated on adequate income support for the long-term care consumer. The long-term care consumer with enough income can always choose to compensate family members (in cash or in kind) for care. The person who needs public subsidy for care (assuming some competence or a competent agent) should have enough money to make purchases plausible and should be able to choose whether to purchase from family members.

Policies should be designed to encourage family care even if it is not mandated. This reinforcement requires better understanding of what kinds of help and support families need and want, and of the best timing for the assistance. Cash payments of various forms would provide funds to pay family members for care or permit them to purchase similar care. Direct payment of family members as PAS providers and in-home workers could also be helpful. Concerns about transforming family care into something unnatural, thus changing the relationship between the consumer and the family member are probably unwarranted. Payment either in cash grants or for services rendered is likely to be applicable only to those low-income families where providing family care may be an insurmountable financial hardship. The trick will be to determine who needs this kind of support without creating yet another bureaucracy.

Regulations and Quality
Regulations are major forces in shaping long-term care. They come in two forms. The obvious component is the rules designed to assure quality by dictating structural, process, and outcome criteria for an individual's care. Equally powerful are regulations that specify who will be eligible for what kind of care under what kind of circumstances. Such rules, often embodied in licensure criteria, end up shaping the service system.

Principles of equity would support the position that all long-term care should be judged by identical standards of quality, but the application of this ideal is complex. If outcomes are emphasized, then it makes sense to argue for a common playing field (as long as adequate adjustments are made for differences in case mix). However, most regulations still address structure and process. Here, common standards will effectively eliminate the very bases of differences in approaches that are the rationale for proposing new forms of care.

The more society can actually hold providers accountable for outcomes, the more it can relent on the standards for structure and process, thereby facilitating the evolution of new forms of care. By extension, holding onto the stringent rules for how care is given in an effort to promote its quality will stultify creativity. The critical question is, How feasible is a quality assurance system based on holding providers accountable for outcomes? Better ways to assess outcomes are continually being developed along with better case-mix adjustment methods. For outcomes to serve the client they need to be sensitive to each client's preferences. Different people will want different ends maximized. Although individualized preference weights may complicate large-scale analysis, it should be feasible to present summary data on how often (or how much) a given provider was able to achieve or approximate the outcomes deemed most salient by its clients.

Outcomes will never be sufficient exclusively. Some outcomes are too important to wait for them to occur. Some aspects of care need to be assured even if their absence does not produce severely bad results. For example, infection control procedures should not be ignored until an infection develops. Likewise, treating consumers with respect and refraining from abusing them should be requirements of the system. It would be inappropriate to rely on a passive complaint system to ensure that such dignity is preserved and that theft and other abuses are purged from the system.

Principles for Change

We have avoided concrete recommendations thus far. Yet we fervently believe that some principles can and must be applied to long-term care. Guideposts are available to indicate whether developments are in a positive direction, and throughout this book we have pointed to some of them. A few of the most important principles are briefly stated below.

1. Long-term care systems are currently imbalanced. Far more public money is spent on nursing-home care than any other form of care. These imbalances need correction.

2. Long-term care programs need to be developed in a way that preserves the dignity and autonomy of those who need long-term care and that allows them to live out their lives in as meaningful a way as possible within their families and communities.

3. Personal care is the bedrock of long-term care services. It needs to be available around the clock every day of the week. The biggest deficit in long-term care in America is the lack of a dependable capability for personal care services across the country.

4. The good long-term care system has options. Consumer choice is an empty slogan if there is no menu to choose from. These options should include a wide range of ways to get service in one's own home and a wide range of residential settings where services can be efficiently received. Consumer direction is important regardless of where the consumer lives and whether the consumer is receiving care from an agency or an independently employed worker.

5. Some form of care coordination seems to be a necessary component of a long-term care system. This care coordination is meant both to serve the individual consumer's interests and respond to the system's interests, which include increasing the supply of high-quality services, keeping the price as low as is consistent with good care, and allocating the services fairly.

6. People who need long-term care also need acute care often and in substantial amounts. At present, many long-term care consumers have imperfect access to good primary care, acute care, and rehabilitation. We need to move beyond slogans that pit a social model against a medical model in order to make it possible for long-term care consumers to get the best of both worlds.

7. If we move to capitated managed care arrangements for long-term care services, they must be designed in such a way that health authorities can manage care without having license to manage people's lives.

8. Congregate residential settings for long-term care must at a minimum offer single-occupancy accommodations as the minimum program standard. This requirement should be phased in for nursing homes as well as assisted living programs and adult foster care programs. Although single occupancy may not be an appropriate worldwide standard, a country as wealthy and as individualistic as the United States should not require that its grandparents and great-grandparents take on roommates or apartment-mates in order to get their necessary care.

9. Regulations should be designed to emphasize what is truly important in the way of process and outcomes and to encourage care providers to improve their own quality. As much as possible, payment incentives should be aligned with the goals sought.

10. Safety must give way as the number one quality indicator, because that is a recipe for oppression of the consumer. Without being foolhardy or encouraging negligent care, long-term care authorities must recognize that complete safety is an unrealistic goal for any population and that excellent health and elimination of injury, disease, and death are impossible goals for the disabled, often sick, often very old people who need long-term care.

11. The family remains at the heart of long-term care. However, some family members cannot or should not be caregivers. Efforts need to be directed toward supporting informal care where it is feasible and desirable, but not to mandating it. Public policies need to recognize the contributions of informal care but not to rely on them.

Conclusion

Long-term care is a set of services that assist people with disabilities secondary to chronic disease or other causes. Given this basic definition, those who provide long-term care should have two general goals: *(1)* to make sure that the underlying disease or the disabilities have been controlled or minimized as much as possible (with referral as needed to acute care programs, rehabilitation programs, and mental health programs) and *(2)* to provide services and help for those people with long-term (perhaps permanent) disability in such a way as to maximize desirable outcomes for the person receiving the long-term care. Put grandiosely, this second goal is that long-term care should promote or not interfere with meaningful lives for the long-term care consumer.

One thing is clear. Publicly supported long-term care services as presently structured and delivered in the United States are woefully inadequate. They depend largely on a service—the nursing home in its typical incarnations—which is hated and dreaded as a lifestyle choice by almost everybody. The substantial investment in the current style of nursing home needs to stop. We are already in the position of a caterer who has stocked up with the wrong kind of provisions and now has refrigerators full of food nobody wants to eat. We take it as an article of faith that Americans have the capability to improve long-term care, just as other societies have done. To do so, we, as a society, must articulate a positive vision of good lives for long-term care consumers. We then must reject any orthodoxies that our common sense tell us stand in the way of achieving the goal.

Glossary

AAPCC (See *Average Adjusted Per Capita Cost*)

Activities of Daily Living (ADL) Basic self-care functions. Inability to perform ADLs is a common trigger for long-term care services and is measured through a variety of ADL scales. The most common ADLs measured are bathing, dressing, using the toilet, transferring in and out of beds and chairs, and eating.

Acute Care All diagnostic, preventive, or curative treatment of illnesses. Includes hospital services and physician services whether delivered to in-patients or outpatients, and all primary care.

ADL (See *Activities of Daily Living*).

Administration on Aging (AoA) The federal agency created in 1965 to administer the Older Americans Act. As of 1992. The Administration on Aging was elevated to a subcabinet level within the US Department of Health and Human Services. It is directed by the assistant secretary for aging in that department.

Adult Foster Care Home A small group home licensed by the state to provide shelter and some care to people with disabilities. Typically adult foster homes are restricted by license as to the maximum number of people they can serve, usually in the range of three to six depending on the state. Sometimes called family care homes or other names.

Advance Directive A statement made by a cognitively intact person about care he or she would wish to have if he or she were temporarily or permanently unable to make a medical decision because of, for example, unconsciousness or cognitive impairment. Advance directives usually take the form of living wills or durable powers of attorney for health. They may be specific about services to be given or withheld (e.g., respirators, intubation, resuscitation), designate proxy decision makers, or both.

Aid and Attendant Program   A financial allowance program established by the Veterans Administration to help veterans who are eligible by dint of their service connection and their disability status to pay for their personal care needs. The beneficiaries may use the money as they see fit, including supporting the care given to them by their spouses.

American Disabled for Attendant Program Today (ADAPT)   This organization was founded in Missouri in 1982. With headquarters in Denver, the national ADAPT program particularly focuses on alternatives to ''warehousing'' people in institutions. To that end, it supports personal attendant services. ADAPT also gave leadership to the passage of the Americans with Disabilities Act. Originally standing for American Disabled for Accessible Public Transport, ADAPT advocates for lifts on buses and access to public transportion. ADAPT functions as a civil rights organization, using a range of organizing techniques, including civil disobedience and non-violent direct action tactics to dramatize and achieve its goals.

AoA   (See *Administration on Aging*)

Area Agency on Aging (AAA)   The designated local program to administer the service functions of the Older Americans Act. The number of AAAs nationwide fluctuates around 660. Each is responsible for implementing the Title III services of the Older Americans Act and the other Older American Act objectives in their Planning and Service Area with budgets that flow from state units on aging. AAAs often have other sources of funding as well. In many states, the AAAs are the central point for long-term care case management and/or management of Medicaid waiver programs and other long-term care programs in the area.

Arizona Long Term Care System (ALTCS)   Arizona's statewide program that provides Medicaid services for low-income people who are nursing home certifiable.

ASPE   (See *Assistant Secretary for Planning & Evaluation, Office of*)

Assistant Secretary for Planning & Evaluation, Office of (ASPE)   A federal agency at the subcabinet level in the United States Department of Health and Human Services that is responsible for a planning and evaluation agenda for the whole department. The Division of Aging, Disability, and Long-term Care within ASPE has funded many of the studies discussed in this book and has recently forwarded the agenda of consumer-directed long-term care for people of all ages.

Assisted Living   A congregate residential care home not licensed or certified as a nursing home that is usually licensed by the state and that provides shelter and care to people with some ADL impairments or needs for routine nursing services. Often, but not always, comprised of apartments with full bathrooms. Services may be provided by staff of the setting, by home care agencies from outside the setting, or both.

Autonomy   Direction of one's own life and decisions affecting one's own life.

Average Adjusted Per Capita Costs (AAPCC)   Term for the per-capita payment received by managed care organizations for each Medicare beneficiary who enrolls in Medicare managed care. The payment received by the managed care organization is established as 95% of the average annual Medicare expenditures in the fee-for-service system in the county where the beneficiary lives, adjusted for age, gender, residence in a nursing home versus in the community, and Medicaid status. AAPCC rates vary a great deal across states and within states.

Birth Cohort   A birth cohort is a group of people who were born within the same year or grouping of years and, therefore, are presumed to share characteristics related to shared historical events and technology as they move through the life cycle. It is common to think of 5-year or 10-year birth cohorts. Gerontologists have difficulty disentangling the effects of age from the effects of the birth cohort to which the older person belongs.

Board-and-Care Home   A generic term for residential care facilities that are not licensed or certified as nursing homes and that typically provide a lighter level of care than nursing homes within a more residentially oriented environment. States use various terms, including residential care facility, in licensing such entities.

Boren Amendment   A federal statute, enacted in 1980 and repealed in 1996, that required states to reimburse nursing homes at a rate sufficient for an efficient provider to run a nursing home that meets quality standards. In many states, the nursing home industry successfully sued the Medicaid program for higher reimbursements under this statute.

Care Coordination   A term sometimes used interchangeably with "case management." Care coordination is sometimes a more favored term when the services being managed are more health-related than socially-oriented.

CASA   (See *Community Attendant Services Act*)

Case Management   A term that refers to the coordination of services on behalf of a group of patients or clients. In long-term care, case management is typically done by social workers or nurses and involves processes of screening, comprehensive assessment, care planning, and plan implementation. Case management for HCBS services has both an advocacy and a gate-keeping component and is often separated from the delivery of service. The term case management is also used for management functions within provider organizations, including managed care organizations providing a comprehensive range of health services; in such applications, case management is usually *not* separated from service delivery.

Case Mix   A term to describe the acuity or need levels of the clientele of a particular program (e.g., the residents of a nursing home, the enrollees in a managed care organization). In long-term care research, case mix adjustment is used so that the outcomes attributed to a program will take into account differences in clientele at entry into the program. Case mix adjustment is also often used to set payment levels for programs or capitation amounts for pre-paid programs.

Cash and Counseling   A demonstration project funded as a partnership of ASPE and the Robert Wood Johnson Foundation in 1995 to demonstrate the effectiveness of cash allocations in lieu of Medicaid or Medicaid waiver services for community-dwelling long-term care consumers. The program is structured as a randomized controlled experiment in four states: Arkansas, Florida, New Jersey, and New York.

Centers for Independent Living (CILs)   A federally-funded program established under the Rehabilitation Act of 1973, as subsequently amended, to create a program of services for people with significant disabilities to promote independence, productivity, and quality of life. The core services are information and referral, independent living skills training, and individual and systems advocacy. A long list of additional services are permissible, including counseling, help securing housing or shelter, rehabilitation technology, mobility training, life skills training, interpreter and reader services, supported living, transportation, physical rehabilitation, employment empowerment, and prostheses. Services may be targeted to specific groups, including children.. In 1998 the CIL supported 250 CILs nationally with at least one in every state. Historically directed towards people under age 65, some CILs are becoming involved with older people with disabilities.

Certificate of Need (CON)   Certification that permits a firm to expand the supply of a particular type of care in situations where the supply is being regulated by the state. Typically a regional or state health unit extends or denies the CON based on a review of the need for more service capacity in a geographic area. CON policies have been widely applied to construction of nursing homes and less frequently to construction of alternative residential settings and licensure of home care agencies.

Channeling Demonstration   A seminal research randomized demonstration that took place in ten states in the early 1980s to demonstrate the cost-effectiveness of community care for people at risk of entering a nursing home. Two models were tested, each in five states: basic channeling, which included case management and money for gap-filling services, and financial control channeling, in which case managers could purchase services for clients up to a maximum amount. The added services were paid for under Medicare and Medicaid, and the research was sponsored by ASPE and AoA.

Chemical Restraints   Use of prescription drugs, particularly psychoactive drugs as a method of behavior control.

Coinsurance   A term for a portion of the charges for a service that are borne by the insured persons themselves. Coinsurance may be expressed as a percentage of the allowable charges or as a fixed amount for a visit. This differs from a deductible, which is a payment that the insured makes before being able to draw upon insurance benefits.

Community Attendant Services Act (CASA)   The Medicaid Community Attendant Services Act, introduced in the United States House of Representatives as HR

2020 by Newt Gingrich in 1997. The bill establishes a required benefit for Qualified Community-Based Attendants Under Medicaid. All Medicaid recipients with ADL impairments would be able to choose between receiving care in a nursing home or other facility or receiving the new benefit in the community. Construed as revenue-neutral.

Community Option Program for Elderly Services (COPES)   The Medicaid waiver and HCBS programs in the state of Washington.

Community Options Program (COP)   Wisconsin's major HCBS program for seniors and people with disabilities. COP refers to its state-funded program and the COP waiver to its Medicaid waiver program.

Consumer-Directed Care   Long-term care where the client (or consumer) has a strong role in planning and directing his or her own individual service and in the establishment of agency pealike. Consumer-directed care is sometimes contrasted to agency-directed care, though the distinction is not part of the definition. At its most pronounced, consumer-direction means that clients select, train, supervise, and fire their care attendants.

Continuous Quality Improvement (CQI)   A process of quality assurance that emphasizes the goal of continuously upgrading the overall performance of a program (as opposed to identifying and eliminating bad performance). Adapted from Japanese industrial practices, CQI approaches entail collection of data on overall performance, identifying areas for attention, and developing strategies at the level of the work group to address the problems. Thus, CQI has a "bottom-up quality" of involving the entire organization in quality improvement, though it also has a "top-down" quality in that the process must be endorsed and supported by the highest echelons of management.

CQI   (See *Continuous Quality Improvement*)

Criminal Record Checks   A process mandated in some states to determine whether personal care workers have criminal records.

Deductible   A payment that insured people must make before their insurance coverage will take effect. Usually a deductible is for a fixed amount of money, though it could be for a period of time during which the insured covers himself or herself.

Dementia   General term for any generalized, irreversible, and usually progressive impairment of cognitive functioning characterized by memory loss and confusion. The most common disease associated with dementia in old age is Alzheimer's disease, followed by strokes. Dementia is also associated with a wide range of other diseases (including Parkinson's disease), with brain injury, and with chronic alcohol problems. Treatable dementia-like conditions, known as pseudo-dementia, may also be caused by prescribed medications, depression, thyroid problems, and a host of other etiologies.

Developmental Disability   A disabling physical or cognitive disability that is incurred at birth or in early childhood. Sometimes, the term DD is also expanded to include mental retardation.

Diagnosis Related Group (DRG)   A disabling classification of Medicare hospital patients that is keyed to discharge diagnosis. All patients are put into a DRG category, and each DRG translated into a fixed amount of money for the hospital stay. Under this prospective payment system, hospitals have an incentive to make stays shorter and to serve hospital patients less intensively in the hospital.

DRG   (See *Diagnosis Related Group*)

Dual Eligibles   People who are Medicare beneficiaries because of age or permanent disability and Medicaid eligible because of income.

EverCare   A managed care plan serving Medicare beneficiaries who reside in nursing homes and who voluntarily enroll in the program. EverCare programs receive the Medicare capitation and are responsible for the entire range of Medicare-covered services. They achieve their efficiencies and their presumed care improvements by vigorous use of nurse practitioners in the selected nursing homes where EverCare is an option.

Extended Care Facility   The original name for the long-term care facilities covered under Medicare, which were viewed as having a rehabilitation capability.

Favorable Selection   The enrollment of people in a capitated managed care system who are likely to use health care less than the average population.

Formal Care   A term that is contrasted to "informal care" given by a long-term care consumer's relatives and friends, usually without compensation. As such it embraces all care delivered by care providers of in-home care or care in congregate settings.

Geriatric Assessment Unit   An older term for Geriatric Evaluation and Management (see below).

Geriatric Evaluation and Management (GEM)   A specialized comprehensive geriatric assessment followed by short-term treatment to stabilize the patient and develop a management plan. The assessments are usually performed by multidisciplinary teams and may include laboratory and x-ray tests as well as administration of standardized scales. GEM programs may be outpatient or in-patient programs.

Geriatrician   A medical specialist who is qualified to care for older people. In the United States, geriatricians are subspecialists of either internal medicine or family practice who have completed additional training and passed a specialty examination.

HCBS   (See *Home and Community Based Services*)

HCFA   (See *Health Care Financing Administration*)

Health Care Facility   (See *Nursing Home*)

Health Care Financing Administration   The federal agency within the United States Department of Health and Human Services that is responsible for the operation of Medicare and Medicaid. The Administrator of HCFA serves as part of the Health and Human Services subcabinet.

Health Maintenance Organization   An organized system of managed care that offers a specific comprehensive package of benefits to an enrolled population for a prepaid fee.

HMO   (See *Health Maintenance Organization*)

Home Care Agency   Any agency that provides services to people in their own homes, including but not limited to those certified as vendors under Medicare. States vary on the kind of licensure they require for home care agencies.

Home and Community Based Services (HCBS)   These services HCBS, include a wide range of long-term care programs that, singly or in combination, might serve as alternatives to nursing home care. The HCBS waiver permits states to use federally matched Medicaid money for a wide range of HCBS services for people who are functionally eligible for nursing homes under the Medicaid program in the state. Usual HCBS services for elderly include home care of various kinds, adult day care, case management, home-delivered meals, medical equipment, home modifications, and payment for services in assisted living, small group homes, adult foster care, or other residential settings. HCBS waivers may be targeted at specific populations such as: seniors, physically disabled, seniors and physically disabled combined, developmentally disabled, mentally ill, traumatic brain injury, children.

Home Health Agency (HHA)   Ordinarily, an agency certified to receive reimbursement as a home health agency under Medicare. The rules for certified health agencies have changed over the years, but certified HHA must offer at least two of six specified services: nursing, physical therapy, occupational therapy, speech therapy, medical social work, and home health aides.

IADL   (See *Instrumental Activities of Daily Living*)

Iatrogenic   A term referring to health problems that are caused by health care itself. Some iatrogenisis (the noun for iatrogenic conditions) is comprised of unavoidable side-effects of health care, such as side effects of medications or complications of surgery. Some iatrogenic problems may have been completely prevented.

ILC   (See *Independent Living Center*)

Independent Choices   A program funded by the Robert Wood Johnson Foundation to promote consumer-direction and choice into long-term care programs for people of all ages and types of disabilities. Programs funded under this initiative include cash options, vouchers, and consumer cooperative organizations, as well as a variety of training and research efforts.

Independent Living Center (ILC)   (See *Centers for Independent Living (CIL)*)

Independent Practice Association (IPA)   An organization that contracts with a managed care plan to deliver services at a single capitation rate. The IPA in turn contracts with individual providers, such as physicians, hospitals, and/or other providers to provide the services either on a capitated or fee-for-service basis.

Independent Provider (IP)   A term often used to connote home care workers and personal assistance workers who are some equivalent of "self-employed" as opposed to being employed by home care agencies. When IP's are covered under Medicaid, they are sometimes paid by the state (after the client authorizes the number of hours), sometimes by the client, and sometimes by agencies designated to act as fiscal intermediaries for the consumer-employers.

Informal Care   Care given by a long-term care consumer's family members and friends, usually without compensation. It is contrasted to formal care, which is delivered by a wide variety of health care providers.

Instrumental Activities of Daily Living (IADL)   A variety of functional tasks associated with independent living. IADL performance areas typically measured include cooking, cleaning, laundry, shopping, taking medicines, using transportation or driving, making and receiving telephone calls.

Intermediate Care Facility (ICF)   A term for a nursing home or part of a nursing home that provides custodial care for people without rehabilitation potential. Until OBRA 1987, ICFs needed to meet less stringent quality standards than skilled nursing facilities (SNFs). Once quality criteria were merged, the Medicare program still pays for nursing facility care only if the resident needs skilled care, whereas Medicaid will pay for intermediate care.

IPA   (See *Independent Practice Association*)

Long-Term Care   Health, personal care, and related social services provided over a sustained period of time to people who have lost or never developed certain measurable functional abilities.

Long-Term Care Facility   (See *Nursing Home*)

Managed Care Organization   Any type of managed care plan, including plans such as health maintenance organizations (HMOs) and preferred provider organizations.

MCO   (See *Managed Care Organization*)

Medicaid   A state-operated and state-administered program that is financed jointly by the state government and the federal government according to a matching formula, and which provides medical benefits for low-income people in need of health and medical care. States operate their Medicaid programs with substantial policy-setting discretion but under general federal guidelines. Medicaid was authorized in 1965 under Title 19 of the Social Security Act.

Medicare A nationwide health insurance program for people 65 and over, for people eligible for social security disability payments for 2 years or more, and for certain workers and their dependents who need kidney transplantations or renal dialysis. The program was enacted in 1965 as Title 18 of the Social Security Act. Under Part A, it covers hospital care and limited nursing home care. Under Part B, it includes physician services, home health care, laboratory services, and medical equipment. Consumers contribute to the costs of Medicare through premiums, deductibles, and copayments as specified under the law.

Medicare-Certified Meeting the standards to bill for reimbursement under Medicare. Separate certification standards and procedures have been developed for the various types of providers that participate in Medicare as providers, including hospitals, nursing homes, home health agencies, hospices, rehabilitation programs, laboratories, and managed care organizations.

Medicare Risk Contracts Also known as *TEFRA HMOs*, this is the mechanism by which a managed care organization enrolls Medicare beneficiaries in a prepaid health care program. The managed care organization receives a capitated payment for each enrollee who voluntarily agrees to have all Medicare services delivered through that mechanism. The managed care organization is at financial risk for providing all services that are part of fee-for-service Medicare to the enrollees.

Minimum Data Set (MDS) A federally-mandated set of data that nursing homes must collect at intervals on all residents of all certified nursing homes. A standard resident assessment instrument (RAI) is used for data collection. Data from the MDS are used to inform careplanning, to provide a basis for external quality surveys and internal CQI (see above), and in case-mix-adjusted reimbursement systems. The MDS was developed as a result of OBRA 1987 (see below). As of May 1998, all nursing homes will be computerized and transmit MDS data to the Health Care Financing Administration.

Minnesota Senior Care Organization (MSHO) An demonstration being conducted under demonstration waivers in Minnesota whereby designated Managed Care Organizations receive capitation from both Medicare and Medicaid for beneficiaries dually eligible for both payment programs and use this combined capitation to deliver all the care that is part of both Medicare and Medicaid.

Morbidity Rates Rates of illness. Morbidity rates may be calculated for specific conditions and be age- and gender-adjusted.

Mortality Rates Death rates.

MSHO (See *Minnesota Senior Care Organization*)

Nurse Delegation A policy that permits licensed nurses to delegate nursing tasks to individuals without a nurse's license without close or continuous supervision of that person. Various states have clarified their nurse practice rules to permit nurses to instruct the delegatee on specific tasks for specific patients and, based on satisfactory performance, authorize them for doing the tasks.

Nursing Home   A residential facility that is licensed as a nursing home by the state. Usually nursing homes are also certified for federal reimbursement under the Medicare and Medicaid program.

OAA   (See *Older Americans Act*)

OBRA (Omnibus Budget Reconciliation Act) 1987   OBRA 1987 are a series of sweeping reforms in nursing home quality assurance enacted in 1987 and gradually implemented over the next decade. The main features were to emphasize outcomes in a system that had largely used structure and process; to create new standards for residents' rights, resident assessment, and quality of care; to clarify that widespread use of physical and chemical restraints are inconsistent with a good quality of life; to mandate nurse's aide training; to revise the inspection process to require observation and interview of residents and their families as part of the input; and to develop enforcement policies that take into account the scope and severity of the particular problems.

Old Age, Survivors, and Disability Insurance (OASDI)   (*See Social Security*)

Older Americans Act (OAA)   A statute enacted in 1965 and subsequently regularly amended. The OAA's major provisions include: a bill of rights for older people (Title 1), a federal responsibility to advocate and coordinate on behalf of the elderly (Title 2), a service capacity for nutritional and other services (including some long-term care services) through a national network of State Units on Aging and Area Agencies on Aging (Title III); training and research on aging (Title 4; employment for seniors (Title V), programs for Native American tribes (Title VI, and a variety of protective programs, including the LTC ombudsman program (Title VII).

Ombudsman   A program mandated by the Older Americans Act, whereby each state establishes a capacity to provide disinterested advocacy and mediation services on behalf of nursing home residents. This is done through responding to complaints and inquiries on a case-by-case basis and system advocacy.

On Lok   The original model program begun in San Francisco's Chinatown area on which the Program of All-Inclusive Care for the elderly is based. On Lot is a capitated, at-risk program that provides full Medicare and Medicaid services to an enrolled group, all of whom are at the nursing home level of need. The program utilizes a day health center and multidisciplinary teams for delivery of primary care and long-term care services to a frail elderly population, supplemented by purchase of hospital care, home care, and nursing home care as needed.

Oregon Project Independence (OPI)   A state-funded program in Oregon that is administered in conjunction with the Medicaid waiver program for HCBS services.

PACE   (See *Program for All-Inclusive Care for the Elderly*)

PAS (See *Personal Assistant Services & PreAdmission Screening*)

Personal Assistant Services (PAS) Services to assist people who have ADL deficiencies with their personal care. PAS may be provided, at state option, as part of the state Medicaid plan. Sometimes PAS is provided through independently employed care providers and is contrasted to care from home care agencies.

Physical Restraints Refers to any device that involuntarily restrains the movements of a long-term care consumer, including chest or trunk restraints (such as Possey vests); hand, waist, or leg ties; chairs that prevent rising (sometimes called geri-chairs); and bed rails.

Post-Acute Care A term used to refer to the care that follows a hospital stay and is usually related to that stay. Medicare covers the following types of post-acute care; rehabilitation center care, skilled nursing home care, and home health care.

Preadmission Screening (PAS) A state program whereby all those who apply for nursing home coverage under Medicaid are first screened to determine whether they need the care and also whether they might prefer an alternative form of care. States vary as to whether they screen only those categorically eligible for Medicaid versus including those who would spend-down to Medicaid within a short period of time of nursing home use; whether they delegate screenings to hospitals; and how integrated the screening is with their HCBS programs.

Preferred Provider Organization (PPO) A collection of providers that have agreed to specific reimbursement schedules and are , therefore, designated as preferred providers under a managed care organization or an insurance plan. Enrollees may go to the physician of his or her choice, even if that physician does not participate in the PPO, but enrollees receive less complete coverage of the costs if they choose providers outside the PPO.

Primary Care Basic or general health and preventive care provided when a patient first seeks assistance from the medical care system. It is also defined as the entry point into the health care system and is generally provided in a physician's office or health care clinic setting.

Primary Care Practitioner A term usually applied to the physician who provides primary care services, such as internists, family physicians, and pediatricians.

Primary Care Provider (PCP) A physician or physician extender (e.g. nurse practitioner, physician assistant) who is designated by a managed care plan or insurer as the gate-keeper for the system. PCPs are responsible for overall management of care and referral to specialists.

Program for All-Inclusive Care for the Elderly This program enabled replications of the On Lot Senior Health Services Program in San Francisco. PACE programs are capitated care organizations that pool Medicare, Medicaid, and private funding sources for dually eligible beneficiaries, all of whom are nursing home certifiable. PACE programs are at financial risk for providing all Medicare and Medicaid services to the enrollees. Characteristic hallmarks of the program are management by a multidisciplinary team including staff physicians, and required or strongly encouraged attendance at day health care centers where medical care and some personal care are provided. Initially organizations could apply to develop PACE sites on a demonstration basis, but the program has now become available under operational waivers.

Proxy Decision Maker   Proxy decision-makers are designated to make decisions for people whose decision-making capability are impaired. The proxy decision-makers may have formal legal authority because they are court-appointed guardians or conservators or they may simply be next-of-kin or readily available relatives who are asked to fill the proxy role.

Quality Adjusted Life Years (QUALYs)   An approach to considering outcomes for health consumers and long-term care consumers that takes into account not only the length of survival but the quality of life during the years that the person survives. Typically disease states and functional status are adjusted for in developing QUALYs measures.

Quality Assurance (QA)   A process to ensure that the quality of care meets an expected threshold. It includes defining quality criteria for quality and standards for performance; assessing whether care accords with the standards; and corrective action when the standards are not met.

Quality Improvement   A process by which long-term care providers attempt to upgrade and sustain the quality of their care. When contrasted to quality assurance, it is often used for an internal process developed by providers as opposed to a process mandated from outside.

Quality of Life   A general term to reflect positive or negative characteristics of a long-term care consumer's life. It is particularly used to refer to congregate care setting, where quality of life is sometimes contrasted to quality of care. Dignity, privacy, social relationships, and social participation are sometimes included as dimensions of quality of life.

Resource Utilization Groups (RUGs)   A case mix system developed for reimbursing nursing homes that takes into account the amount of nursing service time a residents' functional diabilities and other characteristics.

Reverse Mortgage   A financial process by which a person who owns a home can borrow against the value of that home to finance their long-term care.

Robert Wood Johnson Foundation   A charitable foundation located in Princeton, NJ, which was established in 1972 to promote health and health care for all Americans through a grant program. Through its various initiatives, the foundation funds many of the demonstration projects, research projects, and state reform initiatives described in this book.

RUG   (See *Resource Utilization Group*)

SCU   (See *Special Care Unit*)

S/HMO   (See *Social Health Maintenance Organization*)

Skilled Nursing Facility (SNF)   A nursing facility or portion of a nursing facility that meets requirements for Medicare certification.

Social Health Maintenance Organization   This program integrates hospital and physician services with community-based long-term care in a managed, prepaid program. Four S/HMOs were established in 1982 in the first wave of a demonstration program for better integration of acute-care and long-term care; three of those programs are still operational. A second wave of S\HMOs was initiated a decade later to test a different basis for capitation and a more intensive effort to integrate the acute care and long-term care services operationally.

Social Security   A common way of referring to the federally administered Old-Age, Survivors, and Disability Insurance (OASDI) program, which is the national pension system in the United States, established in 1935 and funded through a trust fund established by a payroll tax. The plan has been modified over the years in terms of coverage and benefit levels. Over 90% of households over age 65 receive some income from Social Security, and Social Security is the sole or primary source of income for many American families.

Special Care Unit (SCU)   An area of a nursing home or assisted living facility that is exclusively tailored to serve people with Alzheimer's disease and other dementias. At a minimum an SCU is geographically distinct, but typically they are also characterized by specially designed environments, special programming, and staff who are trained to care for people with dementia.

SSI   (See *Supplemental Security Income*)

SSI Supplements   Required SSI supplements are state supplements to SSI, the amount of which were determined when SSI was implemented as a federal program in 1972 based on each state's previous efforts. Beyond that, states may establish voluntary SSI supplement programs that may be targeted to people with long-term care expenditures or people whose incomes need to be topped to afford housing components of assisted living.

Staff HMO   A staff (or staff-model) HMO is one where the HMOs are employed and salaried by the HMO. This can be contrasted to IPA models (see above).

Subacute Care   Subacute care (which is also called transitional care) refers to the care of persons discharged from hospital who still require active treatment, rehabilitation, or close monitoring. As hospital payment under Medicare was changed to a prospective payment regardless of length of stay, patients were discharged earlier. This care that was formerly provided under a hospital's aegis is now called subacute care. Subacute care can be provided in nursing homes with heavier nurse staffing or in converted facilities that represent former excess hospital capacity.

Supplemental Security Insurance (SSI) A federally-administered cash living allowance for people over age 65 or with severe and permanent disabilities whose incomes, after some disallowances, fall below a specified amount ($484 in 1998).

Surveyor State personnel who inspect nursing homes for licensure and certification are known as surveyors, and their procedures are referred to as a survey.

TANF (See *Temporary Assistance to Needy Families*)

TEFRA HMO The abbreviation for managed care or risk-contracting under Medicare. TEFRA refers to the 1982 Tax Equity and Fiscal Responsibility Act, which first authorized Medicare managed care. (See also *Medicare Risk Contracts*)

Temporary Assistance to Needy Families (TANF) TANF is the "workfare" program that, in 1996, replaced categorical welfare assistance such as Aid to Families with Dependent Children (AFDC). Under TANF, time limits are set for cash benefits and recipients are expected to accept work or be enrolled in training programs.

Title 18 Used synonymously with Medicare, which is Title 18 of the Social Security Act.

Title 19 Used synonymously with Medicaid, which is Title 19 of the Social Security Act.

Title 20 The title of the Social Security Act that began authorizing Social Services Block Grants to states in 1972.

TQM (Total Quality Management) (See *Continuous Quality Improvement (CQI)* above. The terms are used interchangeably.)

Waivers Any authorized exemption of a statutory program.

1115 Waivers Waivers of Medicaid that permit demonstration of new cost-effective delivery of services. The current HCBS waiver program was built on earlier demonstration projects under 115 waivers. Currently 1115 waivers are being used to demonstrate the cost effectiveness of managed care programs for various subgroups of Medicaid clients.

1915© Waivers Waiver under the Social Security Act that allows states that have successfully applied to federal authorities to use matching Medicaid funds with much more flexibility to cover home-and-community based services not ordinarily covered by Medicaid or to waive other Medicaid rules as long as the service recipients are nursing home certifiable. Also known as 2176 waivers.

2176 Waivers (See *1915© waivers*)

222 Waivers   Waivers of Medicare rules that permit demonstration projects to examine the cost-effectiveness of alternative forms of delivering Medicare services.

WID   (See *World Institute on Disabilities*)

World Institute on Disabilities (WID)   A nonprofit organization established in 1983 by leaders in the Independent Living Movement as a vehicle for education, research, and policy making on independent living.

Index

Activities of daily living: *See* ADL

Acute care: viii, 3, 15, 18, 215–30, 304, 307; compared to long-term care, 4, 16, 32; effects on long-term care financing, 56–57, 287; long-term care in, 16; in nursing homes, 165, 167; relationship to long-term care, 215, 289; relationships with long-term care in managed care, 259–62

ADAPT: 130, 307

ADL: 3, 9, 17, 23, 27 *n.*3, 29 *n.*21, 56, 120, 199, 307; assessment of 80–81; in nursing homes, 3, 9, 42–44; in managed care 245, 250–1

Adult day care: viii, 16, 22, 25, 72, 119, 276

Adult foster care: 17, 25, 72, 110, 169, 174–6, 259, 292, 308; relative foster care in Oregon, 139

Administration on Aging (AoA): vi, 45–6, 132, 308

Advocacy: 73, 114, 156 *n.*37, 287

Aid to Families with Dependent Children: 36, 112

AIDS: 11

Alabama: 70

Alaska: 74, 81, 137, 152, 290

Alcohol and drug problems: 13

Alzheimer's disease: vii, 9, 11–13, 19, 58, 67, 81, 114, 120, 139, 151–2, 181; in nursing homes, 167, 170; special care units for, 171–3. *See also* Dementia

Amyotropic lateral sclerosis: 11

Area Agency on Aging: 45, 46, 66, 110, 113, 308; in Oregon, 138–9

Arizona: 178, 237–8, 255

Arizona Long-term Care System (ALTCS): 256, 258, 308

Arkansas: 107, 112, 150

Arthritis: 9

Assessment: 4, 49, 67, 80, 139, 147, 148, 197, 220; comprehensive geriatric assessment, 223, 249; in Germany, 274; in United Kingdom, 277

Assisted living: 17, 51, 72, 82, 161, 169, 179, 259, 308; definition variation, 110, 294; in Oregon, 176–8; pricing of, 177, 298–9, 308

Attendants: 16, 57, 154 n.1, 205. *See also* Personal care assistants

Australia: 74

Autonomy: v, 18, 24–5, 64, 168, 179, 208, 271, 275, 291, 309

Average Adjusted Per Capita Cost (AAPCC): 217, 242, 246, 250

Baby boom generation: 7

Balanced Budget Act of 1997: 109, 239, 243

Bedsores: *See* Pressure sores

Board and care homes: 3, 17, 51, 64, 309. *See also* Assisted living

Boren Amendment: 78–9, 309

Boult, Chad: 11

Brookings Institution: 71

California: 63, 111, 126

California Public Employees Retirement Plan: 55

Canada: 270, 274–6, 278, 281, *n.*9, 300

Cancer: 9, 245